THE UNSTABLE SPINE
(Thoracic, Lumbar, and Sacral Regions)

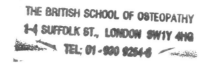
THE UNSTABLE SPINE
(Thoracic, Lumbar, and Sacral Regions)

Edited by

Stewart B. Dunsker, M.D.
Mayfield Neurological Institute
Cincinnati, Ohio

Henry H. Schmidek, M.D.
Professor and Chairman
Section of Neurological Surgery
The University of Vermont College of Medicine
Burlington, Vermont

John Frymoyer, M.D.
Professor and Chairman
Department of Orthopedics and Rehabilitation
The University of Vermont College of Medicine
Burlington, Vermont

Alfred Kahn, III, M.D.
Cincinnati Orthopedic Institute
Cincinnati, Ohio

Grune & Stratton, Inc.
Harcourt Brace Jovanovich, Publishers
Orlando   New York   San Diego   Boston   London
San Francisco   Tokyo   Sydney   Toronto

Grune & Stratton, Inc.
Orlando, Florida 32887

Distributed in the United Kingdom by
Grune & Stratton, Ltd.
24/28 Oval Road, London NW 1

Library of Congress Catalog Number 85-30583
International Standard Book Number 0-8089-1757-9
Printed in the United States of America
86 87 88 89   10 9 8 7 6 5 4 3 2 1

CONTENTS

PREFACE

Interest in the evaluation and treatment of spinal disorders has mushroomed in the past few years. In addition, there has been increasing cooperation between the various specialists who treat these problems. The Joint Spinal Section of The American Association of Neurological Surgeons and The Congress of Neurological Surgeons has sponsored this book and has included neurosurgeons and orthopaedists as both editors and authors so that we could glean the best from both areas of expertise.

In preparing the outline for the book the similarities in problems that affected the thoracic and lumbar spine became apparent immediately. The cervical spine, however, is much more complex and presents many different problems. Indeed it might merit a monograph of its own. In order to highlight similarities in treating disorders in various parts of the spine, we purposely omitted the cervical spine and confined ourselves to discussions of lesions extending from the first thoracic to the last sacral vertebrae.

All the authors reviewed what they considered to be the pertinent and relevant literature. Yet there is great variety in what references were selected. Some authors have focused their attention on a narrow range of topics and others have broadened their reviews to include historical references. There are many and diverse opinions regarding the proper management of some of these pathologic states and each chapter's review of the pertinent literature reflects the authors' bias.

We address the evaluation and treatment of patients with tumors, trauma, and infection. Some of the material is elementary, but we expect that some readers will need the background material to understand the approaches to the various clinical problems. Each author's opinion is not meant to be authoritative or definitive, but to be an acceptable approach to the problem.

Our original intent was to produce a book that would explain surgical techniques of stabilizing the spine. We did not intend to review any clinical series. The chapters by Dr. Walters and Dr. Sundaresan, however, represent an unusual and interesting collection of patients who were well managed. Moreover, they describe the very important aspect of the results of treatment and help the reader identify successful approaches to different problems.

Several chapters duplicate discussions such as the mechanics of injury and emphasize the same points. Similarly, operative techniques are duplicated. The editors have elected to leave the redundancy for numerous reasons. The duplication will allow each chapter to stand alone if read by an individual who wishes to refer to a specific area of the spine. If the book is read in continuity, the common thread between various experts will shine through. Having different authors describe their own techniques allows the reader to capture what appeals to him or her and to identify surgical "pearls."

We recognize that the vast, dynamic, and rapidly changing field of spinal surgery cannot be compressed within the narrow limits of these pages, and that we cannot be completely current with the latest developments. Our only hope is to enlighten.

The editors are indebted to the Joint Section of Spinal Disorders of The American Association of Neurological Surgeons and The Congress of Neurological Surgeons. We are also indebted to Ms. Susan Gay Arkin, Executive Editor, Grune & Stratton, for her patience and for her talents that led to the completion of this monograph. The publisher has been most cooperative in this entire project and the editors are most appreciative. Without the assistance and encouragement of our secretaries, Tina Trimbach, Kathy Devanna, Jean Pang, Antonia Clark, Nancy Briggs and Debbie Brown, this would not have reached fruition.

Stewart B. Dunsker, M.D.
Henry Schmidek, M.D.
John Frymoyer, M.D.
Alfred Kahn, III, M.D.

CONTRIBUTORS

Michael J. Apuzzo, M.D. *Professor, Department of Neurosurgery, University of Southern California School of Medicine, Los Angeles, California*

Linda Brier, R.N., M.S. *Rehabilitation Service, Medical Center Hospital of Vermont, Burlington, Vermont*

Keith Bridwell, M.D. *Assistant Professor, Division of Orthopedic Surgery, Washington University Medical Center, St. Louis, Missouri*

Mark D. Brown, M.D. *Professor of Orthopedics and Rehabilitation and Surgery, University of Miami School of Medicine, Miami, Florida*

William R. Dobkin, M.D. *Instructor, Department of Neurosurgery, University of Southern California School of Medicine, Los Angeles, California*

Frank J. Eismont, M.D. *Associate Professor of Orthopedics and Rehabilitation, University of Miami School of Medicine and Co-director, Acute Spinal Cord Injury Unit, Jackson Memorial Hospital, Miami, Florida*

John W. Frymoyer, M.D. *Professor and Chairman, Department of Orthopedics and Rehabilitation, University of Vermont College of Medicine, Burlington, Vermont*

Joseph H. Galicich, M.D. *Neurosurgical Service, Memorial Sloan-Kettering Cancer Center, New York, New York*

Barth A. Green, M.D.   *Professor of Neurological Surgery, Orthopedics and Rehabilitation, University of Miami School of Medicine, and Attending Surgeon, Veterans' Administration Medical Center, Miami, Florida*

Alfred Kahn, III, M.D.   *Director, Spinal Deformity Center, Good Samaritan Hospital, and Assistant Clinical Professor, Department of Orthopedics, University of Cincinnati Medical Center, Cincinnati, Ohio*

Martin H. Krag, M.D.   *Assistant Professor, Department of Orthopedics and Rehabilitation, University of Vermont College of Medicine, Burlington, Vermont*

Thomas K. Kristiansen, M.D.   *Assistant Professor, Department of Orthopedics and Rehabilitation, University of Vermont College of Medicine, Burlington, Vermont*

Joseph M. Lane, M.D.   *Orthopedic Service, Memorial Sloan-Kettering Cancer Center, New York, New York*

Sanford J. Larson, M.D., Ph.D.   *Professor and Chairman, Department of Neurosurgery, Medical College of Wisconsin, Milwaukee, Wisconsin*

Theodore I. Malinin, M.D.   *Professor of Surgery, Orthopedics and Rehabilitation, and Pathology, University of Miami School of Medicine, Miami, Florida*

Thomas G. Saul, M.D.   *Neurological Surgery, Mayfield Neurological Institute, Cincinnati, Ohio*

H. Scher, M.D.   *Solid Tumor Service, Memorial Sloan-Kettering Cancer Center, New York, New York*

Henry H. Schmidek, M.D.   *Professor and Chairman, Section of Neurological Surgery, University of Vermont College of Medicine, Burlington, Vermont*

Donald A. Smith, M.D.   *Resident, Section of Neurological Surgery, University of Vermont College of Medicine, Burlington, Vermont*

Narayan Sundaresan, M.D.   *Neurosurgical Service, Memorial Sloan-Kettering Cancer Center, and the Neurosurgical Service, St. Luke's/Roosevelt Hospital Center, Columbia University College of Physicians and Surgeons, New York, New York*

Carrie L. Walters, M.D.   *Assistant Professor, Section of Neurological Surgery, University of Vermont College of Medicine, Burlington, Vermont*

Robert G. Watkins, M.D.   *Assistant Clinical Professor of Orthopedics, University of Southern California School of Medicine, Los Angeles, California*

THE UNSTABLE SPINE
(Thoracic, Lumbar, and Sacral Regions)

John W. Frymoyer
Martin H. Krag

1

Spinal Stability and Instability: Definitions, Classification, and General Principles of Management

When a gibbosity seizes persons who have already attained their full growth, it usually occasions a crisis of the then existing disease.

Hippocrates
On Articulations

Deformities of the spine and their affect on neurologic and musculoskeletal function have been well recognized since antiquity. Our understanding of spinal stability, however, has largely evolved since the discovery of roentgenography. Today, we have considerable knowledge of the anatomic and mechanical characteristics of spinal instability as well as its pathologic causes. These topics will be presented in this chapter along with a review of the principles common to the operative and nonoperative management of spinal instability.

SPINAL STABILITY

The basic unit of spinal stability is the motion segment, which White and Panjabi termed the *functional spinal unit* (FSU).[36] This unit includes the two adjacent vertebral bodies, the intervening disc, the facet joints, and the connecting ligamentous structures. Under normal conditions, the FSU is subjected to various external and internal loads (stresses), which are applied from many directions. These stresses produce deformations (strains) of the individual structural elements as well as motion between these elements. The applied loads may be in the form of compression, tension, torsion, or shear (Figure 1-1). Each anatomic unit contributes to the load-bearing capacity of the FSU, although the relative contributions depend upon the direction and the anatomic site to which the load is applied.

In the laboratory, the effect of these loads on the spine and the resultant deformations (strains) can be thoroughly and accurately measured. For example, under

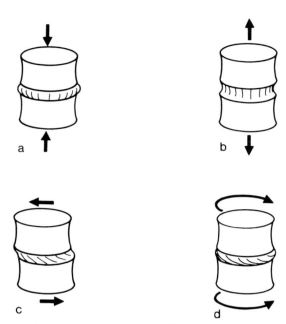

Figure 1-1. Force can be applied to the spine in four directional forms: (A) Compressive loading. Note the bulging of the annulus fibrosis. (B) Tension loading, implying that the annulus actually may become less bulged. This condition is seen in persons subjected to zero gravity, where the disc space height actually increases after prolonged exposure to that environment. (C) Shear forces, which basically are translational changes. (D) Torsional loading. Note that the annular fibers in both shear and torsional loading are placed under considerable stretch and it is likely that this force application is most commonly associated with disruptions of the annulus fibrosis.

compressive loads, the annulus fibrosis bulges, the vertebral endplates deform, and intradiscal pressure increases. If the load continues to increase, the vertebral endplates will fracture before the disc herniates.[30] Approximately 25 percent of a compressive load is shared with the facets; removal of one facet shifts the entire load to the disc.[21] When bending movements are combined with compressive forces, a wide variety of injuries occur to bone and soft tissue.[31] In torsion, the annulus resists approximately 30 percent of the imposed load, with strains generated particularly at the posterolateral corners of the disc.[7] Major strains occur within the lumbar facet joints and their capsules because the perpendicular orientation of these joints is ideally suited to resisting torsional loads. In contrast, the orientation of the cervical facets makes those joints less capable of resisting torsional loads; greater strains are therefore placed upon the capsules, ligaments, and disc. Shear stresses are shared by the discs, the facet joints, and the ligaments, although loading to failure frequently causes fractures about the neural arch.[14] Most tensile stresses are absorbed by the ligaments of the FSU, particularly when the spine is in flexion and extension.

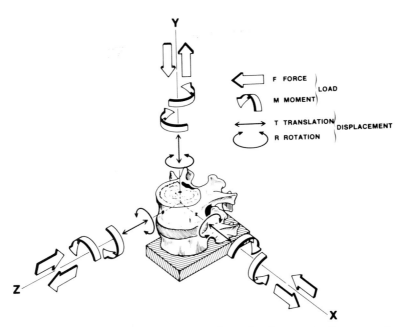

Figure 1-2. Rotations and translations can occur about the three mutually perpendicular axes of any spinal motion segment. By convention these are labeled X, Y, and Z. Note that rotation or translation can occur in two directions about each axis as depicted by the smaller arrows. Applied forces can be made in any of the same directions as the resultant motions and include translational and rotatory forces. In any spinal motion segment, one motion is usually accompanied by a minimum of two other secondary motions. (Reprinted from White AA, Panjabi MM: Clinical Biomechanics of the Spine. Philadelphia, J.B. Lippincott, 1978. With permission of the authors and publisher.)

Imposed stresses also produce motion between structural elements. Although spinal motion is usually described as flexion, extension, lateral bend, and axial rotation, spinal motion is a much more complex event than is suggested by these terms and various combinations of these simple motions can occur simultaneously. This mechanical phenomenon is termed *coupling.*[36] For example, with lateral flexion of the lumbar spine, a small amount of forward flexion and axial rotation also occurs, although the lateral flexion is the "major motion," and the others are the "coupled motions." In general, these motions can be described as rotations about or translations along any one of three mutually perpendicular axes, so that there are six possible components of movement for any single complex motion (Figure 1-2). The specific coupling behavior at a given spinal level is the result of the anatomic configurations of the various components of the motion segment, particularly the facets.

In addition to providing support and transmission of forces, the spine protects neurologic structures. The most catastrophic result of spinal instability is neurologic injury.

Spinal stability is a condition of the spine in which, under physiologic loading, there is neither abnormal strain nor excessive or abnormal motion in the FSU and in which neurologic structures are protected. Although satisfactory, this definition has a number of limitations. First, the spectrum of "normal" spinal motions may increase or decrease with age, physical fitness, and training. For example, the normal preadolescent spine often shows translations or rotations that in an adult would imply instability. Second, spinal stability is not determined by the FSU alone, but also by the musculature, abdominal and thoracic cavity pressures, rib cage support, and fascial envelopes such as the lumbodorsal fascia.[11] Indeed, a cadaveric spine is grossly unstable when separated from its component supportive structures, buckling under axial compressive loads less than the weight of the head.[22] This lack of stability is evident in the collapsing spine seen in patients with paralytic neuromuscular diseases. Third, the material properties of the spine vary between persons as a function of activity, age, density of bone, chemical composition of ligaments, and resiliency of the discs.

SPINAL INSTABILITY

Spinal instability is a condition in which the anatomic elements of the FSU or its supportive structures are disrupted, so that loads that are normally tolerated result in excessive or abnormal spinal motions, displacements, or strains, causing the development of progressive deformities. More difficult than the task of defining spinal instability is determining its presence in a clinical situation. The appearance of the spine on roentgenograms, an analysis of the external forces thought to have produced the instability, the anatomic location of the lesion, and the presence or absence of associated neurologic impairment have been used to attempt to make this determination. Studies of spinal fractures have provided the greatest insight into this problem.

For example, Holdsworth classified instability according to the fracture pattern observed on spinal roentgenograms,[13] defining simple wedge fractures, burst fractures, and extension injuries as stable injuries and shear fractures, rotational fracture-dislocations, and dislocations as unstable injuries. Kelly and Whitesides[17] and Whitesides[37] defined burst injuries as unstable because this type of fracture is commonly associated with a neurologic deficit. Their classification is based on the concept of an anterior (compressive) weight-bearing column and a posterior tension-resisting column. Aided by computed tomographic (CT) scans, McAfee et al.[26] expanded the two-column principle into a three-column principle; the anterior column includes the anterior two thirds of the vertebral body and disc; the middle column comprises the posterior one third of the vertebral body, the annulus fibrosis, and the posterior longitudinal ligaments; and the posterior column includes the remaining posterior structures including the ligaments and facet capsules (Figure 1-3). They suggested compression, axial distraction, and translations in the transverse plane as three forces that are the most common mechanisms of injury. Based on extensive laboratory studies, White and Panjabi[36] developed an even more complex classification based on an analysis of the forces that produced an observed deformity and the three-dimensional coupled motion segment behavior of the spine (Figure 1-4). Their concept of a mean injury vector (MIV) defines both the predominant force along a given axis that results in injury and secondary coupled forces and their resultant effects. Extensive criteria have been developed by these investigators for multiple spinal levels based upon the observed fracture pattern, the angulatory and torsional deformities observed, the response to physiologic loading, and the presence or absence of

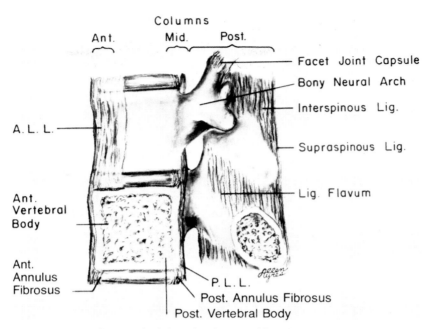

Figure 1-3. The three-column principle. The degree of involvement of these three columns is best determined by computed axial tomography. (Reprinted from McAfee PC, Yuan HA, Fredrickson BE, Lubicky JP: The value of computed tomography in thoracolumbar fractures. J Bone Joint Surg 64A:461–473, 1983. With permission.)

neurologic involvement. Table 1-1 illustrates their analysis based upon the sequential sectioning of supportive structures. Others have characterized specific motion segment instabilities, e.g., the atlantoaxial joints, based upon similar laboratory investigations.[9,27]

The practical ramifications of these studies are that in an acute injury, the deformity, an analysis of the load application, and the presence or absence of neurologic involvement are the best predictors of instability. Complete anatomic knowledge usually can be obtained from standard roentgenograms and CT scans, while in selected cases myelography and multiplanar tomography are useful. Potentially unstable injuries are those in which the injuring forces are less severe or less well understood, in which there is no neurologic involvement, or in which stability is questionable. These conditions are best examined by the application of controlled physiologic stresses. Dynamic radiography (e.g., flexion-extension roentgenograms) can be very useful in defining abnormal motions (Figure 1-5). Controlled traction may also define the extent of injury, particularly in the cervical spine. These same techniques are useful in diagnosing nontraumatic forms of spinal instability.

Spinal instability is associated with a variety of pathologic conditions. Among these, congenital defects most commonly involve the cervical spine, and these may be associated with instability because of deficits of critical bony or ligamentous structures such as the os odontoideum, Klippel-Feil syndrome, and certain chromosomal abnormalities. Spondylolisthesis is the most common such lesion in the lumbar spine. That lesion probably is not present at birth but occurs in adolescence as a result of a

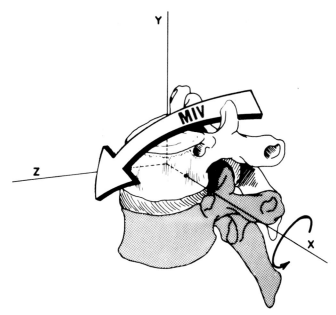

Figure 1-4. The major injury vector (MIV) according to White and Panjabi. Shown here is a bilateral facet dislocation in the cervical spine. Note that the major force application is in translation along the Z axis. An accompanying rotational component is depicted by an arrow about the X axis. Complex and simple fractures may be analyzed according to the forces that have produced the deformity in the three mutually perpendicular planes as shown in Figure 1-2. (Reprinted from White AA, Panjabi MM: Clinical Biomechanics of the Spine. Philadelphia, J.B. Lippincott, 1978. With permission of the authors and publisher.)

congenital predisposition to a fatigue fracture of the pars interarticularis.[39] The instability of a FSU with spondylolisthesis is age-dependent, the adolescent patient being most susceptible to progressive deformity and sometimes to a spondylolisthetic crisis, characterized by severe pain and hamstring spasm. An adult with spondylolisthesis rarely possesses an unstable spine, although destabilization can occur during pregnancy or occasionally after excision of the neural arch (the Gill procedure) and probably in the less common L4-5 isthmic lesion (Figure 1-6). Spondylolisthesis is rarely associated with an acute neurologic deficit, although an acute, traumatically induced spondylolisthesis may be unstable and result in neural injury.

Instability Resulting from Infectious or Inflammatory Processes

Pyogenic infectious diseases, most notably tuberculosis and more rarely fungal diseases, may be associated with progressive spinal instability and deformity. Typically, these processes involve structures of the anterior and middle columns rather than the posterior column.

Table 1-1
Checklist for the Diagnosis of Clinical Instability in the
Lower Cervical Spine

Element	Point Value
Anterior elements destroyed or unable to function	2
Posterior elements destroyed or unable to function	2
Relative sagittal plane translation; 3.5 mm	2
Relative sagittal plane rotation; 11	2
Positive stretch test	2
Spinal cord damage	2
Nerve root damage	1
Abnormal disc narrowing	1
Dangerous loading anticipated	1
Total of 5 or more = unstable	

Adapted from White A, Southwick WO, Panjabi MM: Clinical instability in the lower cervical spine. A review of past and current concepts. Spine, 1:15, 1976.

Rheumatoid arthritis and a variety of other noninfectious inflammatory diseases can also produce instability. In rheumatoid disease, the atlantoaxial joints and cervical spine are involved as a result of the granulomatous destruction of stabilizing ligaments.[4] A peculiar lesion has been documented in ankylosing spondylitis, consisting of a fracture nonunion with instability and progressive deformity.[32]

Instability from Neoplastic Diseases

Most of the structurally significant spinal tumors involve the vertebral body rather than the posterior elements, and the resulting deformities therefore actually involve the anterior weight-bearing column. The propensity for neoplasms to involve the vertebral body most likely is a result of the rich blood supply to that structure. Primary spinal neoplasms are relatively rare; among the more common are osteoid osteoma, osteoblastoma, aneurysmal bone cyst, eosinophilic granuloma, and chordoma. Spinal instability is relatively uncommon in those benign tumors. Malignant primary osseous neoplasms are even more rare, with the exception of multiple myeloma. Virtually all forms of osseous neoplasms have been reported in the spine, most commonly chondrosarcoma and osteogenic sarcoma. In contrast to the relative rarity of those primary neoplasms, multiple myeloma is quite common. Loss of spinal stability may result from a solitary focus or it may be part of a more diffuse syndrome. In diffuse multiple myeloma, a structural weakening is often aggravated by the presence of severe osteoporosis. Despite the relative rarity of most primary neoplasms, they can produce striking instabilities (Figure 1-7).

In contrast to primary neoplasms, secondary neoplasms are common. Currently, the most common metastatic neoplasms are those in the lungs, followed closely by breast cancer. Thyroid and renal neoplasms also have a propensity to metastasize to the spine, and virtually all primary sites have been reported to involve the spine. The magnitude of the resulting instability is a function of the aggressiveness of the tumor, its location, and whether the patient has undergone prior radiation or chemotherapeutic

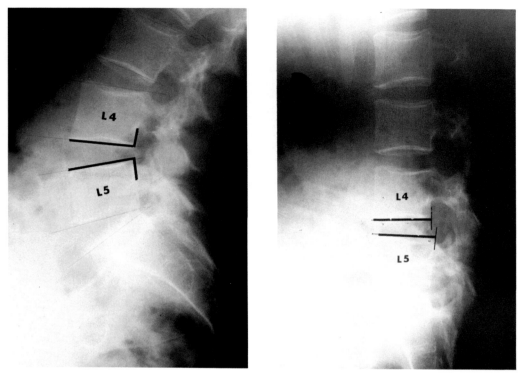

Figure 1-5. These flexion-extension roentgenograms were obtained on a 32-year-old woman with a history of chronic low back pain and recurrent episodes of muscular spasm. She described the sensation of her back "going out of place." Her examination was entirely normal and plain roentgenograms were unrevealing. Note that in extension (A) there is normal alignment of the posterior vertebral bodies of L4 and L5. In forward flexion (B) there is forward translation of L4 and L5 amounting to 4 mm of displacement and a tendency toward asymmetric anterior collapse of the intervertebral disc. The diagnosis is segmental instability (degenerative). This illustrates the importance of obtaining dynamic roentgenograms on patients in whom instability is suspected but not shown by plain roentgenograms.

treatment. It is in this latter group of patients that use of methylmethacrylate for stabilization finds its greatest role.

Instability from Degenerative Diseases

Degenerative spinal instability is most controversial. Knutsson believed that abnormal translations observed on flexion-extension roentgenograms in patients with low back pain were the earliest evidence of a degenerative lesion.[19] Today, the very existence of degenerative instability continues to be questioned. Central to the controversy is the lack of agreed-upon anatomic, mechanical, and radiographic criteria to determine what constitutes a degenerative instability. Because the instability is often subtle, accurate measurements are frequently impossible. Associated pain may further limit spinal motion to such an extent that abnormal motions are not observed. It is not surprising that a high degree of interobserver errors occur when flexion-extension

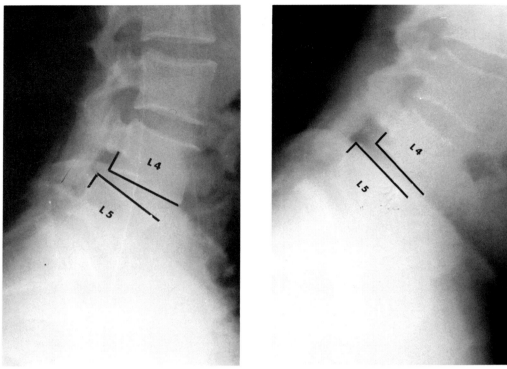

Figure 1-6. This 42-year-old physician had a 20-year history of low back pain with recurrent episodes of pain and spasm. (A) The lateral roentgenogram (Figure 1-6A) demonstrate slight forward slippage of L4 and L5 as well as a very subtle slip of L5 on S1. Oblique roentgenograms demonstrate a defect in the pars interarticularis consistent with spondylolisthesis at the L4-5 and L5-S1 levels. (B) Note that on forward flexion (Fig. 1-6B) there is additional displacement of L4 on L5 and considerable anterior disc space collapse. Spinal fusion resulted in complete cessation of the symptoms. L4-5 spondylolisthesis appears to be more unstable than L4-S1 spondylolisthesis, probably because of the restraining influence of the ligaments attached to the tranverse process.

roentgenograms of a suspected segmentally unstable spine are reviewed by different specialists. Presently, there is no uniformly accepted classification for degenerative instability. In a recent classification, we divided these disorders into five types: translational, rotational, retrolisthetic, postoperative (for example, destabilizing procedures such as total facetectomy), and postoperative occurring above or below a previous spinal fusion.[10] The most commonly used diagnostic test is flexion-extension roentgenography. At least five criteria are currently suggestive of segmental instability: forward translation of the vertebra greater than 3 mm in flexion,[19] asymmetry and disc space collapse between flexion and extension,[18,24] excessive retrolisthesis in extension,[12,20] hypermobility of the motion segment (motion greater than the 90th percentile for a person of a given age and sex),[1,2] and the presence of traction spurs.[25] For adequate films to be obtained, it is often necessary to do selective blocks to reduce the pain level such that a full range of spinal motion can be obtained. Among some of the

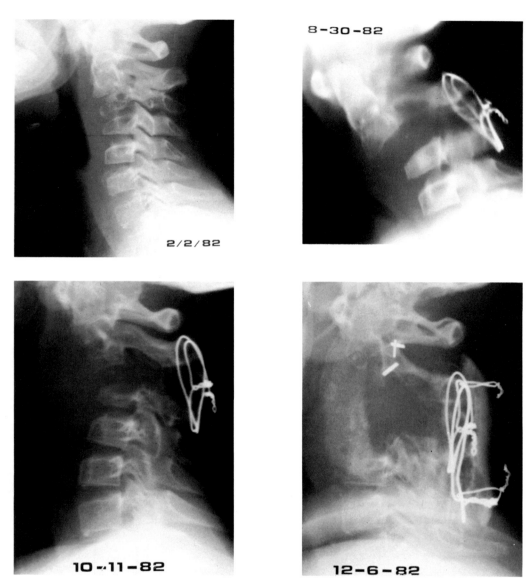

Figure 1-7. A 12-year-old boy with neck pain. (A) The initial roentgenograms demonstrated a destructive lesion of the body of C4. The destruction of the anterior column, combined with the kyphotic deformity, is highly suggestive of instability. A biopsy specimen was interpreted as showing histiocytoma. A posterior fusion was performed based on the presumed benign character of the lesion. (B) Films obtained 6 months later showed striking destruction of the body of C4 and forward translation of C3 on C5. The nonunion of the bone graft also was evident. In retrospect, an anterior fusion might have been more desirable. The child was managed in a halo pelvic stabilization device and a second biopsy was performed. The results indicated a malignant histiocytoma. (C) The tumor subsequently advanced to involve the entire bony structure of C4, including all posterior elements and dissolution of the bone graft. (D) Because of impending neurologic signs, anterior decompression with bone grafting followed by posterior fusion was performed. This provided adequate stabilization until the patient's demise 4 months later from disseminated disease despite radiation and chemotherapy.

10

most promising new methods for diagnosis is the biplanar roentgenogram, which permits calculation of three-dimensional motion abnormalities.[34,38]

In addition to these well-defined pathologic conditions, another large group of spinal instabilities is manifested by progressive deformity of multiple spinal units. These typically occur in childhood and are classified according to the predominant deformity and underlying pathologic cause. The most common lesions involve a scoliotic deformity or kyphus. In addition, children are especially susceptible to destabilization produced by certain surgical interventions, most notably laminectomies. Striking deformities may result in a significant percentage of such patients, particularly if the facet joint capsules are involved in the decompression.

GENERAL PRINCIPLES IN THE TREATMENT OF
SPINAL INSTABILITY

Spinal instability may occur suddenly or gradually. Acute instabilities are usually the result of trauma and the extensive destruction of one or more of the elements that make up the FSU, whereas chronic spinal instability develops slowly and is accompanied predominantly by pain and the late onset of neurologic symptoms. The goals of treatment in both groups are:

1. To ensure adequate healing of the destabilized segment in a position of optimal function.
2. To prevent (and hopefully reverse) neural injury and injury to the other spinal elements.
3. To prevent the subsequent development of a new deformity or progression of a previous deformity.

The specific condition and the affected spinal level dictate whether these goals are achieved by nonoperative management or whether operative stabilization is required. The general factors that influence these therapeutic decisions include:

1. The degree of instability present, as demonstrated by the findings on plain roentgenograms, CT scans, and the associated neurologic history. In more subtle cases, the application of controlled flexion-extension roentgenography or a trial of traction may be necessary to demonstrate the instability.
2. The type of tissue most extensively disrupted. Osseous involvement is made readily apparent by plain roentgenograms as well as the clinical picture. Ligamentous involvement may appear deceptively benign on plain roentgenograms and may not be apparent on CT scans. It is these injuries (e.g., the Chesire lesion) that are least likely to be stabilized by nonoperative intervention and often the most difficult to demonstrate.
3. The risk of subsequent deformity and its attendant complications. Although some lesions will heal even in a deformed position, there remains a high risk of late neurologic or musculoskeletal problems. For example, when there is substantial kyphotic deformity in the cervical spine, progressive increases in kyphosis as well as the development of both central and peripheral neurologic symptoms may often occur. Because such fixed deformities subsequently require complex and difficult operative correction, it is often wiser to consider early stabilization when the deformity is more easily reduced.

4. The balance of risk between operative intervention and the potential for delayed neurologic problems. Most commonly, operative management is chosen when the risk of later neurologic complication is high. This philosophy is particularly applicable to noncompliant patients or to patients who have congenital abnormalities of the upper cervical spine.

5. Socioeconomic and other costs of treatment. Although this consideration is most applicable in acute traumatic injuries, it is also applicable in the case of infectious and neoplastic lesions. There is substantial information that early operative management of unstable spine injuries improves the neurologic outcome, reduces the total cost of care, speeds the rehabilitation process, reduces secondary medical complications, and reduces the psychologic impact of the injury. This general philosophy is by no means uniformly accepted, but it has provided much of the rationale for the operative management of selected cases.

PRINCIPLES OF NONOPERATIVE MANAGEMENT

Numerous methods of nonoperative treatment for spinal instability have been used successfully, including recumbency, gravity reduction, casts, and spinal orthoses. In general, external means of stabilization are most effective in the cervical spine and least effective in the lumbar spine. Johnson et al.[16] have quantified the normal motion allowed and the stabilizing effect of cervical orthoses (Table 1-2). Based on this study, the halo device is shown to provide the most stabilization of any externally applied device. Given practical considerations, providing external stabilization is difficult from the level of T1 to T6; fortunately, however, this level of the spine is infrequently affected because of the stabilizing effects of the rib cage. External support can be provided to the thoracolumbar junction using a brace that depends upon the three-point contact principle, as illustrated in Figure 1-8.[28] Braces that are not based on this principle may limit lateral flexion but are less effective in controlling axial rotation and least effective in limiting flexion and extension.

It has been shown that in the lumbar spine most of the traditional braces and orthotic devices provide minimal stability and may actually accentuate certain motions such as axial rotation.[23,28,29] Recently, Fidler and Plasmans have shown that the range of movement of the lumbar spine is only controllable with a spica cast.[8]

PRINCIPLES OF OPERATIVE MANAGEMENT

Optimal surgical constructs are those which address the major element of the instability and preserve the less injured or normal spinal structures. For example, a complex lesion of the posterior ligaments of the cervical spine is best treated by posterior fusion, whereas a burst fracture of a cervical body would most logically be treated by anterior interbody fusion. In general, posterior approaches to the spine have been preferred in the management of spinal instability in most clinical situations except those conditions in which the major pathologic entity involves the anterior column. The predominant mechanical principle for thoracic and most lumbar injuries has been the concept embodied in the Harrington rod procedure. Cadaveric studies have defined some of the general problems in posterior and anterior spinal fixation. Posterior wire

Table 1-2
Normal Motion Allowed from the Occiput to the First Thoracic Vertebra
(Mean Percentage and 95-Percent Confidence Limits of the Mean)

Test Situation	Number of Subjects (Male/Female)	Mean Age in Years (Range)	Flexion-Extension	Significance	Rotation	Significance	Lateral Bending	Significance
Normal unrestricted (all subjects)	44 (19/25)	25.8 (20–36)	100		100		100	
Soft collar	20 (10/10)	26.2 (20–36)	74.2 ± 7.2	<0.001	82.6 ± 4.6	<0.001	92.3 ± 8.0	0.057 (NS)
Philadelphia collar	17 (9/8)	25.8 (20–34)	28.9 ± 4.7	<0.001	43.7 ± 6.7	<0.001	66.4 ± 10.7	<0.001
Somi brace	22 (7/15)	25.0 (21–31)	27.7 ± 6.6	0.772 (NS)	33.6 ± 6.4	<0.05	65.6 ± 9.4	0.899 (NS)
Four-poster brace	27 (11/16)	25.9 (21–36)	20.6 ± 5.4	<0.05	27.1 ± 3.9	<0.05	45.9 ± 7.5	<0.001
Cervicothoracic brace	27 (11/16)	25.9 (21–36)	12.8 ± 3.0	<0.05	18.2 ± 3.2	<0.001	50.5 ± 7.1	0.063 (NS)
Halo with plastic body vest	7 (6/1)	40.0 (20–48)	4		1		4	

* Significance reported is the probability value of one brace or collar compared with the test situation directly above, using the paired t test. For example, flexion-extension in the soft collar was significantly different from normal unrestricted motion ($P < 0.001$) and the Philadelphia collar was significantly better in restricting flexion-extension than the soft collar ($P < 0.001$), whereas the Somi brace was similar in effectiveness to the Philadelphia collar ($P = 0.772$).
Adapted from Johnson RM, Hart DL, Simmons EF, Ramsby GR, Southwick WO: Cervical orthoses: A study comparing their effectiveness in restricting cervical motion in normal subjects. J Bone Joint Surg 59A, 332–339, 1977.

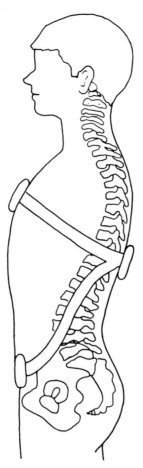

Figure 1-8. The three-point contact principle is illustrated by this brace. Two points of attachment contact the pubis and sternum with the third point of contact directly overlying the injured area, in this case a compression fracture. By using these three points of contact, the straightened posture of the spine can be maintained.

fixation, particularly when limited to the spinous processes, has significant problems with the wires cutting out of the spine and fatigue failure of the metal.[28] Although there have been favorable reports on the use of Weiss springs, particularly in kyphotic lesions, these have less stability than other forms of instrumentation, particularly in axial rotation, and have recently been modified to correct this deficiency. Stauffer and Neil[33] and Jacobs et al.[15] have compared the stabilizing effects of multiple forms of internal fixation. The greatest degree of stabilization is provided by the Harrington distraction system, which embodies the "fuse-short, rod-long" concept. Correction of the spinal deformity occurs fairly predictably,[5] provided that the anterior longitudinal ligament is intact. There is, however, a growing body of evidence that anterior decompression and stabilization may be more effective in reversing partial neurologic lesions, particularly at the thoracolumbar junction.[3] In the cervical spine, adequate stability is provided by effective means of supplementary external fixation such as the Rogers' fusion. An anterior bone graft provides greater strength when the vertebral endplates are left intact and the orientation of the cortices of the graft is perpendicular to the disc space.[35]

The other goal of surgical intervention is to maintain the corrected and stabilized spinal unit, and this is best achieved with the use of autogenous graft materials. Methylmethacrylate is appealing because it achieves instant stabilization and avoids the additional morbidity associated with obtaining the graft. Since this material is strongest in compression and weakest in tension, its optimal use is in the replacement of anterior rather than posterior structures. Under certain conditions, where bone fusion is difficult to obtain or life expectancy is short, methylmethacrylate may be used; however, it usually should be supplemented with an autogenous bone graft.[6]

SUMMARY

Spinal stability is dependent on the structural integrity of the functional spinal unit and its surrounding muscular, fascial, and cavity support structures. Instability occurs when there is a loss of structural integrity in either the functional spinal unit or the adjacent spinal support elements. Such destabilization results in excessive or abnormal motion, abnormal strains upon the various elements of the FSU, and risk of neurologic injury. The clinical detection of instability may be obvious when there is major involvement of the anatomic elements of the FSU. Factors that help determine the presence and magnitude of instability include a knowledge of the forces that produced it, the pattern of anatomic involvement as determined from plain roentgenograms and CT scans, and the presence or absence of neurologic signs and symptoms. When spinal instability is not clearly evident, application of controlled physiologic stresses, most commonly flexion-extension roentgenography, may often demonstrate the unstable condition.

The classification of spinal instability is based upon the underlying pathologic process that produced it. A broad range of congenital, inflammatory, neoplastic, degenerative, and traumatic conditions, as well as iatrogenic factors are associated with spinal destabilization.

Principles of treatment are directed toward ensuring adequate stabilization in an anatomic position, the prevention of later deformity, and the protection of neurologic elements. This objective may be met by nonoperative treatment, although there are certain fundamental limitations in bracing, particularly in the lumbar spine. Often, surgical intervention is chosen for complex anatomic and socioeconomic reasons. Surgical stabilization may be achieved by a variety of surgical constructs and fixation devices. In general, such devices should always be supplemented by autogenous bone grafts, although certain conditions, for example, neoplasms, may require the use of bone substitutes such as methylmethacrylate.

REFERENCES

1. Aho A, Vartiainen O, Salo O: Segmentary mobility of the lumbar spine in anteroposterior flexion. Ann Med Intern Fenn 44:275, 1955
2. Allbrook D: Movements of the lumbar spine column. J Bone Joint Surg 39B:339, 1957
3. Auden U, Lake A, Nordwall A: The role of the anterior longitudinal ligament in Harrington rod fixation of unstable thoracolumbar spinal fracture. Spine 5:23, 1980
4. Bland JH: Rheumatoid arthritis of the cervical spine. J Rheumatol 1:319, 1974
5. Bradford DS, Akbarnia BA, Winter RB, Seljeskog EL: Surgical stabilization of fracture and fracture dislocations of the thoracic spine. Spine 2:185, 1977
6. Clark CR, Keggi KJ, Panjabi MM: Methylmethacrylate stabilization of the cervical spine. J Bone Joint Surg 66A:40, 1984

7. Farfan HF: Mechnical Disorders of the Low Back. Philadelphia, Lea & Febiger, 1973

8. Fidler MW, Plasmans CMT: The effect of four types of support on the segmental mobility of the lumbosacral spine. J Bone Joint Surg 65A:943, 1983

9. Fielding JW, Cochran G van B, Lawsing JF, Hohl M: Tears of the transverse ligament of the atlas. A clinical and biomechanical study. J Bone Joint Surg 56A:1683, 1974

10. Frymoyer JW, Selby DK: Segmental instability: Rationale for treatment. Spine 10:280, 1985

11. Gracovetsky S, Farfan HF, Lamy C: A mathematical model of the lumbar spine using an optimized system to control muscles and ligaments. Orthop Clin North Am 8:135, 1977

12. Hagelstam L: Retroposition of lumbar vertebrae. Acta Chir Scand (Suppl) 143, 1949

13. Holdsworth FW: Fractures, dislocations and fracture-dislocations of the spine. J Bone Joint Surg 52A:1534, 1970

14. Hutton WC, Stott JRR, Cyron BM: Is spondylolysis a fatigue fracture? Spine 2:202, 1977

15. Jacobs RR, Nordwall A, Nachemson A: Reduction, stability and strength provided by internal fixation systems for thoracolumbar spinal injuries. Clin Orthop 171:300, 1982

16. Johnson RM, Hart DL, Simmons EF, Ramsby GR, Southwick WO: Cervical orthoses. A study comparing their effectiveness in restricting cervical motion in normal subjects. J Bone Joint Surg 59A:332, 1977

17. Kelly RP, Whitesides TE: Treatment of lumbodorsal fracture-dislocations. Ann Surg 167:705, 1968

18. Kirkaldy-Willis WH, Farfan HF: Instability of the lumbar spine. Clin Orthop 165:110, 1982

19. Knutsson F: The instability associated with disc degeneration in the lumbar spine. Acta Radiol 25:593, 1944

20. Lehmann T, Brand R: Instability of the lower lumbar spine. Paper presented at the Eighth International Society for Study of the Lumbar Spine, Toronto, 1982. Orthop Trans 7:97, 1983

21. Lorenz M, Patwardhan A, Vanderby R: Load bearing characterisitcs of lumbar facets in normal and surgically altered spinal segments. Spine 8:122, 1983

22. Lucas DB, Bresler B: Stability of the ligamentous spine. Biomech Lab Report #40, University of California, San Francisco, 1961

23. Lumsden RM, Morris JM: An in vivo study of axial rotation and immobilization at the lumbosacral joint. J Bone Joint Surg 50A:1591, 1968

24. MacGibbon B, Farfan HF: A radiologic survey of various configurations of the lumbar spine. Spine 4:258, 1979

25. Macnab I: The traction spur—An indicator of segmental instability. J Bone Joint Surg 53:663, 1971

26. McAfee PC, Yuan HA, Fredrickson BE, Lubicky JP: The value of computed tomography in thoracolumbar fractures. J Bone Joint Surg 64A:461, 1983

27. Mouradian WH, Fietti VG Jr, Cochran GV, Fielding JW, Young J: Fractures of the odontoid: A laboratory and clinical study of mechanisms. Orthop Clin North Am 9:985, 1978

28. Nagel DA, Koogle TA, Piziali RL, Perkash I: Stability of the upper lumbar spine following progressive disruptions and the application of individual internal and external fixation devices. J Bone Joint Surg 63A:62, 1981

29. Norton PL, Brown T: The immobilizing efficiency of back braces. Their effect of postures and motion of the lumbosacral spine. J Bone Joint Surg 39A:111, 1957

30. Perey O: Fracture of the vertebral end-plate in the lumbar spine: An experimental investigation. Acta Orthop Scand (Suppl) 25, 1957

31. Roaf R: A study of the mechanics of spinal injuries. J Bone Joint Surg 42B:810, 1960

32. Simmons EH, Goodwin C: Spondylodiscitis: A manifestation of ankylosing spondylitis. Presented at the Annual Meeting of the International Society for the Study of the Lumbar Spine, April, 1983. Orthop Trans 7:460, 1983

33. Stauffer ES, Neil JL: Biomechanical analysis of structural stability of internal fixation in fracture of the thoracolumbar spine. Clin Orthop 112:159, 1975

34. Stokes IAF, Wilder DG, Frymoyer JW, Pope MH: Assessment of patients with low back pain by biplanar radiographic measurement of intervertebral motion. Spine 6:233, 1981

35. White AA, Hirsch C: An experimental study of the immediate load bearing capacity of some commonly used iliac bone grafts. Acta Orthop Scand 42:482, 1971

36. White AA, Panjabi MM: Clinical Biomechanics of the Spine. Philadelphia, J.B. Lippincott, 1978

37. Whitesides TE: Traumatic kyphosis of the thoracolumbar spine. Clin Orthop 128:78, 1977

38. Wilder DG, Seligson D, Frymoyer JW, Pope MH: Objective measurement of L4-5 instability: A case report. Spine 5:56, 1980

39. Wiltse LL, Widell EH, Jackson DW: Fatigue fracture: The basic lesion in isthmic spondylolisthesis. J Bone Joint Surg 57A:17, 1975

Michael J. Apuzzo
Robert G. Watkins
William R. Dobkin

2

Biomechanics of the Neural Axis

Excursion of the vertebral column through its normal functional range produces extreme physiologic deformation from the mesencephalon to the filum terminale. In order to understand how the spinal cord adapts to these stresses, it is necessary to analyze the morphologic, physical, and architectural properties of the normal spinal cord.[1] This will provide a basis for comprehending the pathologic processes that act upon the thoracic spinal cord. Since these elements of neural mechanics are not only a function of anatomic and physiologic alterations of the neural elements but are also related to impairment in the vascular supply of these structures, an understanding of the anatomy of the blood supply to the major spinal neural axis is critical.[2,4]

The arterial blood supply to the cervical portion of the thoracic spinal cord originates from tributaries of the subclavian artery, while branches of the intercostal arteries supply the midthoracic and thoracolumbar segments. With the exception of the intradural branches of the vertebral arteries, all other blood vessels supplying the thoracic cord pass through the intervertebral foramina. These segmental arteries accompany each anterior and posterior root. Their presence originally led Willis to propose the concept of a symmetrical metameric arterial blood supply to the spinal cord. The classic dissections of Adamkiewicz and Kalzi, however, not only disproved this thesis, but also yielded insight into the true nature of the blood supply to the spinal cord. They stressed that certain preferential radicular arteries are larger and supply the cord as the anterior and posterior radiculomedullary arteries. At the cord these arteries are distributed in an anterior and posterior anastomotic chain.

The anterior spinal artery runs in the median fissure the entire length of the cord and is composed of an anastomotic chain of ascending and descending inosculating branches arising from multiple radiculomedullary arteries. The diameter of the anterior spinal artery varies as a function of its proximity to a major arterial feeder, being largest in the lumbar enlargement and smallest in the midthoracic region. The posterior arterial system is less developed in its longitudinal pattern, and unlike the anterior system with its few critical arterial channels, it receives small radiculomedullary branches at almost every interspace. The paired posterolateral channels are often totally replaced by a posterolateral vascular plexus.

The arterial distribution within the cord is essentially composed of a peripheral system from radicular branches of the pia mater, which supplies the superficial structures and the white matter tracts; and a central system, which vascularizes the central areas, the gray matter, and the innermost aspects of the deep white matter.

In contrast to the variability that exists in the segmental afferent arterial supply to the neural axis, the intramedullary disposition of arterial channels appears more constant. There is a range for the number of anterior sulcal arteries, however, and this probably reflects unequal growth of the various segments of the spinal cord. This relative deficiency of anterior sulcal arteries, particularly in the midthoracic region, is also a function of the relative lack of metabolically active gray matter in this section of the spinal cord. In the cervical cord there are five to eight anterior sulcal arteries per centimeter; the lumbosacral region has five to twelve vessels per centimeter, while in the midthoracic region there are only two to five vessels per centimeter. Because of the limited number of afferent vessels in the midthoracic region, their field of vertical coverage is more extensive; in the thoracic region this may span 3 cm, while in the cervical and lumbosacral regions it is at most 1.2 and 1.7 cm, respectively. Unlike the longitudinal capillary anastomoses, which occur within the gray matter, only a few nonfunctional anastomoses exist between these central arteries and the juxtaposed circumferential pial plexus.

The structural arrangement of the cord circulation therefore produces three functionally distinct zones: (1) the cervical and upper thoracic region, (2) the midthoracic region, and (3) the thoracolumbar region. Direct radiculomedullary branches to the midthoracic segment are few and blood flowing caudad from the upper thoracic region and cephalad from the low thoracic and lumbar regions contributes to this segment, which constitutes the largest and most critical "watershed area"— T3–T7. Likewise, the microcirculation of the midthoracic cord has the fewest number of penetrating arteries and therefore the largest field for each vessel to cover. The characteristics of the macrocirculation and the microcirculation of the midthoracic spinal cord therefore make it extremely vulnerable to a wide variety of lesions.

Microangiography of the human spinal cord has defined alterations that may occur in the microcirculation under both physiologic and pathologic stresses. With axial tension over a mass disposed anteriorly or from the direct effect of a large mass impinging anteriorly or anterolaterally, the cord is widened and flattened. As a consequence, the arteries from the pial plexus supplying the anterior and posterior columns become mildly tortuous, while those vessels supplying the superficial aspects of the lateral columns experience greater impairment, becoming elongated with a consequent decrease in their diameter. Branches from the central arteries supplying the lateral gray matter are similarly stretched lengthwise and compromised. The clinical manifestations of these ventrally situated masses therefore often involve functional impairment of the lateral coriticospinal tracts. The frequent loss of pain and tempera-ture sensation up to a level well below the region of the lesion indicates that the lateral aspects of the spinothalamic tracts, supplied by the pial mesh, are also involved. A mass located to one side of the cord will produce stress side to side. This characteris-tically interferes with the function of the lateral columns adjacent to it, probably by direct compression rather than on a vascular basis. The difference seen here between ventral and lateral masses probably stems from the shape of the canal and location of the roots, ligaments, and so forth.

The state of the vessels within the cord also will undoubtedly influence the reaction of the spinal cord to mechanical deformation. Minimal compression of an arteriosclerotic vessel may produce catastrophic changes; such compression might be tolerated by a younger pliant vessel.

SPINAL CORD MECHANICS

Anatomic Correlates

The fibers of the spinal cord are arranged in three patterns: folds, spirals, and a rhomboid network. The rigid collagen fibers within the epipial region encircle the entire cord as a monolayer rhomboid network and therein produce its chief structural support. This geometric and topographic configuration of collagen fibers allows for extensive axial translation of the spinal cord. Furthermore, it is through modulation of this complex mechanical array that the cord is able to adapt to certain mechanical deformations without compromising function.

The dentate ligaments tether the epipial layer to the adjacent dura mater. When stress is applied to the cord, either in axial or tranverse planes, deformation of the dentate ligaments occurs, partially through alteration of the geometry of their collagen meshwork. Contrariwise, when forces are distributed in the dura mater, they can secondarily impart tension to the spinal cord through their dentate attachments and thereby produce physiologic and pathologic sequelae.

The myelin sheath of the axis cylinders in the spinal cord consists of a spirally coiled lamella, which is composed of a bilayered lipid membrane. When the cord lengthens in flexion, it has been assumed that the coiled arrangement of the lamella provides the axis cylinders protection against damage precipitated by axial traction. Although no strict definition exists, it is possible that the myelin sheath itself accomodates to cord lengthening through axial extension of the coiled lamella. When the spinal cord shortens, histologic observations have shown that the axis cylinders fold in irregular spirals. Because of these three-dimensional foldings, the cross-sectional area of the axis cylinders and myelin increase, although the specific morphologic alterations are not well defined.

Microscopic examination of transverse sections of the spinal cord demonstrates numerous clefts containing vessels. The walls of these channels buttress and protect the vessels against mechanical damage. Like the epipial surfaces of the cord, these spaces have a rhomboid array of collagen, which accommodates certain movements but tends to resist excessive forces. As the cord shortens, these spaces remain patent because of the presence of these fibers. As the cord is stretched, the axially distributed nerve and glial fibers tend to centrifigally compress the vessels, whereas the mesenchymal network that runs transversely or parallel to the channel offers resistance to this compression.

The anterior spinal artery occupies a fairly protected position in the anterior median fissure. When a cord affected by an anteriorly disposed mass is stretched, all arteries running anteroposteriorly in the cord are also protected from compression as long as these mechanical forces are moderate. However, an increase in transverse tension resulting from elongation of the spinal canal tends to reduce the lumina of the arteries running transversely and thus produces neurologic injury.

In true compression it is chiefly those lateral branches of the central arteries running in the axial direction that are exposed to harmful overstretching; the sagittal branches of the central arteries that have been telescoped in extension are at first elongated within the normal range, but when the local tension is great enough, they rupture. Experimental cord compression in cadavers disclosed that tearing of vessels will take place when compression has reduced the anteroposterior diameter of the cord to slightly more than 20 percent.

Transmission of Tension in Soft Tissues of the Spinal Canal

Stretching and displacement of the dura mater within the spinal canal follows the physical principle known as Saint Venant's Law. This rule describes the distribution of axially directed traction at a point on the border of an elastic cylinder. This force is distributed around a cylinder in such a fashion that at a distance not exceeding two times the diameter of the cylinder, all points along the circumference of the cylinder will experience equal forces and therefore are equally displaced. The effect is the same irrespective of the material of which the tube is composed as long as the geometry of the tube is undisturbed. The dural tube, however, may not always be a perfect cylinder.

In cadaver experiments anteroposterior and lateral flexion of the thoracic spine resulted in stretching of the convex side of the dural tube, while relaxation and reduplication of the dura occurred on the concave side. In cadavers, where the only component of cerebrospinal fluid pressure is hydrostatic, infoldings of the dura mater were produced. Any tensile force applied to the convex side was immediately transmitted, whereas when such a force was applied to the concave side the slack first had to be taken up. In living subjects, dilatation of the arachnoid membrane and dura by CSF pressure produced a low uniform pretension in the dura, inhibiting the phenomenon of dural infolding and promoting immediate transmission of any additional tension over great distances. Scarring in the epidural displacement layer can result in permanent fixation of the dura in extension and result in alteration of dural mechanics. It is important to recognize this possibility during neurosurgical procedures undertaken to reduce stress on the cord and dura.

The local tension set up in various sections of the dura by pathologically increased angulation between two or more vertebrae or several large protrusions in the spinal canal is additive. Since the caudal end of the dura is firmly anchored in the sacral canal, the aggregate tension in the cervical cord and possibly also the thoracic dura is transmitted to the lumbar region.

Effect of Tension on the Spinal Cord

Under certain conditions the functional integrity of the spinal cord may be compromised by adverse mechanical tension exerted on either the nervous tissue itself or on its supporting structures. Breig[1] has outlined four types of mechanical action that may have an adverse impact on the spinal cord and its integument: (1) a unilateral thrust from without, (2) a multilateral thrust from within, (3) pinching or clamping, and (4) concentration of tension in intact nerve fibers around an intramedullary fissure.

A unilateral thrust is usually exerted by a structure located anteriorly or anterolaterally to the spinal cord; the pathologic force is generated by stretching of the spinal cord tracts during flexion of the spine. As long as the tract remains slack, the spinal cord will usually not be exposed to a thrust from any structure protruding into the spinal canal. Similarly, a multilateral thrust from within is exerted by a firm intramedullary lesion or structure, especially when flexion produces stretching of the tract.

In a bilateral pincer or clamping action on the cord, one of the contact surfaces is either a pathologic structure in the spinal canal or the margin of a displaced vertebral body; the other surface is the canal wall. The pincer or clamping actions are augmented during extension of the spine when the cross-sectional area is minimized. They are also intensified by the normal protrusion of the soft tissues into the canal.

Although it appears that great dissimilarity exists between the four mechanisms cited by Breig, histologic and microangiographic examinations have shown that the nerve fibers, blood vessels, and supporting tissues can be overstretched in various segments of the spinal cord. Unilateral as well as multilateral thrusts give rise to both a transverse and an axial tensile component. The forces in all four of these situations have been shown experimentally to result in constriction of nerve fibers and functional impairment. This attenuation of fiber cross-sectional area occurs where the cross-sectional diameter of the fiber is the smallest—a point midway between the nodes of Ranvier. Furthermore, it is precisely in this region where rupture of the fiber tends to occur. The stress set up in the cord by the pincer mechanism obviously produces little derangement in the longitudinal plane. Experimental studies have shown that when the anteroposterior diameter of the cord is reduced by 20 to 25 percent of its normal value, the axial tension in these structures is so great that rupture of the nerve fibers and blood vessels will probably occur initially in the central region of the cord. The magnitude of the pincer force will ultimately determine the degree of damage.

The forces involved in unilateral and multilateral thrusts and in notch stress around intramedullary fissures are considerably weaker than that produced by a pincer mechanism, and the resulting stress fields have a different configuration. In contrast to the limited range of the pincer action, in unilateral and multilateral thrusts the forces are transmitted over considerable distances and therefore can result in damage remote from the source of the tension. In the case of unilateral thrust the neurologic symptoms are caused by the axial tension in the nervous system; it is this component that constricts the nerve fibers and myelin sheaths and distorts the axoplasm.

The axial and tranverse tensile forces to which the nervous and vascular elements are subjected in the case of a unilateral or a multilateral thrust can result in an increase in the tensile forces around the end of a fissure. This can be eliminated by slackening of the cord.

When considering the nature of the stress induced in the cord by a pincer action, it is reasonable to assume that by removing one of the responsible pincers or clamping structures the tension can be removed. This can be done in certain situations with bilateral laminectomy.

In addition to nerve fibers, the blood vessels of the spinal cord are subjected to tension in the four mechanical situations noted earlier. The potentially great axial tension in the part of the tract exposed to a pinching mechanism or clamping action can lead to such severe stretching of the vascular elements, especially those located centrally in the medullary tissue, that they too may be ruptured. Less extreme tension may result in narrowing of the vessels, especially the small descending and ascending branches of the central arteries; the detrimental effect of this will be aggravated if their lumina are already reduced by fibrosis. The consequent reduction of the blood supply to the nerve fibers may further impair their function.

The tension set up in the vessel in any of the four mechanical situations should be released by appropriate functional measures—the tension caused by a pincer action by protective bilateral laminectomy, and that caused by unilateral and multilateral thrust by cervicolodesis or another surgical procedure that reduce axial strain.

The ability to analyze the response of the central nervous system to specific extrinsic stimuli has become possible with the advent of computer signal averaging techniques.[3] This instrumentation was necessary since the induced evoked potentials were several orders of magnitude less than the background electrical noise, which is composed mainly of the signals recorded by an EEG but also of nonneural electrical activity. This tehnique has particular application in monitoring manipulations of the midthoracic spine, the spinal canal, and its contents.

Elucidation of the anatomic correlates responsible for somatosensory evoked potentials (SEPs) has received considerable interest. Gliblin as well as Halliday and Wakefield recorded evoked potentials from scalp electrodes after shock pulse peripheral nerve depolarization in patients with a wide variety of spinal cord disorders. They found that abnormal loss of vibratory and joint position sense corresponded with abnormal SEPs. They concluded that the dorsal columns were requisite for transmission of evoked potentials through the spinal cord. Recordings of SEPs initiated in this fashion were made by several investigators on patients undergoing spinothalamic cordotomies. The absence of any impact on cortical SEPs after cordotomy implied that the spinothalamic tract was not necessary for spinal cord transmission of these SEPs. Chapman, however, has shown that stimulation of pain endings with laser light of insufficient intensity to produce tissue damage can induce a SEP that is transmitted through the spinothalamic tract.

The electrical potentials with the shortest latency recorded after somesthetic stimulation at the wrist occurred within 15 msec; at the ankle they occurred within 32 msec. They are of small amplitude since they represent far-field potentials or potentials recorded at a distance from their source. As a consequence of the distance these potentials must travel through a volume conductor composed of various tissues and CSF, it is difficult to exactly localize their source. It would appear that these potentials reflect summation action potentials from peripheral nerves and lemniscal tracts. A contribution from postsynaptic potentials generated in the brain stem nuclei of these sensory systems probably occurs as well. The cortical or near field potentials generated in the postcentral sulcus neurons has a latency of about 20 msec after median nerve stimulation at the wrist. In the thoracic spinal cord, we are concerned not only with the absolute latencies of all the supraspinal SEPs, having all been proportionately delayed in transit through a damaged spinal cord, but also with the increased time interval between the shortest latency responses and those in the caudal brainstem.

Spinal cord function has been further evaluated by recording of evoked potentials by both invasive and noninvasive techniques. Intrathecal conduction times from the lumbosacral enlargement to the cervical cord are reported to be from 30 to 50 msec. Cracco et al. have described a noninvasive technique for recording a triphasic evoked potential wave that is demonstrated from electrodes placed over the proximal cervical spinal cord. The conduction velocity of this evoked potential ranged from 60 to 80 msec. Although numerous elements of the cord contribute to this evoked potential, it is thought to originate primarily in the dorsal funiculus. Application of this technique allows for more accurate identification of the location of spinal cord compromise than does evaluation of SEPs.

Intraoperative recordings of SEPs have been done for a variety of lesions affecting both the spinal cord and the spine. They have proved to be useful both in preventing untoward manipulation of the spine during surgical positioning and in tempering surgical dissections. Furthermore, they have been employed as a means to prevent overdistraction when Harrington rod instrumentation is used for corrective scoliotic surgery. Also, recordings from epidural electrodes implanted during surgery for myelopathy induced by spondylosis have suggested that the degree of conduction abnormalities encountered at surgery may correlate with eventual resolution of the myelopathy.

Therefore, the contribution of evoked potential recordings in patients harboring lesions of the thoracic spine is three-fold. First, somatosensory evoked potentials will allow assessment of the degree of involvement of the dorsal columns. Second, spinal evoked potentials can help localize that segment of the cord that is compromised. Third, intraoperative recordings, whether from electrodes over the spinal cord or over the brain, will prevent unacceptable surgical positioning, may prevent overzealous surgical dissections, and appear to be helpful in elucidating the maximum distracting forces that can safely be induced during stabilization procedures. In addition, the degree of dysfunction recorded at surgery over the involved segment of abnormal nervous tissue may suggest the future course of spinal cord recovery. However, the exact clinical role for the use of evoked potentials has not been fully established.

REFERENCES

1. Breig A: Adverse Mechanical Tension in the Central Nervous System. New York, John Wiley & Sons, 1978
2. Lazorthes G, Gouaze A, Zadeh JO, Santini JJ, Lazorthes Y, Burdin P: Arterial vascularization of the spinal cord. J Neurosurg 35:252, 1971
3. Macon JB, Poletti CE, Sweet WH, Ojemann RG, Zervas NT: Conducted somatosensory evoked potentials during spinal surgery: Clinical applications. J Neurosurg 57:354, 1982
4. Turnbull IM: Microvasculature of the human spinal cord. J Neurosurg 35:141, 1971

Theodore I. Malinin
Frank J. Eismont
Mark D. Brown

3

Materials Used in Spine Stabilization

The spinal column is considered to be unstable when it can no longer maintain normal anatomic alignment of one of its motion segment units (comprising adjacent vertebrae with their neural arches and intervertebral disc, facet joint capsules, and ligaments), protect the neural elements within the spinal canal, support the body in an erect position, or allow for normal motion.[54] Spinal instability can be the result of severe degenerative disease of the motion segment unit, involving either the intervertebral discs, the posterior elements, or both. It can also occur with trauma, tumor, or infection resulting in destruction of the anterior, posterior, or both columns of the spine. Under these circumstances it is the goal of the clinician to restore alignment, stabilize the spine, and maintain or restore normal function.

Stabilization of the spinal column can be achieved either by various external support devices or, more effectively, by direct internal fixation of the spine. Various traction devices have been found effective in treating the cervical spine, but their use in the thoracic and lumbar spine has been largely disappointing. In general, the lower the lesion, the less effective is splinting of the spine.[21] Thoracic and lumbar supports such as braces and corsets provide at best only partial immobilization of the spine to which they are applied.[58] Among these devices, a custom-made polypropylene thoracolumbosacral orthosis is probably the most effective. Motion is often increased in segments of the spine adjacent to the ends of such orthoses.[43] The plaster body jacket used with considerable frequency several decades ago is now used but rarely. The "halo" brace adequately immobilizes the cervical spine,[44] but it is not effective for thoracic or lumbar instability unless combined with upright rods connected to either an external pelvic orthosis or to internal pelvic fixation.[11,34]

These difficulties with external stabilization of the thoracic and lumbar spine have led to the development of methods and devices for internal stabilization of the spine. The materials used for internal stabilization include metal instrumentation, polymethylmethacrylate cement, and cadaver and autogenous bone grafts.

SPINAL FUSION

Successful arthrodesis of the spine achieves permanent internal fixation of the spinal column. Rigid arthrodesis is only rarely produced without bone grafts being interposed between the vertebral bodies or superimposed on exposed bone of the vertebral column. For this purpose, two types of bone grafts—autografts and allografts—are available. The most frequently used grafts are grafts of autologous bone. The advantages of using the patient's own bone are obvious, but these are counterbalanced by limitations in the quantity and occasionally the quality of bone that is available. In many circumstances, adequately prepared bone allografts work as well as autogenous bone grafts,[37] and they have the advantage of anatomic versatility.

Autografts of Bone

As early as 1911, Albee advocated fusing the spine in children with Pott's disease with autologous struts obtained from the tibia.[1] Tibial bone is still occasionally used, but corticocancellous bone taken from the ilium is now by far the most frequently used autograft. When placed in an environment with a good blood supply, these grafts act as scaffolding for the growth of new bone and induce osteogenesis from surrounding mesenchymal cells. Whether or not these grafts actively contribute cells to bone formation currently is an unresolved question. The use of autografts is limited by the quantity and dimension of the graft and by the morbidity associated with obtaining the grafts. In addition, autografts in patients with osteoporosis may be structurally weak and unable to provide initial structural support for the spine.

Autogenous bone may be harvested from various portions of the ilium. Curved tricortical struts can be taken from the top of the ilium, straight corticocancellous strips are available from the lateral aspect of the ilium, and cancellous bone in copious amounts can be taken from the posterior and superior aspects of the iliac crest. If longer and structurally stronger grafts are needed, they can be obtained by taking sections of the ilium or the middle portion of the fibula. In the case of the fibula, care must be exercised not to divide the interosseous membrane at the distal fourth of the fibula, since this would make the ankle unstable. Ribs are also excellent sources of bone with good osteogenic potential, but they are often structurally weak and do not provide as much support as may be needed. Rib grafts with a vascular pedicle have been used recently as anterior struts in reconstructing the thoracic and thoracolumbar region. These heal rapidly, hypertrophy when placed under stress, and provide good structural support with time.

The presence of periosteum on an autologous bone graft is not essential for its successful transplantation. Some investigators believe that the cells die in a transplanted autograft and the graft is subsequently repopulated by cells derived from the surrounding tissues. Other investigators, however, argue that osteocytes in cancellous bone survive transplantation, in which case care should be taken to avoid injuring these cells. Exposure to air with subsequent dessication decreases cell viability. Prolonged exposure to saline, elevation in temperature, many chemical agents, and antibiotics are lethal to bone cells.[4,47] Empirical observations show that bone autografts survive for five to six hours in blood-soaked gauze sponges. Marx et al. have shown that iliac cancellous bone and marrow cells can survive up to four hours of storage in saline or Ringer's lactate.[40]

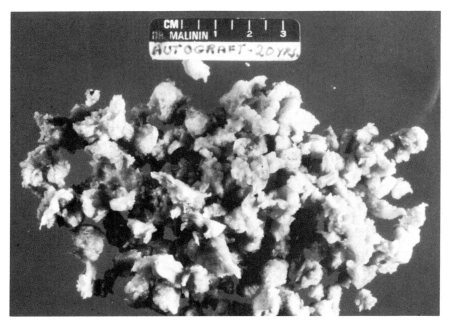

Figure 3-1. Hypertrophic bone overgrowth removed 20 years after fusion of the lumbar spine with an autologous bone graft.

The healing of bone autografts is similar to the healing of fractures. In the early stages of repair, a similar process occurs in both cortical and cancellous autografts. After the initial "clean-up" phase in autograft repair, the primitive mesenchymal cells differentiate into osteogenic cells. Cancellous bone is replaced in uniform manner throughout its thickness. In cortical grafts the replacement process is spotty; the periphery becomes pitted and replaced with new bone rather uniformly, but the interior is replaced in an irregular fashion. These differences in the bone replacement patterns of cancellous and cortical bone account for the more uniform and quicker incorporation of cancellous autografts.[20] Despite the widespread use of bone autografts in spinal surgery, little is known about the biomechanical properties of these transplants or of the physical properties of the fusion mass.

In the lumbosacral spine, a 95-percent fusion rate can be anticipated after posterolateral iliac bone grafts are placed across the transverse processes and the lateral surfaces of the superior facets at the lumbosacral junction. At the L4 and L5 levels, a rate of about 85 pecent can be expected.[48] In general, throughout the spine, the rate of nonunion increases as the number of segments being fused increases and the union rate increases as the degree of spine immobilization is increased either by internal or external fixation. A factor associated with a poor rate of fusion is the placement of the graft on the tension side of the spine. This is seen when posterior spinal fusion is performed over a kyphosis of greater than 50 degrees.[58]

Complications encountered with autologous bone grafts include resorbtion, collapse of the graft under compression, pseudoarthrosis, or bone mass overgrowth (Figure 3-1).[18,32] Spinal stenosis may develop after posterior spinal fusion at the site of pseudoarthrosis or wherever the bone graft has been placed over an area of decompression.[57] This complication has not been reported after anterior interbody fusion.

Allografts of Bone

Bone allografts used in spinal surgery are usually preserved by either freezing or freeze-drying. Bone banking has made these allografts readily available for surgical procedures involving stabilization of the spine.[37] There are, however, distinct differences in the healing behavior of autogenous grafts and allografts. With allografts, new bone forms more slowly and vascular penetration proceeds at a much lower pace than in autografts. The factors that create this discrepancy relate to the nonviability and possibly the antigenicity of the graft.[38]

Frozen Bone Allografts

The storage of bone at about −20°C in conventional freezers is popular because it requires only placement of the graft into generally available freezers. However, at this temperature ice crystals grow continually and eventually destroy the bone. Therefore, bone grafts can be stored in such freezers only for a limited period of time. No precise data are available to indicate the maximum storage time for bone grafts maintained at this temperature. Recommendations vary from 3 months to 1 year. Wilson[56] has reported a high failure rate with grafts stored for over a year, while Brown et al.[6] reported satisfactory incorporation of grafts stored for 6 months or less. In addition to disruption by ice crystals, freezing injury is caused by other factors, which may include chemical injury, dehydration, and metabolic aberrations. The latter result from storage at temperatures at which some enzymes may continue to function. It is necessary, in order to obtain near cessation of biochemical activity, to store tissues at close to −100°C.

Solid carbon dioxide (−70°C), also known as dry ice, was commonly used for storing bone grafts. Mechanical freezers that approximated the temperature of dry ice superceded dry ice. For reliable long-term storage, however, it is necessary to reduce the temperature to approximately −120°C. At this temperature ice crystals cannot develop and all enzymatic activity stops. Temperatures this low are obtained through the use of cryogenic gases. Liquid nitrogen, which boils at −196°C at atmospheric pressure, provides an ideal temperature at a reasonable cost. Another desirable property of liquid nitrogen is its inertness. Unlike carbon dioxide or other solvents used as cooling media, liquid nitrogen does not react with the materials with which it comes into contact, has no effect on the pH of frozen tissue, and vaporizes without a residue.

A review of the biologic effects of freezing and thawing of tissues emphasizes that the tissue cells are killed by the process and that frozen bone allografts do not contain living cells. The mechanism of freeze–thaw injury is complex.

Freeze-Dried Bone Allografts

Freeze-drying is a more complicated procedure than storing bone in the frozen state and it does produce tissue alterations.[39] The advantage of freeze-dried bone, however, is that it can be stored at room temperature. Freeze-drying may also have the desirable effect of reducing the antigenicity of bone. Although the mechanism is unknown, objective evidence of such a reduction in tissue graft antigenicity has been adequately demonstrated by laboratory studies.[26] The destruction of viable cells in the allograft as the result of the freeze-drying process may be a factor.

The preparation of freeze-dried grafts by the authors involves removing the grafts from frozen storage, rapidly unwrapping them in a sterile field, and placing the grafts on the shelf of a freeze dryer, the chamber of which has been sterilized with ethylene oxide and then ventilated. The shelf is precooled to −40°C. After the door of the freeze dryer is closed, a vacuum pump and condenser are turned on. The shelf temperature is maintained at −40°C for ten days, and the condenser temperature is kept between −60 and −70°C. After ten days the refrigeration to the shelves is turned off and the shelves are warmed to 25°C. The vacuum in the freeze dryer chamber is maintained between 200 and 100 mtorr for the first day of the cycle. It is then reduced to less than 100 mtorr (usually 30–50 mtorr) for the remainder of the drying cycle. At the end of the freeze-drying cycle, a port equipped with a bacterial filter is opened and the chamber is brought to atmospheric pressure. The freeze-dried bone is removed from the chamber, pieces of tissue are taken for bacteriologic culture, and the containers with the allografts are sealed under a vacuum.

Before its implantation, the freeze-dried bone graft must be rehydrated by immersion in saline, which facilitates cutting, drilling, or shaving the graft. Freeze-drying significantly alters the biomechanical properties of bone; unreconstituted freeze-dried bone will shatter easily and grafts that are inadequately reconstituted are brittle and fracture easily. Fortunately, the biomechanical properties of such bone are almost completely restored with adequate rehydration.[38]

Sources of Allografts

Bone allografts are obtained from cadaver donors. The risk of transmitting disease by transplanting tissues obtained from cadavers is of concern; however, the potential threat of infecting a recipient can be minimized if tissue allografts are excised from selected donors under sterile conditions, subjected to standard forms of processing, and adequately monitored for microbiologic activity.[36] Bones are excised from donors free of known infectious or malignant diseases or diseases of unknown etiology that may be potentially transmissible. The bone grafts are removed within 24 hours of death from bodies that have been refrigerated.

During the excision of bone, multiple tissue samples are submitted for bacteriologic analysis. Blood is obtained from the vena cava by a catheter threaded through the greater saphenous vein and subjected to aerobic and anaerobic culture. Serologic tests for the presence of syphilis, hepatitis B antigen, and HTL VIII-Ab are also performed. After the excision of the tissue grafts, a complete autopsy is performed on the donor cadaver.

The isolation of microorganisms from normally sterile cadaver tissues obtained less than 24 hours after death indicates an antemortem infection. If bacteriologic evidence of such an infection is conclusive, the tissues from a contaminated donor are discarded. Even after a careful screening of available clinical histories, tissues from 10 to 15 percent of donors at the University of Miami Tissue Bank have been discarded. Unsuspected cases of malignant disease found at autopsy and laboratory indications of the presence of hepatitis accounted for roughly one third of these. The remainder were discarded because of bacterial contamination.

The incidence of infections associated with transplanted bone allografts has been reported by Tomford et al.[49] An analysis of 303 cases revealed an infection rate comparable with that of procedures using autogenous bone. An analysis of data on patients receiving allografts at our institution has produced similar conclusions.

Chemosterilized, Autolysed, Antigen-Extracted Allogeneic Bone Allografts

Chemosterilized, autolysed, antigen-extracted allogeneic (AAA) bone allografts are excised without sterile precautions and are then subjected to autolytic digestion in the presence of sulfhydryl enzyme inhibitors, and antigen extraction by chloroform-methanol, which also sterilizes the grafts. This process is followed by partial demineralization in 0.6N HCl at 2°C. The grafts are preserved by freeze drying. Chemosterilized, autolysed, antigen-extracted allogeneic bone allografts have been used successfully as a substitute for autologous bone grafts. However, AAA grafts have been used only as cortical bone grafts or cortical bone chips. Because of demineralization, the bone grafts cannot be used for structural support.[50]

Xenografts

The literature contains many references to xenografts treated to make the grafts biologically acceptable. These include boiled calf bone, so-called *os purum*, bone with extracted organic matrix, Kiel bone, and Boplant. None of these have withstood the test of time and their use in the United States largely has been abandoned.

When examined after several years of implantation, xenogeneic bone grafts in the spine generally have remained either unchanged or surrounded by chronic inflammatory cells or both (Figure 3-2).

Metallic Internal Fixation Devices

Metallic internal fixation devices for stabilizing the spine were developed primarily for correcting spinal deformities and are used in patients who will also undergo posterior or anterior spinal fusion. Harrington devised the first universally accepted method of internal fixation for the treatment of spinal deformity.[30] It was initially thought that this system would permanently stabilize the spine without arthrodesis. However, when the rods were used alone they frequently broke and the hooks became disengaged.[31] Current practice involves stabilizing the spine with Harrington compression or distraction instrumentation in conjunction with a posterior fusion with bone grafts.[29] Although introduced as a method of treating spinal deformity, Harrington instrumentation has been used for stabilizing and fusing the thoracic and lumbar spine for unstable fractures, fracture-dislocations, spinal tumors, and spinal infections.[12,25]

The implantable Harrington instrumentation is made of stainless steel. The hardness of the steel used gives a tensile strength of 130,000 to 140,000 psi. The force that can be constantly applied to the spine is limited by the device itself and by the vertebrae that receive the hooks. With properly placed hooks and healthy vertebrae, a force of approximately 136 kg can be applied.[31] However, forces that exceed 35 to 40 kg are seldom used.[42]

A distraction rod will provide a distracting force for approximately 12 to 18 months

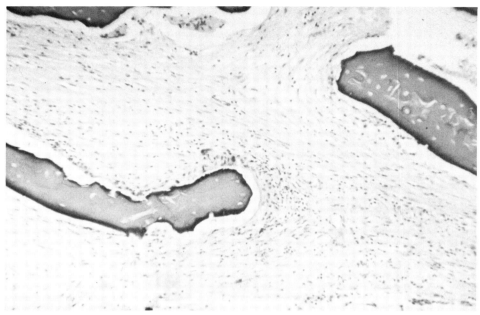

Figure 3-2. A bovine xenograft used for fusion of the lumbar spine. Virtually unchanged 15 years after implantation, the xenograft is surrounded by dense fibrous connective tissue and chronic inflammatory cells. (Hemotoxylin and eosin stain: ×100).

but it will eventually break.[30] The stainless steel distraction rod is designed to withstand at least 3.5 million undulations at forces of up to 30 kg of stress per undulation before breaking. During normal activity, an average man with an instrumented spine will subject it to between 7,000 and 10,000 undulations a day.

Dwyer instrumentation was developed to provide stability to the spine during anterior fusion. Dwyer instruments are made of titanium and consist of vertebral plates, swaging clamps, a tension apparatus, and cannulated screws. Titanium was chosen for the Dwyer instrumentation not only because of its strength and inertness, but also because of all implantable metals, titanium is the only metal ductile enough to be formed into a cable. The maximum tension that can be applied by the Dwyer apparatus is 40 kg. Swaging produces a force of 1600 to 2000 kg between the cable and the screw heads. Under laboratory testing conditions, a force of 140 kg is needed to break the cable; a force of a little less than half that much is required to cause the cable to slip through the screw head. Although biomechanical studies comparable with those performed on Harrington instrumentation have not been performed on Dwyer instrumentation, clinical experience suggests that stress relaxation exists in both systems,[42] although cables are much more fatigue resistant than rods. Internal fixation with Dwyer instrumentation is relatively poor. Since flexible cables can only resist tensile forces, stability is achieved solely by compression of one vertebral body on another. The weakest part of the Dwyer system is at the metal–bone interface, with screw pull-out not uncommonly occurring at the end vertebrae, especially in osteoporotic patients. The frequency of this problem can be diminished by inserting polymethylmethacrylate cement into the screw holes before inserting the screws in patients with a high risk of developing screw pullout.[15]

In 1975, the Dwyer system was modified by Zielke et al. and termed the ventral derotational spondylosis (VDS) system.[59] This system, compared with posterior fusion and Harrington instrumentation, achieves good correction while requiring fusion of a shorter segment of the spine.[14] The VDS system is made of stainless steel and the screws are slotted rather than cannulated. The screws are inserted into the bodies of the vertebrae through circular washers and plates. Instead of a flexible cable, a 3.2-mm (1/8-inch) diameter solid rod is used. Collared hex nuts are used to lock the rod in place.

SEGMENTAL SPINAL INSTRUMENTATION

The term *segmental spinal instrumentation* (SSI) has been applied to several methods of spine segment stabilization, but it is now primarily used to describe a metal implant attached to several contiguous vertebrae.[2,3,16] The most popular and versatile SSI is the so-called ''L'' rod instrumentation (LRI). The advantage of LRI over all other SSIs is that it requires neither cast nor brace for external support after the operation.

Luque segmental spinal instrumentation is designed to apply corrective forces to the spinal segment at each level. The corrective forces are generated by two stainless steel ''L'' rods, which are wired to both sides of the posterior neural arch. The rods are contoured to achieve the desired degree of correction. The diameters of Luque rods are 4.8 mm (3/16 inch) and 6.4 mm (1/4 inch). The most common failure with the system is wire breakage, although rod breakage has also been reported.

Laboratory studies on animal spines showed that compared with the Harrington method, Luque instrumentation offers an advantage because stress inherent with the Harrington hook is avoided. When a spine is instrumented with Luque rods and wires, acute failure occurs by fracture-dislocation of the spine at the end of the instrumented segment.[41] Two 4.8-mm-diameter Luque rods, when attached to the spine, could be bent by applying a force of 53 kg. A much greater force was needed to bend a single 6.4-mm Harrington rod segmentally wired to the spine.[53]

Luque rods have been used for segmental spinal stabilization in patients with malignant disease.[22] To lessen the chance of wire breakage, doubled 16-gauge wire was used to secure each of the rods in place at each level. This double wire technique is also recommended for corresponding traumatic spine instability.

Luque reported on 316 patients with spinal afflictions other than scoliosis. He provided neither a detailed description of the results nor of the technique but advocated inserting either a rectangular rod or a C-shaped rod in patients with markedly unstable spines to help prevent axial collapse.[35]

ACRYLIC CEMENT

Methylmethacrylate or polymethylmethacrylate, commonly referred to as ''bone cement,'' is an acrylic polymer. Methylmethacrylate monomer is a volatile liquid with a characteristic odor that polymerizes spontaneously, but very slowly, into a hard

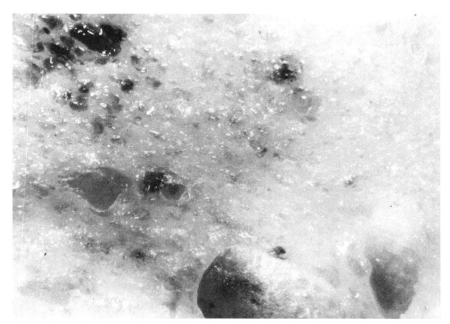

Figure 3-3. A section through methylmethacrylate showing the porosity and bubbles in the cement. (×25).

resin. Polymerization of methylmethacrylate is accelerated by ultraviolet light and by heat. To prevent spontaneous polymerization of the monomer, hydroquinone, which is a polymerization inhibitor, is added to the cement. In the case of "self-curing" acrylic material, polymerization is initiated chemically, usually by the addition of dimethylparatoluidine.

Self-curing acrylic cement is prepared in granular form to which is added powdered activator. The liquid portion is methylmethacrylate monomer, to which is added the initiator. When the liquid is added to the powder and mixed with it, the activator and the initiator polymerize, which then binds together the granules of polymer. Microscopically, the cement consists of aggregates of small spheres of polymer. Polymerization is an exothermic reaction, with a ball of cement 5 cm in diameter transiently reaching approximately 90°C in the center as it sets.[7]

The use of acrylic cement to stabilize the spine was reported by **Knight in 1959**.[33] Because it liberated very little heat, he chose self-curing acrylic cement, which took 24 hours to harden.

Biomechanical analysis of acrylic cement used to bind vertebral bodies in a laboratory setting was undertaken by Whitehill et al.[55] The findings of this study led to the prediction of a high incidence of fixation failures if polymethacrylate acrylic cement preparations were used to produce instantaneous posterior fusion. Wang showed in a laboratory model that fixation of the spine with acrylic cement resulted in failure to regain normal structural strength in extension.[51]

In practice, methylmethacrylate does not form a homogeneous polymer mass. Sections of acrylic cement removed from patients and examined under a microscope

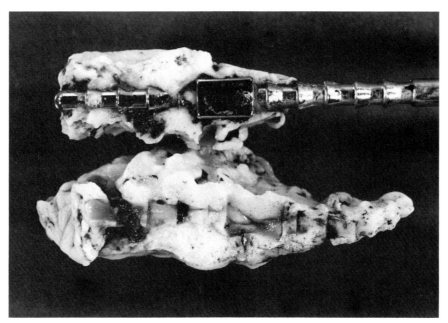

Figure 3-4. Methylmethacrylate in combination with a Harrington rod removed from a patient after being implanted for over a year. Note the space around the metal and the crevices in the methylmethacrylate filled with blood and granulation tissue.

show numerous cavities and bubbles (Figure 3-3). The surface of the cement mass has irregularities, crevices, and cracks. In addition, it is usually pitted. The cement itself does not form a strong bond with the metal imbedded in it. Eventually tissue elements grow into the spaces between the cement and the metal (Figure 3-4). The porosity of acrylic cement, coupled with the irregularities of its surface, are the features that are responsible for the eventual fragmentation of the cement mass (Figure 3-5).

Clinically, methylmethacrylate has been used primarily in the cervical spine, but even in this location the numbers of cases reported are relatively small and the follow-up short. In patients with metastatic disease to the spine, methylmethacrylate has been used to replace bone elements of vertebrae destroyed by the tumor or those that have been resected.[8]

A review of posterior stabilization with methylmethacrylate in 14 patients with metastatic lesions of the cervical spine was provided by Dunn.[13] He reported two failures of fixation. On portmortem examination in two additional patients a failure at the bone–cement interface was found.

The experience accumulated to date indicates that methylmethacrylate has a rather limited application in stabilization of the thoracic and lumbar spine. Its main use has been in palliative surgery for metastatic disease. Whenever possible, however, ancillary reinforcement of the acrylic by either Harrington or Knodt rods is recommended.[28]

Methylmethacrylate may be safely used to maintain and recreate vertebral spaces after the bone elements have been destroyed by tumor; however, methylmethacrylate does not produce arthrodesis, and because of its physical properties, the construct will

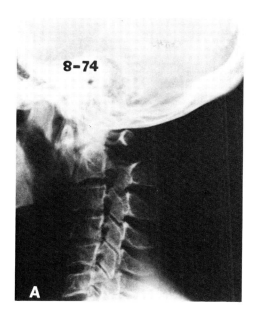

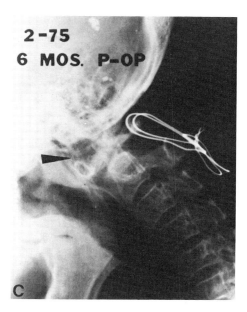

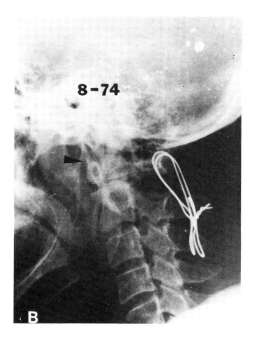

Figure 3-5. (A) This lateral roentgenogram of the cervical spine demonstrates posttraumatic C1-2 subluxation in a patient with rheumatoid arthritis. Surgical stabilization was recommended since the patient was symptomatic. (B) In surgery, the C1-2 subluxation was reduced to correct anatomic position and wires were used to secure the posterior arch of C1 to the posterior arches of C2 and C3. No bone graft was used and the wires and posterior spinal elements were covered with methylmethacrylate. (C) At 6 months after surgery, it is apparent that the reduction has been lost secondary to failure of the bone–cement interface. This can often be seen with the use of methylmethacrylate in the posterior approaches to the spine since the bone–cement bond is strongest in compression and weakest in tension. (Reprinted from Epps CH: Complications in Orthopedic Surgery. Philadelphia, J.B. Lippincott, 1978. With permission.)

eventually fail.[17] Since the pain relief produced by stabilization with methylmethacrylate is immediate and it does not interfere with irradiation,[28] its use is an attractive option for patients with vertebral body metastases with a limited healing potential and a limited life expectancy.

CLINICAL APPLICATIONS

Posterolateral Fusion

When fusion is indicated through the posterior approach, posterolateral intertransverse process fusion with autogenous bone grafts is the most commonly performed procedure. This has been a frequently used method for arthrodesis of the lumbar spine because of the high fusion rate, low morbidity, rapid convalescence, and lack of associated development of spinal stenosis or pars defects after fusion. Mechanical studies show posterior bilateral lateral fusion to provide more rotational stability than either anterior interbody or pure posterior fusion. The most common indication for this operation has been fusion in conjunction with decompression of the lumbar spinal canal or neural foramina for spinal stenosis or spondylolisthesis. This in situ fusion of the lumbar spine is appropriate for minor degrees of instability. It is less appropriate for moderate or severe instability, in which cases instrumentation is routinely used to supplement the fusion.

Arthrodesis of the Spine in the Presence of Spinal Instrumentation

Arthrodesis of the thoracic or lumbar spine with spinal instrumentation is most commonly performed for a variety of congenital or developmental deformities such as scoliosis or for an unstable spinal fracture-dislocation requiring open reduction and internal fixation. Instrumentation also is often used when treating severe spinal instability resulting from tumor or infection.[24] The objective of inserting instrumentation in all of these cases is to correct the deformity and to maintain the vertebral column in the corrected position. The instrumentation used to realign the thoracic and lumbar spine must be supplemented with a bone fusion, otherwise the fixation devices will probably fatigue and break. The use of methylmethacrylate has been suggested instead of bone grafts to reinforce the instrumentation since this provides immediate stabilization. The cement, however, has a limited longevity, and once it begins to break down, the stabilization it provides is lost. Methylmethacrylate is therefore used preferentially in cases of spinal instability secondary to malignant tumors in patients with a life expectancy of less than 1 year.

The posterior fusion technique must include the destruction of the articular cartilage of the facet joint with packing of cancellous bone into the facet joint; adequate debridement of the soft tissue attachments to the bone, i.e., the facet joint capsules, tendon insertions and ligaments; and decortication of the host bone surfaces. Corticocancellous autogenous bone taken from the iliac crest in adequate quantity is the graft material usually used for rapid bony incorporation and formation of a fusion mass in the thoracic and lumbar spine from the posterior approach.

Crushed corticocancellous allografts have been used successfully in conjunction with rigid posterior spine instrumentation in treating adolescents with thoracic and lumbar spinal deformities.

Anterior Fusion of the Spine—Single and Multiple Levels

Anterior spinal fusion is used to treat vertebral body destruction or anterior neural compression that can only be safely and adequately removed through an anterior approach. These conditions are often seen after trauma, tumor (benign and malignant), and infections. The techniques for these procedures is described in Chapters 0, 0, and

0; attention here will be devoted to the materials used for accomplishing stabilization in these operative procedures.

Autologous bone is available for anterior fusion; its main limitation is the size of tricortical iliac bone grafts, ribs, or fibulas. Tricortical bone grafts offer significant structural stability because of the three cortical surfaces, however, 6 to 8 cm is usually the maximum length obtainable from one side of the ilium. Rib autografts have the disadvantage of lacking significant strength although several of these can often be impacted adjacent to one another in order to improve the structural support. Fibula autografts have the advantage of being straight and extremely strong, but they have the disadvantage of slow incorporation; it takes approximately 2 years for the bone to completely revascularize.[19] Also, because of the cortical nature of fibular autografts they are not appropriate for use in cases of pyogenic infection. Cortical bone will often act as a sequestrum and source of late persistent infection because of its slow revascularization (Figure 3-6).

The use of allografts to replace several anterior vertebral bodies in the spine is extremely attractive because of their ready availability and little size restriction (e.g., entire femoral or tibial shafts can be used to span several segments). Fibular, ilial, and rib allografts are available in longer lengths than can be easily obtained from the patient (Figure 3-7); however, these allografts require 2 years or more to become vascularized even though they are solidly incorporated at the allograft–host interface in a period of several months.

Polymethylmethacrylate is particularly useful for anterior reconstruction of the spine, since in the thoracic and lumbar areas it is loaded in compression and it is inherently strongest in resisting compressive forces. This material can be used either with anteriorly placed Harrington rods or Steinmann pins or screws inserted into the adjacent vertebral body. Because methylmethacrylate eventually fails at the bone–cement interface in tension and because of its tendency to fragment over time with repeated axial compression, its use should be restricted to patients with a life expectancy of less than 1 year. Because of the tendency of methylmethacrylate to act as a foreign body and to locally suppress white blood cell chemotaxis and the ability of lymphocytes to kill bacteria, its use is contraindicated in the presence of infection.[45,46]

A vascularized rib graft may be used in the anterior column (Figure 3-8). This technique requires thoracotomy. The resected rib remains attached to its muscle and vascular supply and as a result incorporates faster than most bone grafts and tends to hypertrophy with time, making its original lack of structural support less important. When used in conjunction with an allograft, the allograft provides needed structural support and the rib provides early incorporation. With this vascularized autograft-allograft combination, the amount of time the back must be braced postoperatively is lessened, making the procedure comparable with the other more routine types of stabilization.

It should be emphasized that just as in posterior spine instrumentation systems, bone fusion must be used in conjunction with anterior instrumentation systems in order to prevent eventual fatigue failure of the metal. Also, the long-term effects of these systems, particularly on adjacent organs and vascular structures, is not yet known. Considering these unknowns, the benefits that may accrue from the added stability achieved with anterior systems must be balanced against a more routine anterior decompression and fusion combined with a posterior stabilization with instrumentation.

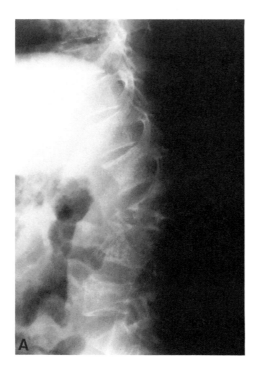

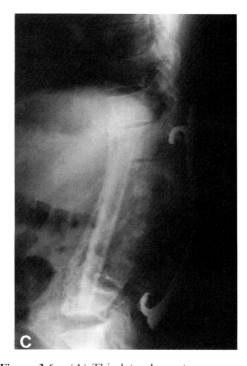

Figure 3-6. (A) This lateral roentgenogram of the lumbar spine shows nearly complete destruction of the L1, L2, and L3 vertebral bodies secondary to tuberculosis. (B) This CT scan demonstrates bilateral abscesses of the psoas muscle as marked by the arrows. (C) The patient was treated with combined anterior debridement of the spine, drainage of the abscesses, and fusion from T11 to L5 and posterior fusion over the same levels. An autogenous fibular bone graft was used anteriorly as well as autogenous iliac crest bone grafts both anteriorly and posteriorly. At 3 years after surgery, there is excellent incorporation of the bone grafts. If this had been a pyogenic infection rather than a tuberculous infection, the use of fibula would not have been recommended because of the slow rate of revascularization and its tendency to act as a nidus of recurrent infection. If this had been a pyogenic infection, the use of autogenous rib grafts would have been the preferred treatment because of their more rapid revascularization.

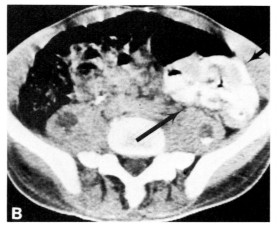

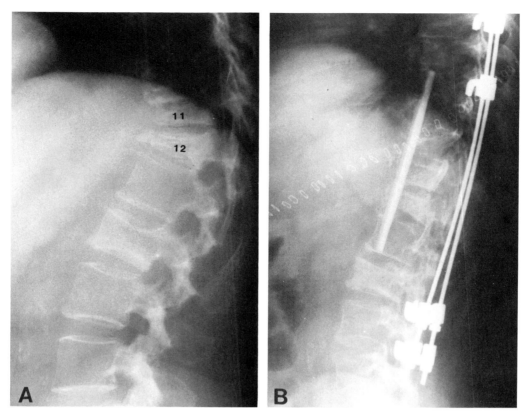

Figure 3-7. (A) This patient with severe osteoporosis fell and sustained multiple severe compression fractures at the T10, T11, and T12 levels. When the patient was in the upright position, this increased to a 90-degree kyphosis, hence demonstrating the severe instability present. (B) A lateral roentgenogram from the immediate postoperative period shows the 20-cm length of cortical allograft used to provide anterior structural support to the spine. It would have been most difficult to obtain this length of autogenous cortical bone from the patient except by removing the majority of her fibula.

Interbody Fusion

Anterior

Anterior interbody fusion, regardless of whether the approach is intraabdominal or retroperitoneal, requires a large volume of bone graft to stabilize the spine. Anterior interbody fusions have been performed most commonly as salvage procedures where a posterior approach is difficult or contraindicated.

There is some disagreement regarding the success rate with anterior fusions. This is attributed primarily to what had been defined as a successful result.[27] Paradoxically, about one half of patients with clinical success have radiologic evidence of nonunion and, vice versa, one half of patients with clinical failures achieve arthrodesis.[23]

Autologous grafts used for anterior interbody fusions are either full-thickness sections of the ilium or segments from the fibula. With ilium, two grafts are placed parallel, longitudinally with the cortex facing anteriorly and laterally. The grafts are

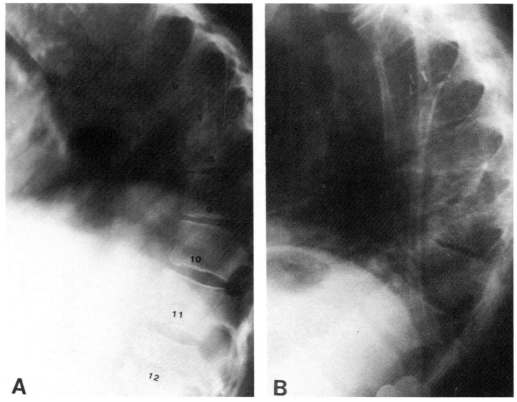

Figure 3-8. (A) This lateral roentgenogram of the thoracic spine shows a severe kyphosis in a patient who has had multiple anterior and posterior operations on her spine with subsequent pseudoarthrosis, posterior spine infection, and chronic pain because of the residual instability. Posterior osteotomies and instrumentation were felt to be contraindicated because of the presence of recurrent and chronic infection. (B) The patient's chronic spine pain was alleviated by performing an anterior fusion in situ using a vascularized rib graft spanning six vertebral levels. The main advantage of this type of graft is that it incorporates rapidly at the ends of the graft and that it will hypertrophy over a period of time and hence provide the needed support for the spine. At 2 months after the fusion, the patient's chronic back pain was markedly improved.

impacted in the interbody spaces widened anteriorly by hyperextension of the spine. Fibular grafts can placed axially, in several sections, with the cut surfaces facing the superior and inferior vertebral endplates.

Complications with autologous grafts are most likely to occur when the ilium from which the grafts are taken is osteopenic. Since the bone in osteopenic grafts is soft, it cannot support the weight transmitted through the vertebral column and frequently collapses. In such circumstances, it is advisable to use biomechanically stable allografts. Watkins et al.[52] have retrospectively reviewed the cases of 55 patients who underwent anterior interbody fusions with autologous iliac grafts or with allografts of iliac bone. They reported no significant difference in the fusion rates between patients receiving autografts, allografts, or a combination of the two.

LaRocca popularized filling of the intervertebral disc space with several segments of the fibula placed in a vertical position. Preliminary unpublished reports indicate that the fusion rates with autografts and those of freeze-dried allografts are comparable.

Posterior Lumbar Interbody Fusion

Posterior lumbar interbody fusion (the PLIF operation)[9] is used to achieve anterior spinal interbody fusion of the lumbar spine through a posterior approach to the disc space. Cloward now uses full-thickness iliac grafts, which are driven into the interspace, two grafts on each side, to fill the disc space completely. An analysis of 97 consecutive cases with a 30-year follow-up with 9 patients undergoing fusion with autologous grafts and 88 patients undergoing fusion with frozen allografts showed collapse or partial absorption of the graft in 14 patients and pseudoarthrosis in 3 patients.[10] A fusion rate of approximately 80 percent is achieved if one level is fused and 70 percent if two or more levels are fused with this technique.[5] The fusion rate is the same regardless of whether the patient's own bone or allografts are used.

REFERENCES

1. Albee IH: Transplantation of a portion of the tibia into the spine for Pott's disease. JAMA 57:885, 1911
2. Allen BL, Jr, Ferguson RL: The Galveston technique for L-rod instrumentation of the scoliotic spine. Spine 7:276, 1982
3. Allen BL, Jr, Ferguson RL: The Galveston technique of pelvic fixation with L-rod instrumentation of the spine. Spine 9:388, 1984
4. Bassett CAL: Clinical implications of cell function in bone grafting. Clin Orthop Rel Res 87:56, 1972
5. Brown MD: Lumbar spine fusion. In Finneson BE: Low Back Pain. Philadelphia, J.B. Lippincott, 1980, p. 381
6. Brown MD, Malinin TI, Davis PB: A roentgenographic evaluation of frozen allografts versus autografts in anterior cervical spine fusions. Clin Orthop Rel Res 119:231, 1976
7. Charnley J: Acrylic Cement in Orthopedic Surgery. Baltimore, Williams & Wilkins, 1970, p. 23
8. Clark CR, Keggi KJ, Panjabi MM: Methacrylate stabilization of cervical spine. J Bone Joint Surg 66A:41, 1984
9. Cloward RB: The treatment of ruptured intervertebral disc by vertebral body fusion. Ann Surg 136:967, 1952
10. Cloward RB: Spondylolisthesis: Treatment by laminectomy and posterior interbody fusion. Clin Orthop Rel Res 154:74, 1981
11. DeWald RL, Ray RD: Skeletal traction for the treatment of severe scoliosis. J Bone Joint Surg 52A:233, 1970
12. Dickson JH, Harrington PR, Erwin LD: Results of reduction and stabilization of the severely fractured thoracic and lumbar spine. J Bone Joint Surg 60A:801, 1978
13. Dunn EJ: The role of methylmethacrylate in the stabilization and replacement of tumors of the cervical spine. A project of the Cervical Spine Research Society. Spine 2:15, 1977
14. Dunn HK: Spinal instrumentation. In Evarts CM (ed): AAOS Instructional Course Lecture, vol 32. St. Louis, C.V. Mosby, 1983, p. 209
15. Dunn HK, Bolstad KE: Fixation of Dwyer screws for the treatment of scoliosis. J Bone Joint Surg 59A:54, 1977
16. Dwyer AF, Schafer MF: Anterior approach to scoliosis. J Bone Joint Surg 56B:218, 1974
17. Eismont FJ, Bohlman HH: Posterior methylmethacrylate fixation for cervical trauma. Spine 6:347, 1981
18. Eismont FJ, Simeone FA: Bone overgrowth (hypertrophy) as a cause of later paraparesis after scoliosis fusion. J Bone Joint Surg 63A:1016, 1981
19. Enneking WF, Burchardt H, Puhl JJ, Piotrowski G: Physical and biologic aspects of repair in dog cortical bone transplants. J Bone Joint Surg 57A:237, 1975
20. Enneking WF, Morris JL: Human autologous cortical bone transplants. Clin Orthop Rel Res 87:28, 1972
21. Finneson BE: Low Back Pain. Philadelphia, J.B. Lippincott, 1980, p. 234
22. Flatley TJ, Anderson MH, Anast GT: Spinal instability due to malignant disease. J Bone Joint Surg 66A:47, 1984

23. Flynn JC, Hoque A: Anterior fusion of the lumbar spine. J Bone Joint Surg 61A:1143, 1979

24. Fountain SS: A single stage combined surgical approach for vertebral resections. J Bone Joint Surg 61A:1011, 1979

25. Fresch JR, Leider LL, Erickson DL, Chou SN, Bradford DS: Harrington instrumentation and spine fusion for unstable fractures and fracture dislocations of the thoracic and lumbar spine. J Bone Joint Surg 59A:143, 1977

26. Friedlaender GE, Strong DM, Sell KW: Studies on the antigenicity of bone. I. Freeze dried and deep frozen bone allografts in rabbits. J Bone Joint Surg 58A:854, 1976

27. Goldner JL, McColum OE, Urbaniak JR: Anterior disc excision and interbody spine fusion for chronic low back pain. In American Academy of Orthopedic Surgeons Symposium on the Spine. St. Louis, C.V. Mosby, 1969, pp. 111

28. Harrington KD: The use of methylmethacrylate for vertebral body replacment and anterior stabilization of pathologic fracture dislocations of the spine due to metastatic malignant disease. J Bone Joint Surg 63A:36, 1981

29. Harrington PJ, Dickson JH: An eleven year clinical investigation of Harrington instrumentation. Clin Orthop Rel Res 93:113, 1973

30. Harrington PR: Instrumentation in structural scoliosis. In Graham D (ed): Modern Trends in Orthopaedics. London, Butterworths, 1967, p. 93

31. Harrington PR: Technical detail in relation to the successful use of instrumentation in scoliosis. Orthop Clin North Am 3:49, 1972

32. Kestler OC: Overgrowth (hypertrophy) of lumbosacral grafts causing a complete block. Bull Hosp Joint Dis 27:51, 1966

33. Knight G: Paraspinal acrylic inlays in the treatment of cervical and lumbar spondylosis and other conditions. Lancet 2:147:1959

34. Kostiuk J, Tooke M: The application of pelvic pins in halo-pelvic distraction—an anatomical study. Spine 8:35, 1983

35. Luque E: Segmental spinal instrumentation. Spine 7:256, 1982

36. Malinin TI: Organization of a tissue bank—University of Miami experience. Proceedings of the 1977 meeting of the American Association of Tissue Banks. Rockville, MD, 1978, p. 79

37. Malinin TI, Brown MD: Bone allografts in spinal surgery. Clin Orthop Rel Res 154:68, 1981

38. Malinin TI, Thompson CB, Brown MD: Freeze-dried tissue allografts in surgery. In Karow AM, Pegg DE (eds): Organ Preservation for Transplantation. New York, Marcel Dekker, 1981, p. 677

39. Malinin TI, Wu NM, Flores A: Freeze-drying of bone for allotransplantation. In Friedlaender GE, Mankin HJ, Sell KW (eds): Osteochondral Allografts. Boston, Little, Brown, 1983, p. 181

40. Marx RE, Snyder RM, Kline SN: Cellular survival of marrow during placement of marrow cancellous bone graft. J Oral Surg 37:712, 1979

41. McAfee PC, Werner FW, Glisson DA: Biomechanical analysis of spinal instrumentation systems in thoracolumbar fractures—a comparison of traditional Harrington distraction instrumentation with segmental spinal instrumentation. Spine 10:204, 1985

42. Mears DC: Materials in Orthopaedic Surgery. Baltimore, Williams & Wilkins, 1979, p. 484

43. Norton PL, Brown T: The immobilizing efficiency of back braces. J Bone Joint Surg 39A:1, 1957

44. Perry J, Nickel VL: Total cervical spine fusion for neck paralysis. J Bone Joint Surg 41A:37, 1959

45. Petty W: The effect of methylmethacrylate on bacterial phagocytosis and killing by human polymorphonuclear leukocytes. J Bone Joint Surg 60A:752, 1978

46. Petty W: The effect of methylmethacrylate on chemotaxis of polymorphonuclear leukocytes. J Bone Joint Surg 60A:492, 1978

47. Puraren J: Reorganization of fresh and preserved transplants. An experimental study in rabbits using tetracycline labeling. Acta Orthop Scand (Suppl) 92, 1966

48. Stauffer RN, Coventry MB: Posterolateral lumbar spine fusion. J Bone Joint Surg 54A:1195, 1972

49. Tomford WW, Starkweather RJ, Goldman MH: Study of the clinical incidence of infection in the use of banked allograft bone. J Bone Joint Surg 63A:244, 1981

50. Urist MR, Dawson E: Intertranverse process fusion with aid of chemosterilized autolyzed antigen-extracted allogeneic (AAA) bone. Clin Orthop Rel Res 154:97, 1981

51. Wang GJ, Lewish GD, Roger SI, Jennings RL, Hubbard SL, Mehaurin CA, Stamp WG: Comparative strengths of various anterior cement fixations of the cervical spine. Spine 8:717, 1983

52. Watkins R, Springer D, Wiltse L, Champonx, J Schlitz J: Anterior interbody fusion of the lumbar spine: A review. Presented at the 52nd Annual Meeting of the American Academy of Orthopedic Surgeons, Las Vegas, 1985, p. 58

53. Wenger DR, Carollo JJ, Wilkerson JA, Jr, Wauters K, Herring JA: Laboratory testing of segmental spinal instrumentation versus traditional Harrington instrumentation for scoliosis treatment. Spine 7:265, 1982

54. White AA, Panjabi MM: Clinical biomechanics of the spine. Philadelphia, J.B. Lippincott, 1978

55. Whitehill R, Reger S, Weatherup N, Werthmuller C, Bruce J, Gates P, Rollins G: Biomechanical analysis of posterior cervical fusion using polymethacrylate as an instantaneous fusion mass. Spine 8:368, 1983

56. Wilson PD: Follow-up study of the use of refrigerated homologous bone transplants in orthopedic operations. J Bone Joint Surg 37A:307, 1951

57. Wiltse LL: The place of spinal fusion in intervertebral joint disease. In American Academy of Orthopedic Surgeons Symposium on the Lumbar Spine. St. Louis, C.V. Mosby 1981, p. 152, 177

58. Winter RB, Moe JH, Wang JF: Congenital kyphosis. J Bone Joint Surg 55A:223, 1973

59. Zielke K, Stunket R, Duquesne J, Beaujean F: Ventrale derotationspondylose. Orthop Prax 11:562, 1975

Alfred Kahn, III

4

Current Concepts of Internal Fixation

The concept that operations on the spine designed to produce stability depend on a solid arthrodesis began with reports of such procedures by Hibbs[15] and Albee.[1] Since that time, it has remained axiomatic that solid fusion is required in the treatment of instability of the spine, and in current surgical practice instrumentation of the spine is a frequent adjunct to spinal fusion. This approach dates from Harrington's demonstration that spinal instrumentation could be used to correct and stabilize a deformity and that it could be safely performed on patients with a scoliotic deformity.[13,14] Since Harrington's landmark article, the use of posterior instrumentation to produce spinal stability has become routine, and several methods of anterior spinal stabilization currently are used in correcting spinal deformities.[9,10] This chapter reviews some of these devices and the biomechanical mechanisms by which they act.

Internal fixation provides a means for correcting a spinal deformity and is of equal benefit in the early mobilization of patients undergoing extensive spinal surgery. The implant that provides the greatest amount of stability to the spine in all planes of motion theoretically is the one preferred, and laboratory analyses of these devices have demonstrated how the implants react under various modes of stress, e.g., compression, bending, and rotatory forces. These laboratory circumstances are suspect, however, since the optimal rigidity required to provide the ideal environment for bone healing or fusion is unknown. Small amounts of motion may in fact stimulate the healing process in bone and therefore may be beneficial.

All spinal segments have complex coupled motion and six degrees of freedom. Kaufer[17] has noted that certain anatomic features influence the degree of freedom for each segment. There are six directions of motion in the thoracolumbar spine (flexion, extension, right lateral bending, left lateral bending, right torsion, and left torsion) and certain anatomic features influence the amount of freedom of each spinal segment. In the thoracic spine, the paired ribs restrict lateral bending, flexion, and extension of the spinal segments, although there is little restriction to torsion. The lumbar spine, having

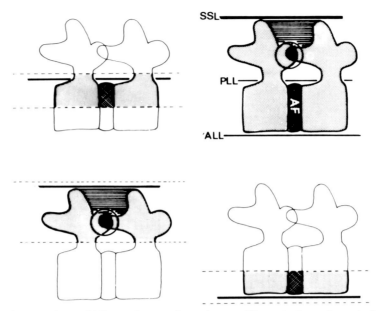

Figure 4-1. The anterior, middle, and posterior columns. The anterior column is formed by the anterior longitudinal ligament (ALL), the anterior annulus fibrosis (AF), and the anterior part of the vertebral body. The posterior column is formed by the supraspinous ligament (SSL), the interspinous ligament (ISL), capsule (C), and the ligamentum flavum (LF) along with the posterior vertebral arch. The middle column is formed by the posterior longitudinal ligament (PLL), the posterior annulus fibrosis, and the posterior wall of the vertebral body. (Reprinted from Denis F: The three-column spine and its significance in the classification of acute thoracolumbar spinal injuries. Spine 8:817, 1983. With permission.)

large vertebral bodies and posterior elements that are widely spaced, has the potential for large arcs of motion. White and Panjabi[31] have noted that these motions are not pure and that some degree of coupling exists so that there may be flexion coupled with rotation, extension coupled with bending, and so forth. Any system designed to stabilize the spine must take into account this potential for motion. The surgeon must also recognize that the integrity of the soft tissue as well as that of the bony spine can influence the degree to which the vertebrae may act when different forces are applied. For example, in dealing with a Chance fracture, distraction forces should be avoided since there may be total disruption of the ligamentous complex about the spine; a distraction force in this instance would further destabilize the spine and potentially increase the neurologic damage, whereas compression applied over the injured segment reduces this fracture and maintains it in a corrected position, minimizing the possibility of further neurologic injury. Nearly all forms of instrumentation depend on an intact osteoligamentous complex. In analyzing this, Denis[5] has introduced the concept of viewing spinal stability in terms of three columns: the anterior, middle, and posterior columns (Figure 4-1). The anterior column is formed by the anterior longitudinal ligament, the anterior annulus fibrosis, and the anterior part of the vertebral body. The posterior column is formed by the supraspinous ligament, the interspinous ligament capsule, and the ligamentum flavum, along with the posterior vertebral arch. The

Table 4-1.
The basic modes of failure of the three columns of the spine in the four
major types of spinal injury

Type of Fracture	Column		
	Anterior	Middle	Posterior
Compression	Compression	None	None or distraction (severe)
Burst	Compression	Compression	None
Seat-belt type	None or compression	Distraction	Distraction
Fracture-dislocation	Compression rotation shear	Distraction rotation shear	Distraction rotation shear

middle column is formed by the posterior longitudinal ligament, the posterior annulus fibrosis, and the posterior wall of the vertebral body.

The basic modes of failure in the three columns in the four major types of spinal injury are delineated in Denis's study (Table 4-1). This model permits a more accurate categorization of the type of fracture, thereby making decisions regarding therapeutic indications possible on a rational basis.

POSTERIOR INSTRUMENTATION

Harrington Instrumentation

The Harrington system consists of either distraction rods or compression rods. Distraction rods apply axial forces through two sublaminar hooks attached to the rods by means of a hub on one end and a ratchet locking mechanism on the other. The compression system consists of a thinner threaded rod; compression is applied by small nuts threaded onto the rod above each hook (Figure 4-2). The Harrington distraction hook–rod complex functions through two different mechanisms to provide correction of a spinal deformity: a pure distraction force and three-point fixation (Figure 4-3). It is through spinal distraction and the application of bending movements that spinal alignment can be changed. This was demonstrated by Flesch et al.[11] as being the mechanism of reduction of burst fractures of the spine using distraction forces.

The anterior longitudinal ligament is extremely important with regard to maintaining the integrity of the spine, since it serves to prevent overdistraction of the spine during trauma and serves to help reduce fractures in which fragments are attached to the ligament itself. Disruption of the anterior longitudinal ligament associated with a fracture-dislocation of the spine is therefore a contraindication to the use of pure distraction instrumentation.[32] Without the hinge effect produced by the anterior longitudinal ligament for the system to work against, the neural elements are distracted with potentially disastrous results. For this reason, Murphy and Southwick[23] and Yocum et al.[34] have advocated the use of compression instrumentation in the treatment of spinal instability. Compression instrumentation in combination with distraction instrumentation is useful not only because of the increased rigidity it provides, but also because it can prevent overdistraction; in addition, the three-point bending forces

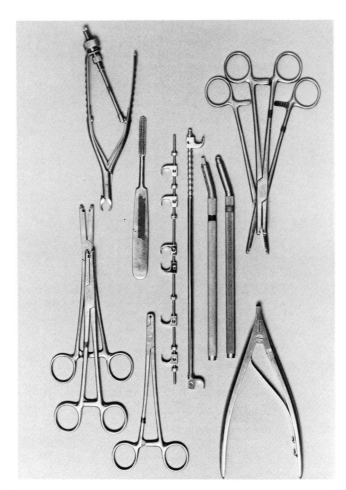

Figure 4-2. A Harrington distraction rod (right center) and compression rod (left center). The distraction rod has two hooks attached by means of a ratchet locking mechanism on one end and a hub holding the hook on the opposite end. The compression rod is a thinner threaded rod, the hooks being held in place by nuts behind each of the hooks on the rod. Surrounding the rods are instruments used to place the rods (clockwise from upper right corner): hook-holding forceps for the distraction rod; hook inserters; distraction device; compression rod holding forceps; hook-holding forceps for the compression rod; nasal rasp for turning the compression rod nuts; small bone holding forceps, also for turning the compression rod nuts.

provided by the compression system are greater than those provided by the Harrington distraction system (Figure 4-4).[32]

It was Harrington's belief that his original system, which included both distraction and compression instrumentation, should be used in most cases where instrumentation was deemed necessary, whether it be to correct a spinal deformity or to stabilize a fracture; the compression rod was thought to augment the strength and holding potential of the distraction rod.[27] This concept was substantiated by Simmons,[27] who experimented with the vertebral columns of calves and various forms of internal fixation.

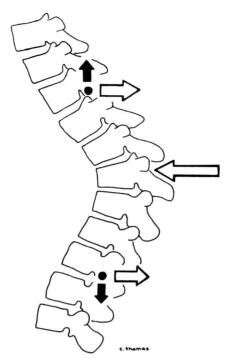

Figure 4-3. The forces applied by a Harrington distraction rod. The small black arrows represent the distraction forces; the large white arrows represent forces of three-point fixation. (Reprinted from White AA, Panjabi MM (eds): Clinical Biomechanics of the Spine. Philadelphia, J.B. Lippincott, 1978, p 434. With permission.)

White and Panjabi[32] have noted that the change in the position of each individual vertebra between the ends of the rod is dependent upon the bending moment produced at the center of rotation for the various vertebrae. Correction will occur when the centers of rotation are between the rod and the concavity of the curve. The deformity can be exaggerated, however, when the centers are between the rod and the convexity of the curve (Figure 4-5). The rationale for the use of combined Harrington compression and distraction instrumentation is further illustrated in Figure 4-6. Among the variations in this technique is the "rod-long/fuse-short" principle. The advocates of this technique believe that the inclusion of a greater number of spinal segments increases early spinal stabilization. The detractors of this technique cite its need for greater exposure; the increased morbidity of rod removal, which is necessary at a later date; and potential adverse effects on the unfused facet joints. Waugh[28] demonstrated that the maximum corrective force that can be produced with Harrington distraction instrumentation is dependent on the stress concentration at the hook in the upper lamina, and that this force will lessen with time in a patient. Nachemson and Gosta Elfstrom[24] demonstrated in a small series of patients with idiopathic scoliosis with nonrigid curves that

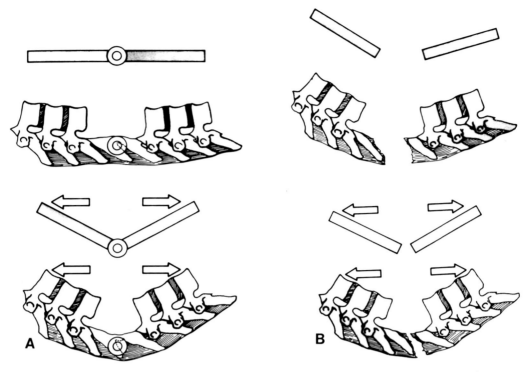

Figure 4-4. (A) The anterior longitudinal ligament, the intertransverse ligaments, bone, or posterior ligamentous structures can serve as a hinge. For obvious reasons the spinal cord should not be a hinge. (B) With no hinge, it is impossible to change the angle between the limbs of a deformity with an axial force. The two portions tend to separate. (Reprinted from White AA, Panjabi MM (eds): Clinical Biomechanics of the Spine. Philadelphia, J.B. Lippincott, 1978, pp 434–438. With permission.)

distraction forces of 20 to 40 kg resulted in corrections of 55 to 70 percent. The force that was transmitted through the Harrington rods diminished with time. After 10 days, there was a stabilization of forces that equaled about one third of the maximum force applied during the operation.

Technique for Harrington Instrumentation

Harrington distraction instrumentation.[22] After the appropriate areas are exposed, the hook sites must be selected. The upper hook will sit within the joint while the lower hook will reside under the lamina. All ligamentous and capsular material is removed from the upper hook site (Figure 4-7). The inferior part of the superior facet is cut at an oblique angle with a small osteotome. A No. 1251 hook is inserted into the joint by tilting it forward so that it is properly placed against the pedicle. After it meets the pedicle, it is impacted gently. The No. 1251 hook is removed and is replaced with either a dull unflanged hook (No. 1253) or with a dull flanged hook (No. 1262). Whichever hook is used is then impacted gently into the pedicle.

The lower hook is dull (No. 1254) and is inserted under the superior edge of the

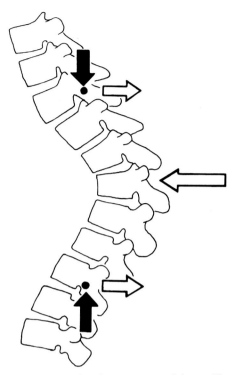

Figure 4-5. The forces created by a Harrington compression rod. The three white arrows represent the forces caused by the three-point bending of the spine as the Harrington rod is inserted between the two hooks. The black arrows are the compressive forces applied when the nuts are tightened. (Reprinted from White AA, Panjabi MM (eds): Clinical Biomechanics of the Spine. Philadelphia, J.B. Lippincott, 1978, p 434. With permission.)

lamina (Figure 4-8). The ligamentum flavum, the most inferior part of the inferior facet, and the superior laminar edge are removed. The hook is then inserted. If a facet fusion is needed, the joint is prepared by stripping it of soft tissue as was done above, and the bone graft is impacted into the joint before the rod is attached to the hook (Figure 4-9).

An outrigger may be used to facilitate stabilization of the spine while the intervening joints are prepared and the laminar surfaces are decorticated in preparation for bone grafting. After decortication and facet fusion are completed, the outrigger is removed and the distraction rod inserted. Only experience can dictate how much to distract the spine, but the alignment of the spine can be inspected on intraoperative roentgenograms to help avoid overdistraction of a fractured segment. At times, a combination of compression and distraction rods is advantageous. Whereas the distraction hooks are inserted into the joint and under the lamina, the compression rod

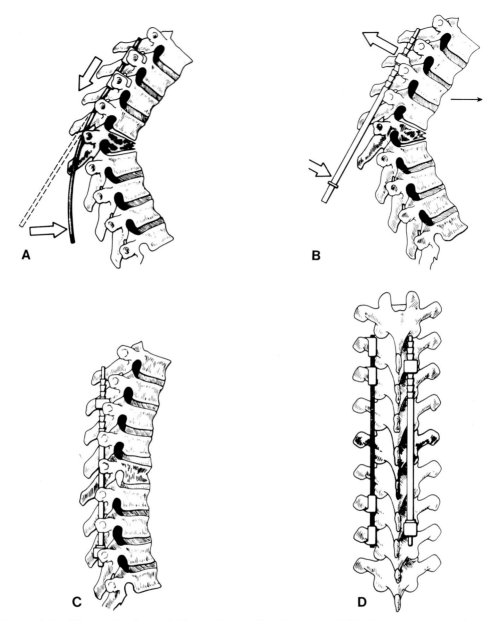

Figure 4-6. The rationale and biomechanics for the use of Harrington compression and distraction rods. (A) The compression rod is relatively flexible and may not be helpful in correcting a deformity. (B) The distraction rod is about five times as stiff as the compression rod. It applies a strong couple to the deformity and is likely to correct it. The rod is then attached and serves as a splint to maintain the correction. It is not used as a distractor. (C) The compression rod is then applied to stabilize the two parts of the kyphos in their correct position. (D) Frontal plane rotation is small because of the short distance between the two rods and is restricted by the buttressing of the spinous processes against the stiff Harrington rod. (Reprinted from White AA, Panjabi MM (eds): Clinical Biomechanics of the Spine. Philadelphia, J.B. Lippincott, 1978, p 436. With permission.)

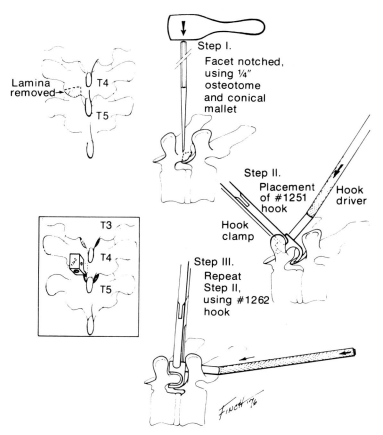

Figure 4-7. Preparation for the insertion of the upper hook of a Harrington assembly. (Step I) A small (1/4-inch; 0.6-cm) osteotome is used to cut the inferior portion of the superior facet at a slightly oblique angle. The facet joint is then easily identified and its most medial margin delineated. (Step II) A No. 1251 hook is inserted into the facet interspace. The hook should be tilted forward at least 45 degrees to ensure proper placement and to prevent the hook from improperly engaging the superior facet. (Step III) Once the hook has engaged the pedicle, it can be driven in with a light mallet. This sharp hook is then removed and a flanged hook, No. 1262, is inserted and driven into the pedicle. (Reprinted from Moe JH, Winter RB, Bradford DS, Lonstein JE: Scoliosis and Other Spinal Deformities. Philadelphia, W.B. Saunders, 1978, p 492. With permission.)

hooks attach to the transverse processes. Compression rods are supplied in two sizes: 1/8th inch and 5/11th inch. The latter size is more flexible and easier to use.

The hooks are placed under the transverse processes at the junction of the process and the lamina (Figure 4-10). The hooks have a sharp edge and should be inserted several times to cut the costotransverse ligaments so the hooks seat easily (Figure 4-11). Inferior to T11 there are no suitable transverse processes and the hooks must be placed under the lamina as close as possible to the facet joints.

After the hook sites have been prepared, the threaded rod with the hooks attached

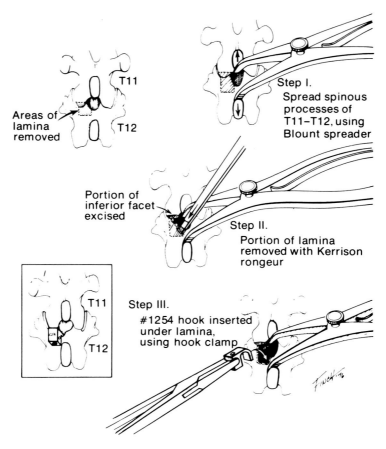

Figure 4-8. Insertion of the lower hook (No. 1254) assembly for Harrington distraction instrumentation. (Step I) It is best to curette out the ligamentum flavum from its attachment to the lamina. It is helpful to remove the most inferior portion of the inferior facet in order to better outline the limits of the ligamentum. A sharp curette or a knife can then be used to completely remove the ligamentum flavum and thus expose the dura. It is helpful to use a Blount spreader to obtain a wider exposure of this area. (Step II) Portions of the lamina are removed with a Kerrison rongeur, producing a flat margin that extends to the pars interarticularis. It is easiest to prepare the facet joint at this level and pack it with cancellous bone before insertion of the Harrington outrigger or the Harrington rod. Insertion of the Harrington outrigger between the two hooks is demonstrated. Facet fusion is carried out. (Reprinted from Moe JH, Winter RB, Bradford DS, Lonstein JE: Scoliosis and Other Spinal Deformities. Philadelphia, W.B. Saunders, 1978, p 493. With permission.)

is inserted. The inferiorly placed hooks are inserted first. Six or more hooks may be used in a compression assembly. The compression system is also tightened using rod holders and spreaders. The hooks are tightened by means of locking nuts. After the nuts are tightened, the threads adjacent to the nuts are crushed to prevent the nuts from loosening (Figure 4-12).

In a patient with a kyphotic deformity, two compression rods may be needed. If so,

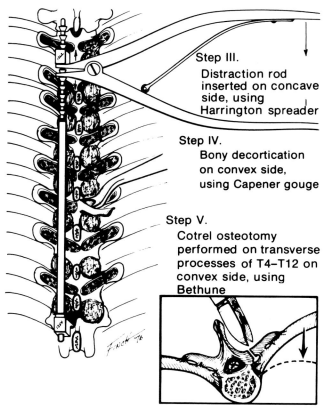

Step III.

Distraction rod inserted on concave side, using Harrington spreader

Step IV.

Bony decortication on convex side, using Capener gouge

Step V.

Cotrel osteotomy performed on transverse processes of T4–T12 on convex side, using Bethune

Figure 4-9. After the concave side of the curvature is completely decorticated and a distracting rod is inserted on the concave side with a Harrington spreader (Step III), bony decortication is carried out on the convex side (Step IV). A Cotrel osteotomy completes the procedure (Step V). A Cotrel transverse process osteotomy is performed if a rib hump elevation greater than 1.5 cm is present before surgery. The transverse processes are osteotomized as vertically as possible at their base with a sharp rib cutter and then hinged superiorly and laterally, allowing the rib to fall forward at the costovertebral articulation. (Reprinted from Moe JH, Winter RB, Bradford DS, Lonstein JE: Scoliosis and Other Spinal Deformities. Philadelphia, W.B. Saunders, 1978, p 495. With permission.)

the joints between the rods should not be fused, since this would interfere with the correction of the deformity.

Segmental Spinal Instrumentation

Segmental spinal instrumentation was first advocated by Luque and Cordosa in 1976,[20] and refers to a system that fixes the spine at each level of the segment to be instrumented rather than only at each end as in Harrington instrumentation. When compression is added to the Luque system, it then is closer to being a segmental system. Luque's original procedure consisted of attaching sublaminar wires to a Harrington distraction rod, thereby producing both axial and tranverse fixation. This system frequently failed because the Harrington rods invariably fractured at the

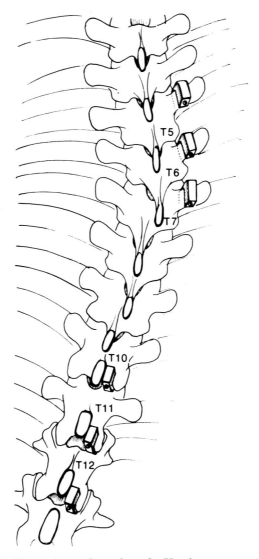

Figure 4-10. Insertion of a Harrington compression assembly. (Step I) No. 1259 hooks are inserted temporarily around the transverse processes of T5, T6, and T7 on the convex side, creating a bed for later permanent insertion. (Reprinted from Moe JH, Winter RB, Bradford DS, Lonstein JE: Scoliosis and Other Spinal Deformities. Philadelphia, W.B. Saunders, 1978, p 497. With permission.)

56

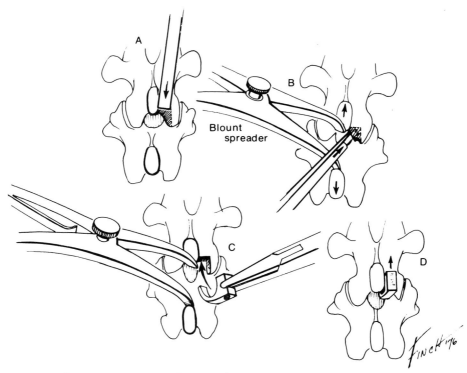

Figure 4-11. (Step II) A portion of the lamina on the convex side of T10, T11, and T12 is removed with an osteotome, gouge, and rongeur to facilitate insertion of the No. 1259 hooks. (Reprinted from Moe JH, Winter RB, Bradford DS, Lonstein JE: Scoliosis and Other Spinal Deformities. Philadelphia, W.B. Saunders, 1978, p 498. With permission.)

ratchet–rod junction as a result of a stress riser created by the stepoff in rod diameter at the point where the ratchets start at the upper end of the rod. A single smooth rod was then tried. This was replaced by a double smooth rod system so that forces could be applied to both the convex and concave sides of a scoliotic curve. The rods were then bent into an "L" shape to prevent their rotation and migration (Figure 4-13); however, as a result of the compressibility of the L-rod system and because they provided minimal torsional stiffness, a C-shaped rod and then a rectangular rod replaced these earlier designs for use in trauma and in tumors (Figure 4-14). Based on these studies, Luque developed the following principles:

1. Rigid internal fixation of the spine must be segmental.
2. A concave rod and a convex rod in contact with the lamina produce, with an intervertebral disc, a three-point fixation that acts as a coupled force to resist lateral and rotational strains.
3. To avoid fatigue and migration of rods, the distraction ratchet must be eliminated and an L-shaped bend should be introduced, thus fixing the end of the rods to a predetermined spinal segment.
4. Arthrodesis is enhanced by rigid internal fixation.

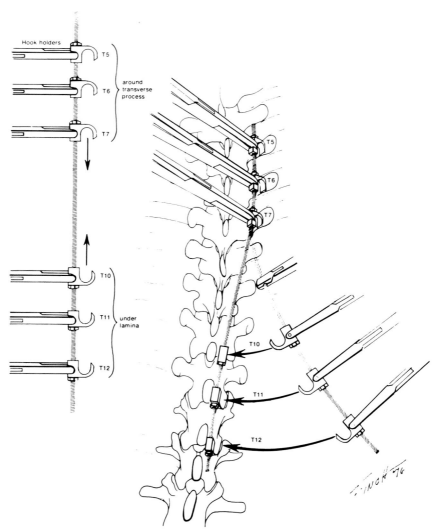

Figure 4-12. After the transverse processes and laminae have been prepared, a threaded rod with the appropriate size hooks is inserted. It is generally easier to insert the cranially directed hooks first followed by insertion of the caudally directed hooks in a single step. After the hooks are securely in place, they may be tightened with either a wrench or a spreader placed between a rod holder and a hook holder. The nasal elevator can then be used to tighten the nut between the hook holder and the rod holder after the distraction has taken place. After maximal contraction, the threads adjacent to the nut are crushed with a clamp to prevent the nut from loosening. (Reprinted from Moe JH, Winter RB, Bradford DS, Lonstein JE: Scoliosis and Other Spinal Deformities. Philadelphia, W.B. Saunders, 1978, p 498. With permission.)

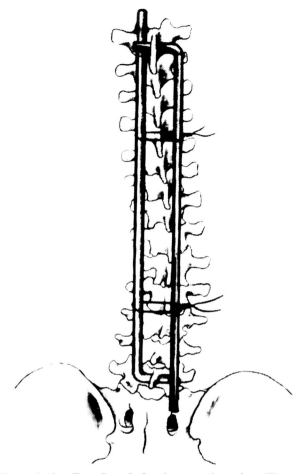

Figure 4-13. Two L rods in place on the spine. The rods have not been wired sublaminarly. (Reprinted from Luque ER: Segmental Spinal Instrumentation: Surgical Technique. Zimmer, Inc., 1980.)

5. Arthrodesis occurs without external support when rigid internal fixation of the spine, decortication, and facetectomy are performed.

6. In unstable spines, where the vertebral body has been resected or where distraction must be used as a method of correction, fixing the length of the area to be segmentally instrumented should be done by inserting either a rectangular or a C-shaped rod.[18]

The Technique of Ferguson and Allen for Segmental Spinal Instrumentation

According to the technique of Allen and Ferguson,[2] the spine is prepared by subperiosteal dissection of all soft tissues from the posterior elements and the spinous processes are removed (to be used as bone grafts). The bases of the spinous processes

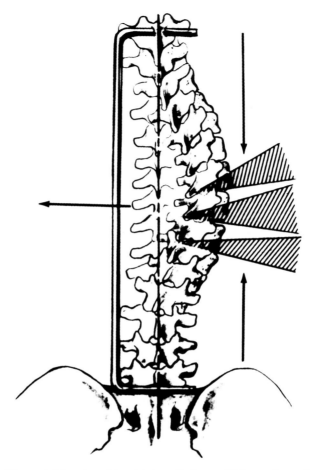

Figure 4-14. A rod bent into a C shape. This configuration would be used for trauma and tumor work where compressibility of the system would be detrimental. (Reprinted from Luque ER: Segmental Spinal Instrumentation: Surgical Technique. Zimmer, Inc., 1980.)

are left protruding as much as possible since they prevent migration of the rods across the midline of the spine (Figure 4-15). Next, the ligamentum flavum is removed. This ligament is thinner in the dorsal than in the lumbar spine. Once the space between the paired ligamenta flava has been visualized, it is possible to put a small angled Kerrison rongeur underneath it and remove it piecemeal (Figures 4-16 and 4-17).

The facet joints are not removed before excision of the ligamenta flava because of bone bleeding. The bleeding can obscure visualization of the spinal canal. At this point, doubled 25-cm lengths of 18-gauge wire are passed sublaminarly. A double bend is placed in each wire so that a loop is created (Figure 4-18). The tip of the loop is then introduced into the spinal canal, with care being taken to ensure that the wire is kept snugly against the under surface of the lamina. It should be possible to pass the wire beneath the lamina with only fingertip pressure (Figure 4-19). There should be no

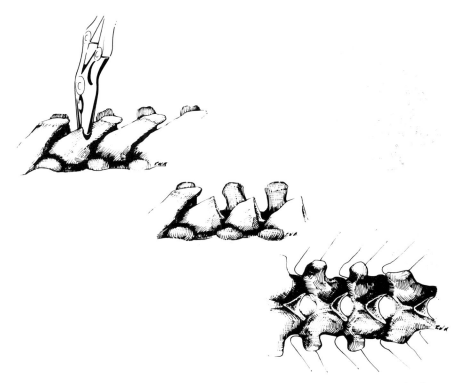

Figure 4-15. In segmental spinal instrumentation, a rongeur is placed vertically over the interlaminar space and the bone is cut to expose the ligamentum flavum. As much of the base of the spinous process is preserved as possible because the rods will be fixed against this bone. (Reprinted from Allen BL, Ferguson RL: The Galveston technique for L-rod instrumentation of the scoliotic spine. Spine 7:276, 1982. With permission.)

resistance; if any resistance is met, the wire should be removed and the interspace inspected.

Once the wire has been passed beneath the lamina and through the next interspace, an assistant grabs the wire tip with a wire-holding forceps. Again, with the wire kept snugly against the undersurface of the lamina, the wire is gently pulled through the canal so that equal lengths of wire are left on either side of the lamina.

At this point the tip of the loop is cut and one wire is pulled to each side of the spine. The wires are bent so that they exit the spine in the midline where the canal is largest (Figure 4-20).

After all the wires have been passed sublaminarly, an L-rod is bent and cut to an appropriate length. The bend should conform to the final correction that is planned. Normal postural curves (i.e., kyphosis and lordosis) should also be incorporated.

Generally, the convex rod is placed first. The L portion of the rod is secured at one end of the spine, and the wires are sequentially secured over the rod. Once the rod has been secured as far as the apex of the deformity, it must be pushed into contact with the lamina at the opposite end of the curve. This rod functions as a lever arm, reducing the deformity. The wires are tightened sequentially by twisting them down over the rod (Figure 4-21).

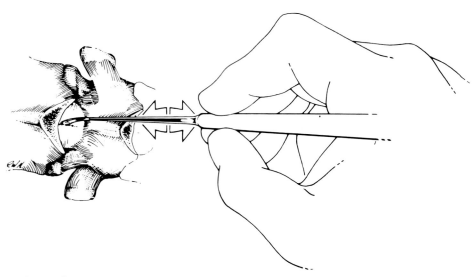

Figure 4-16. Segmental spinal instrumentation. The paired ligamenta flava are separated and each ligamentum is freed from the tissues in the neural canal. A No. 4 Penfield dissector is swept carefully across the deep surface of the ligamentum on the right and left sides through the midline plane. The ligamentum flavum is removed on both sides of all laminae to be instrumented. (Reprinted from Allen BL, Ferguson RL: The Galveston technique for L-rod instrumentation of the scoliotic spine. Spine 7:276, 1982. With permission.)

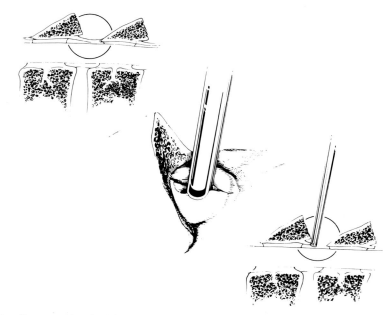

Figure 4-17. Segmental spinal instrumentation. The interspaces are now ready for excision of the ligamentum with Kerrison punches (the largest size that can be fitted into each particular space). (Reprinted from Allen BL, Ferguson RL: The Galveston technique for L-rod instrumentation of the scoliotic spine. Spine 7:276, 1982. With permission.)

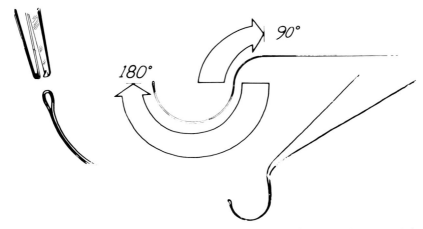

Figure 4-18. Segmental spinal instrumentation. A second bend is placed in the hook in the wire with an arc of about 90 degrees. This will allow the wire to enter the neural canal almost vertically. (Reprinted from Allen BL, Ferguson RL: The Galveston technique for L-rod instrumentation of the scoliotic spine. Spine 7:276, 1982. With permission.)

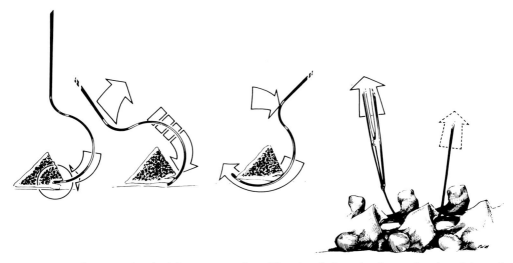

Figure 4-19. Segmental spinal instrumentation. The tip of the wire is gently placed into the neural canal at the inferior laminar edge in the midline. The wire is rotated so that the tip is pointed cephalad; it is then advanced 5 to 6 mm, allowing the tip to clear the sublaminar origin of the ligamentum flavum. The tails of the wire are lifted and pulled to keep the wire snugly against the undersurface of the lamina, and the tip is rolled so that it emerges above. (Reprinted from Allen BL, Ferguson RL: The Galveston technique for L-rod instrumentation of the scoliotic spine. Spine 7:276, 1982. With permission.)

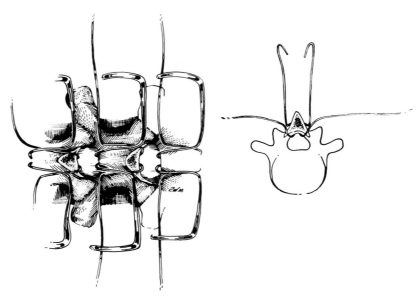

Figure 4-20. Segmental spinal instrumentation. An assistant places the wire clamp with the tooth placed in the loop. The surgeon then pulls the wire with the clamp (while also grasping the tail of the wire) until it is positioned beneath the lamina with half its length protruding above and half below. The tip of the wire is cut and one length is placed to the right side and the other to the left side of the lamina. Each single wire is crimped. All of the wires in the intercalary spinal segment are placed in this manner. Double wires are used at the cephalad and caudad laminae in the instrumented segment. (Reprinted from Allen BL, Ferguson RL: The Galveston technique for L-rod instrumentation of the scoliotic spine. Spine 7:276, 1982. With permission.)

The concave rod is then attached. Again, it is cut to appropriate length. The rod ends should overlap so that the wires incorporating the L portion of one rod incorporate the straight end of the opposite rod. On the concave side, both ends of the rod are attached and then the wires are attached from either end toward the midportion of the curve with manual pressure to further reduce the deformity (Figure 4-22).

The spinous process should not be removed at the inferior aspect of the fusion. A 3/16th-inch drill hole can be made through the spinous process so that the inferior L rod can be stabilized through this portion of the vertebra, thereby eliminating migration of the rod. Likewise, at the superior end of the fusion, the spinous process should be left as long as possible and notched on either the superior or inferior surface to provide stability and prohibit migration.

Secure fixation to the pelvis can also be obtained with the segmental spinal instrumentation of Allen and Ferguson (Figure 4-23). However, appropriate bends must be made in each rod before their insertion into the pelvis (Figure 4-24). Once the rods are bent and the spine is instrumented, there will invariably be slight rotation of the rods. A fusion can then be performed (Figure 4-25). This should be taken into account when the rods are bent before instrumentation.

In order to compare the efficiency of segmental spinal instrumentation with Harrington instrumentrations, Wenger and Carrollo performed loading experiments on four groups of instrumented spines.[29,30] Included were simple Harrington distraction

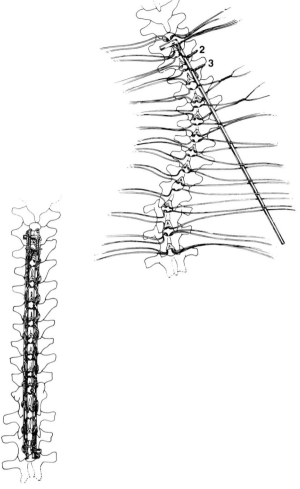

Figure 4-21. Segmental spinal instrumentation. Two rods are implanted in all straightforward operations for scoliosis. The initial rod is used to obtain most correction; the second rod is used to increase the strength of the instrumentation. When the initial rod is placed in the convex side of the scoliotic curve, the deformity is said to be corrected by the convex rod technique, which is a method that is useful in the correction of dorsal curves. The initial rod is fastened to the upper region of the scoliotic curve with the short limb of the rod placed transversely across the lamina of the second vertebra above the curve. Wires 2 and 3 are tightened by twisting, leaving the end wires until last if possible. The rod is levered to the spine, with the wires secured sequentially as the rod contacts the successive laminae. (Reprinted from Allen BL, Ferguson RL: The Galveston technique for L-rod instrumentation of the scoliotic spine. Spine 7:276, 1982. With permission.)

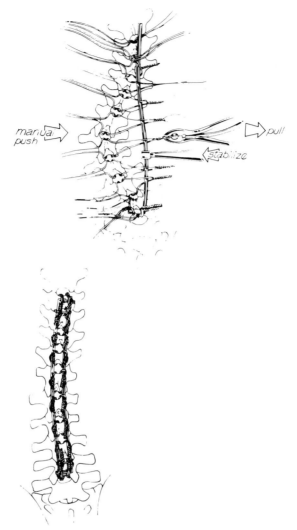

Figure 4-22. Segmental spinal instrumentation. Lumbar scoliosis is more easily corrected by a concave rod technique. The initial rod is placed with its short limb passing transversely across the lamina of the lowermost vertebra to be instrumented. It should pass through a hole at the base of the spinous process or through a notch cut vertically into the spinous process. The inferior double end of the wire on the concave side and the wires to the laminae of the vertebrae above and below the curve with which the rod in is contact are twisted. The spine is reduced to the rod with either manual correction or the wire tensioner device. An assistant can effect manual correction by applying appropriate pressure on the trunk while the surgeon pulls the wires beneath the laminae of the apical vertebra. When maximum correction has been obtained, the wires immediately above and below the apical wires are twisted; the other wires in the area of the deformity are then secured. (Reprinted from Allen BL, Ferguson RL: The Galveston technique for L-rod instrumentation of the scoliotic spine. Spine 7:276, 1982. With permission.)

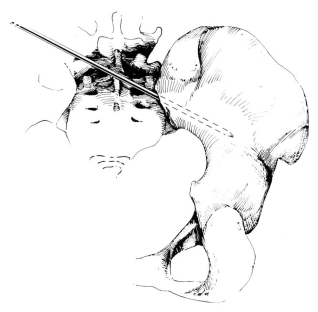

Figure 4-23. Segmental spinal instrumentation. A guide pin is driven along the transverse bar of the ilium. The site at which the pin enters should be just before the sacroiliac joint at the level of the posterior iliac spine; the pin is left in place to serve as a guide for shaping the rod. (Reprinted from Allen BL, Ferguson RL: The Galveston technique for L-rod instrumentation of the scoliotic spine. Spine 7:276, 1982. With permission.)

instrumentation, Harrington distraction and compression instrumentation with transverse approximators, single 1/4th-inch Harrington distraction instrumentation with 18-gauge sublaminar wires, and Luque segmental instrumentation with 3/16th-inch double L rods and 18-gauge sublaminar wires. In tests of longitudinal compression loading, the Harrington distraction instrumentation failed at 94 pounds, the Harrington distraction-compression instrumentation and Harrington distraction instrumentation with sublaminar wires failed at approximately 180 pounds, and the Luque L-rod instrumentation failed at 134 pounds. In addition, only the L-rod system did not fail at the metal–bone interface, whereas the other systems all disengaged from the spine because the hooks cut through the instrumented vertebrae (Figure 4-26). In tests of rotational stability, each of the systems was found to be more stable than the single Harrington distraction rod system, which failed in rotation because the sublaminar hooks cut through the hook–bone interface at a lesser force than did the Luque system or the Harrington rod system with sublaminar wires. Adding the Harrington compression system to the Harrington distraction system added only a slight increase in stability on torsional testing.

The fallacy of these biomechanical studies performed in vitro is that spinal instrumentation in vivo fails because of repetitive small forces being applied in many different modes. A closer approximation to these events resulted when Nasca et al.[25]

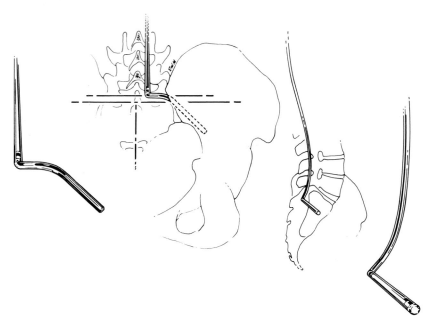

Figure 4-24. Segmental spinal instrumentation. Two bends are made in the rod: (1) at the point at which the rod exits the ilium to place it parallel with the surface of the sacrum; and (2) at the point at which the rod reaches the sacral spinous processes and runs cephalad. The first bend is made between the sacral and spinal portions of the rod with two sleeve benders. The other bend is made between the iliac and sacral portions of the rod approximately 1 to 2 cm lateral to the first bend. The bend is made easily with the pelvic rod bending clamp and a sleeve bender in combination. Secondary spinal contours and lateral deviations may now be bent into the rod as desired. The pelvic pin is removed and the iliac portion of the rod is driven into the hole. (Reprinted from Allen BL, Ferguson RL: The Galveston technique for L-rod instrumentation of the scoliotic spine. Spine 7:276, 1982. With permission.)

developed a method of cyclic torsional loading to study implant failure. These investigators found that both Harrington and Luque systems performed well with no structural failures and that the Luque system resisted axial compression in the sagittal plane but was less stable than the Harrington system in the coronal plane.

The routine use of sublaminar wires to reinforce spinal instrumentation is still controversial, primarily because of the greater risk of neural injury. In centers accustomed to this procedure, however, it is indeed safe. Shufflebarger et al.[26] reported 234 consecutive cases of idiopathic adolescent scoliosis treated by sublaminar wiring; there were no instances of neurologic compromise. Winter[33] reported 100 cases of posterior instrumentation with sublaminar wiring performed without neurologic problems.

Aside from neural injury, other problems may arise, one of which has been noted by many advocates of segmental spinal instrumentation, namely, fatigue fractures of the stainless steel wire used in the construct. In the author's series, of 37 adults followed for over 1 year with SSI without external orthotic support 30 percent were found to have broken wires at at least one level. In 73 children followed for over 1 year

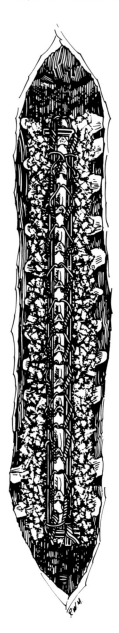

Figure 4-25. The Galveston fusion technique obviates the need for decortication and facet excision. A large amount of graft material is the key. Cancellous bone is usually harvested from the posterior iliac crest or both crests; one or both fibulae can be used as well. In patients with a significant rib hump, posterior thoracoplasty additionally provides a large volume of bone as well as improving the cosmetic result. The grafts are placed lateral to the rods along both sides of the spine and to the tips of the transverse processes. (Reprinted from Allen BL, Ferguson RL: The Galveston technique for L-rod instrumentation of the scoliotic spine. Spine 7:276, 1982. With permission.)

treated by SSI without postoperative immobilization, 12 percent were found to have at least one wire broken. Typically the wires break within the first 3 months after insertion. As a result, Allen and Ferguson[2] have advocated the use of certified cobalt-nickel alloy wires (ASTM F-562) for both the 3/16th-inch Luque L-rod and the sublaminar wires. Since using this alloy, I have had no wire failures in 32 cases of adolescents followed for over 1 year, although among 16 cases involving adults with scoliosis followed for over 1 year, two wire failures have occurred. As a result, all of

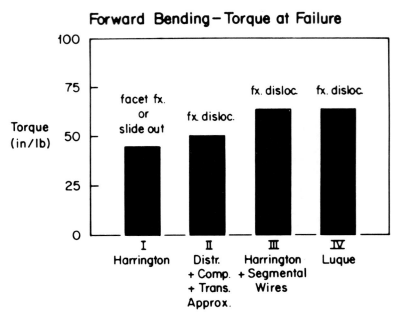

Figure 4-26. Results of tests in forward bending. The addition of various types of segmental fixation improves the ability of the instrumentation to withstand an acute forward bend. The mode of failure is listed at the top of the respective columns. (Reprinted from Wenger DR, Carrollo JJ: Laboratory testing of segmental spinal instrumentation versus traditional Harrington instrumentation for scoliosis treatment. Spine 7:265, 1982. With permission.)

our adult patients are now immobilized for at least 6 months postoperatively in addition to our use of the more rigid alloy rods and wires for internal fixation.

White and Panjabi[31] advocated the use of dual Harrington distraction rods to correct kyphotic deformity secondary to fracture, and Luque has suggested the same principle in correction of kyphosis resulting from trauma or disease (Figure 4-27). In both instances, distraction forces and bending movements are used. Distraction rods act through the application of pure distraction forces axially and by elongating the spine through the intact posterior elements. The facet joints on the posterior aspect of the spine act as a fulcrum through which each vertebra on the concavity is extended as the spine is straightened. With segmental spinal instrumentation, the only distraction force comes from the inherent elongation of the spine that occurs with the straightening procedure. White and Panjabi emphasized that pure distraction forces are dangerous with this type of deformity and should be avoided.

Harrington Instrumentation with Sublaminar Wiring

While Harrington distraction instrumentation with sublaminar wiring has been condemned by Luque because of rod failure, others have condemned it because of neurologic damage caused by rotation of the hooks into into the spinal canal. The proponents of this technique[12] have reported good results in patients treated with double Harrington distraction instrumentation and sublaminar wiring. Neurologic recovery in matched series of surgically treated and non-surgically treated patients did

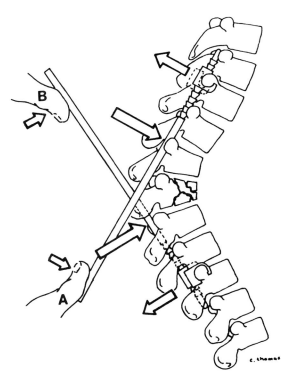

Figure 4-27. The simultaneous use of two Harrington distraction rods to correct a kyphotic deformity. These rods, which are about five times as stiff as the compression rods, can be used to create two effective correcting couples to each end of a kyphotic deformity. This is actually a four-point bending system. One rod is placed in the traditional manner with the upper hook placed as for correction of scoliosis. This rod exerts a couple on the upper segment of the spine through a force applied by the lower finger (A). The second rod is placed on the other side in an inverted position. It exerts a correcting couple to the lower portion of the spine through a force applied by the upper finger (B). This technique has the practical advantage of providing good control and corrective forces (couples) to both portions of the deformity. (Reprinted from White AA, Panjabi MM (eds): Clinical Biomechanics of the Spine. Philadelphia, J.B. Lippincott, 1978, p. 437. With permission.)

not seem to improve with early spine reduction and stabilization, but patient mobilization and its intended benefits were improved. Postoperative bracing and casting were felt to be necessary to prevent instrument failure before the advent of sublaminar wiring. In 17 patients followed for 9 to 30 months with thoracic and thoracolumbar fractures, Gaines had no instrument failures and solid fusion with early mobilization without benefit of external support.[12]

The Luque system with either double L rods or a single rectangular rod may be used to treat the fractured unstable spine. It is my feeling that Harrington distraction instrumentation with sublaminar wiring is the preferable construct. In 23 cases of trauma treated with dual Harrington distraction instrumentation and sublaminar wires, there have been no cases of instrument failure in cases followed from 3 to 42 months. Five of these 23 patients had complete lesions and did not recover; four had partial

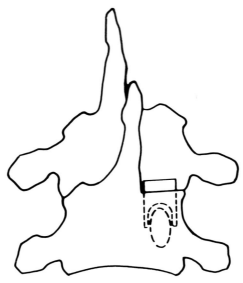

Figure 4-28. Interspinous segmental spinal instrumentation. The upper hook is seated as follows: a transverse osteotomy is made through the inferior facet. The direction of this cut should be slightly oblique in a caudal and lateral direction. The osteotomized facet site is prepared for hook placement with a sharp bifid hook, which grasps the pedicle. The blunt bifid hook is then inserted and its rotational stability assessed. The lower hook site is prepared in exactly the same way as for standard Harrington instrumentation. (Reprinted from Drummond DS, Keene JS: Interspinous Segmental Spinal Instrumentation: Surgical Technique. Zimmer, Inc., 1984.)

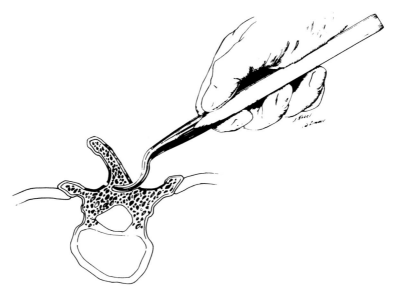

Figure 4-29. Interspinous segmental spinal instrumentation. Insertion of the implant is begun by creating holes in both sides of the spinous process. First the cortical bone is penetrated with a sharp Zuelzer awl. These two holes are then joined with a curved awl. To penetrate good bone but avoid the spinal canal, the hand should be kept close to the lamina during passage of the awls. Only one button-wire implant is inserted from the concave side to the convex side at the uppermost and lowermost segments. At each intervening level the hole through the base of the spinous process should be made large enough so that two implants can be passed in opposite directions. (Reprinted from Drummond DS, Keene JS: Interspinous Segmental Spinal Instrumentation: Surgical Technique. Zimmer, Inc., 1984.)

lesions, three of whom recovered completely; and 14 patients were neurologically intact. All patients were braced for 6 months. When reducing spinal fractures, one should depend partially on distraction forces, and levering on the posterior elements to obtain three-point fixation should be avoided since further damage to neural elements can occur.

Interspinous Segmental Spinal Instrumentation (ISSI)

While the biomechanical advantages of more secure fixation with sublaminar wiring have been demonstrated, the potential risk of this procedure has prompted the development of another segmental wiring system. In the Wisconsin system, interspinous segmental spinal instrumentation, each vertebra is segmentally wired to an overlying rod without the wires entering the spinal canal.[6,7] The technique uses paired

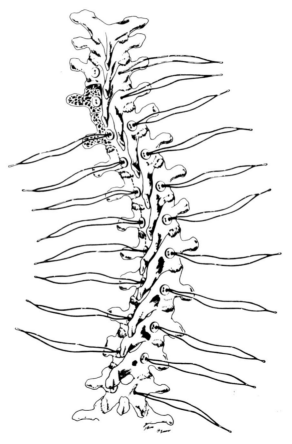

Figure 4-30. Interspinous segmental spinal instrumentation. After the wires are passed through the hole in the opposite button of the pair, the buttons are pulled snugly against the base of the spinous process and shaped there with a round-ended tamp. (Reprinted from Drummond DS, Keene JS: Interspinous Segmental Spinal Instrumentation: Surgical Technique. Zimmer, Inc., 1984.)

button–wire implants, which are anchored to the base of the spinous process. Two rods are used. The first rod is a malleable Luque segmental spinal instrumentation rod that is bent into a "C" shape. The "C" spans the full length of the segment to be instrumented. It is placed on the convex side of the curve. The second rod is a Harrington distraction rod that is placed in the concavity of the curve (Figures 4-28, 4-29). The wires are then tied over each of the rods after they are passed through the spinous process and secured on either side of the process by a button that increases the pull-out strength of the wire through the bone (Figure 4-30). It is critical to use the base

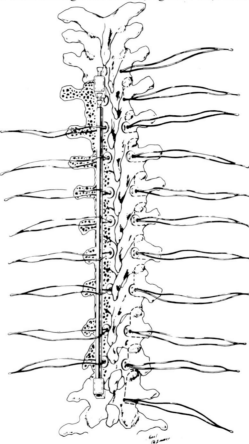

Figure 4-31. Interspinous segmental spinal instrumentation. A careful posterior and facet joint fusion is now done on the concave side of the curve. Only the posterior elements lateral to the button should be decorticated. After carefully contouring the distraction rod for physiologic kyphosis and lordosis, the rod is passed through the open ends of the wire of the implant on the concave side of the curve and inserted into the upper and lowoer hooks. Initial correction is then accomplished by distraction. (Reprinted from Drummond DS, Keene JS: Interspinous Segmental Spinal Instrumentation: Surgical Technique. Zimmer, Inc., 1984.)

of the spinous process and not the middle or tip with this system since this provides maximum strength for the implant construct. Special awls have been developed to create holes at the bases of the spinous processes for passage of the wires (Figures 4-31, 4-32, 4-33). McCarthy used a dog model to show that ISSI was as strong as sublaminar wiring.[21] Drummond et al.[6,7] also reported that ISSI was biomechanically as strong as sublaminar wiring. They compared a matched group of patients treated with Harrington

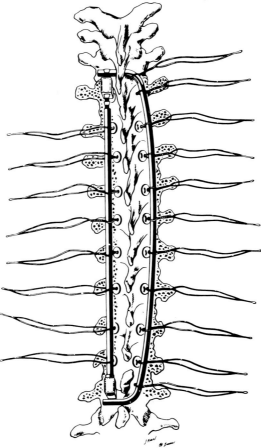

Figure 4-32. Interspinous segmental spinal instrumentation. A 3/16th- or 1/4th-inch Luque rod in now contoured. A right-angled bend is made at the upper and lower end of the rod. These bends should be long enough to span the canal and thus prohibit rotation toward it. The upper limb should lie adjacent to the upper edge of the bifid hook and pass under the ratchet system of the contralateral distraction rod. The lower limb of the Luque rod should lie adjacent to the lower edge of the distal hook. The contoured rod is then introduced into its proper location. The rods are then sequentially tightened from the apex caudally and cephalad. (Reprinted from Drummond DS, Keene JS: Interspinous Segmental Spinal Instrumentation: Surgical Technique. Zimmer, Inc., 1984.)

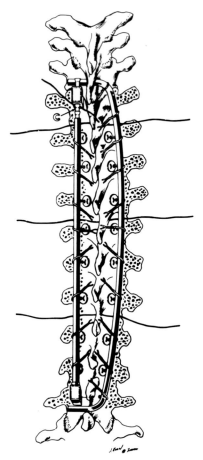

Figure 4-33. Interspinous segmental spinal instrumentation. The instrumentation is then completed by tying down the wires on the distraction rod on the concave side of the curve. (Reprinted from Drummond DS, Keene JS: Interspinous Segmental Spinal Instrumentation: Surgical Technique. Zimmer, Inc., 1984.)

instrumentation with those treated by ISSI. They found that hospitalization time was decreased by five days with ISSI. In addition, they noted that while the initial correction was approximately the same with both systems, the loss of correction was less in the patients treated with ISSI.

When there is compression or disruption of the middle column of the spine, some degree of distraction is usually necessary to reduce the fracture; therefore, the Harrington system offers an immediate advantage. If a Luque system is used, distraction might be used intraoperatively. If distraction is not used, ventral decompression might be necessary.

ANTERIOR SPINAL INSTRUMENTATION

The first modern anterior spinal instrumentation technique was developed by Dwyer et al.[9,10] Their system was developed for the correction of scoliosis and applied compressive forces to the convexity of the scoliotic spine. This was accomplished by means of transvertebral screws linked by a heavy cable under tension. While there is much support for the use of this type of instrumentation in scoliosis, there is little use for it in the treatment of instability of the spine for fractures, since it requires an intact spine complex in order to function properly.

Several newer forms of instrumentation have recently been fashioned. Dunn et al.[8] have developed a rigid fixation technique that can be used when anterior approaches to the spine are necessary. Two systems have basically been developed: one for trauma and a second for large vertebral resections (e.g., tumors) or for correction of spinal deformity. This instrumentation has the advantage of being able to fix the length of the segment to be stabilized without depending on intact support from any of the osteoligamentous structures surrounding the spine. The design of the implant system was influenced by biomechanical studies performed by Dunn and his coworkers. They could obtain satisfactory stability when fixing to only one level above and one level

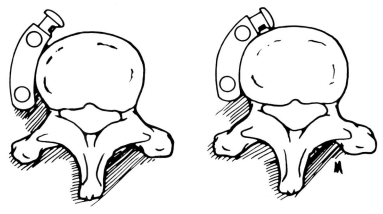

Figure 4-34. Anterior spinal instrumentation. Vertebral body bridges are selected to accomplish the best fit to the curve of the adjacent vertebra. These vertebral body bridges are sized according to the radius of the curvature of their inner portion. They range from 17 mm to 23 mm. The holes for the rods are interchangeable between any size bridge. (Courtesy of Harold K. Dunn, MD)

below a fracture site if they used two rods linked together by a pair of curved bridges, each affixed to vertebral bodies at two points at least 75 degrees apart on the circumference of the vertebral body. Dunn's system uses a transvertebral screw through a metal bridge on the posterolateral side of the vertebral body with a staple providing fixation at a point 75 degrees away on the metal bridge. The two bridges, one above the fracture and one below, are then linked by means of threaded rods, which can be used to fix the length of the segment to be stabilized. In Dunn's experience, the need for external support and the need for combining the procedure with a posterior one have been obviated (Figures 4-34 through 4-39).

Arena et al.[3] reported on 17 patients followed for an average of 29 months using this form of stabilization. They obtained a solid fusion in 11 of 12 patients with fractures followed a minimum of 1 year. One patient developed a nonpainful pseudoarthrosis, and the remaining five patients, all of whom had metastatic disease, demonstrated a progression of their deformity until the time of their deaths. The authors concluded that the Dunn device serves as a *useful adjunct in the anterior approach to the thoracic and lumbar spine and that two-stage procedures for the treatment of fractures could be eliminated by the single anterior instrumentation device advocated by Dunn.*

One of the major advantages of an anterior approach to the spine is that *fewer vertebrae need to be fused.* A posterior approach for fracture treatment requires that at least two levels above and below the fracture site be included in the construct, whereas Dunn instrumentation saves two segments from being involved in the fusion. This is particularly important in the lumbar spine, where normal postural curves should be saved if at all possible in order to prevent later problems. If a patient has a burst fracture

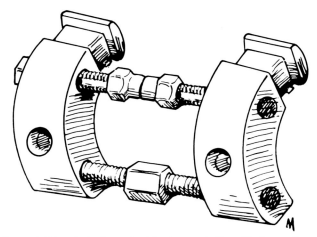

Figure 4-35.   Anterior spinal instrumentation. Rods are then chosen to complete the assembly of the system. In general about 1 cm of distraction is the most that will be needed. The vertebral body bridges are initially connected with the right-hand or left-hand threaded posterior rod. The most anterior rod is then added and as it is slipped between the two vertebral body bridges the two lock nuts are positioned. The assembled implant is placed on the vertebral bodies and a screw starter is used to penetrate the cortex of the vertebral body. (Courtesy of Harold K Dunn, MD)

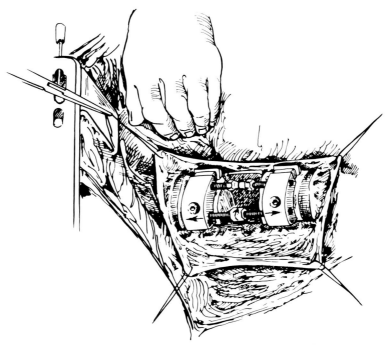

Figure 4-36. Anterior spinal instrumentation. The proper length of the screws is determined by simply using a screw to measure the distance across the vertebral body. The vertebral body screw is self-tapping and goes across the body roughly parallel to the posterior longitudinal ligament. The screw should penetrate the cortex on the far side of the vertebral body. With the two vertebral screws in place the posterior right-hand or left-hand threaded rod is turned to distract and reestablish the height of the posterior longitudinal ligament. (Reprinted from Dunn HK: Instrumentation for the Anterior Spine: Surgical Technique. Zimmer, Inc., 1984.)

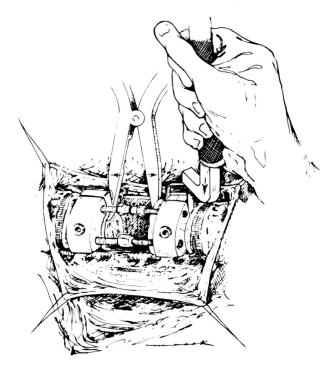

Figure 4-37. Anterior spinal instrumentation. A spreader is placed anteriorly and the kyphosis is corrected. The vertebral body staples are driven into place. These staples are self-locking and cannot be removed once they are driven past the clip on the vertebral body bridge. (Reprinted from Dunn HK: Instrumentation for the Anterior Spine: Surgical Technique. Zimmer, Inc., 1984.)

at L3, it would be possible to instrument from L2 to L4 with the Dunn instrumentation. In a posterior approach, one would have to instrument down to L5. This would leave only the lumbosacral junction to bear all the stresses of pelvic tilt. On a theoretical basis at least, requiring the lumbosacral joint to absorb the entire increased stress load as opposed to dividing it between the lumbosacral joint and another mobile segment would have to increase the wear and tear at that joint considerably, thereby producing long-term disability.

My experience with the device is limited to four cases, which have been followed for over 1 year. Two patients had burst fractures treated with an anterior approach without posterior instrumentation, one patient had a metastatic lesion from breast disease and died approximately 1 year postoperatively, and the other patient had a metastatic lesion also from the breast and is still alive. In all cases, fibular strut grafts were used in addition to the Dunn instrumentation and in none of these cases did the instrumentation fail.

Recent reports to the manufacturer have indicated problems with this implant. The aorta in some cases has been found to lay over a portion of the buttress plate. Aneurysm formation has therefore been postulated. While the biomechanical principles of the

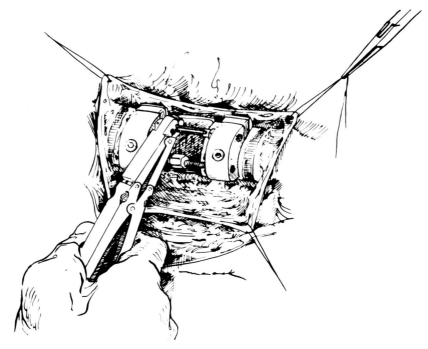

Figure 4-38. Anterior spinal instrumentation. The two nuts on the anterior rod are tightened and the system is secured by crimping the skirt on these two nuts. (Reprinted from Dunn HK: Instrumentation for the Anterior Spine: Surgical Technique. Zimmer, Inc., 1984.)

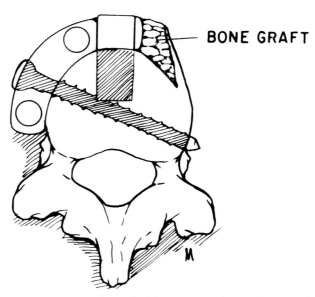

BONE GRAFT

Figure 4-39. Anterior spinal instrumentation. A bone graft can then be added in an osteoperiosteal sleeve, which has been created on the far side of the bridge at each level. (Reprinted from Dunn HK: Instrumentation for the Anterior Spine: Surgical Technique. Zimmer, Inc., 1984.)

Dunn System remain sound, this potential disastrous complication should obviate its use in its current design.

Three other anterior implants are also available. These all consist of two rods that extend a single level above and below the site of injury. The systems include the double Hall-Dwyer solid rod, the Kaneda implant, and the Bradford implant.[4,9,10,16] Each of these devices acts as a strut, helping to prevent collapse when there is a significant anterior instability although they all react poorly to torsional loading and require either posterior instrumentation or significant additional external support.

REFERENCES

1. Albee FH: Transplantation of a portion of the tibia into the spine for Pott's disease—A preliminary report. JAMA 57:885, 1911
2. Allen BL, Ferguson RL: The Galveston technique for L-rod instrumentation of the scoliotic spine. Spine 7:176, 1982
3. Arena MJ, Cotler HB, Cotler JM: The Dunn device for anterior stabilization of the thoracic and lumbar spine. Scoliosis Research Society Meeting, New Orleans, LA, October, 1983 (abstr)
4. Bradford DS, McBride G: Thoracic lumbar spine fractures with incomplete neurologic deficit—Correlative study on the adequacy of decompression versus neurologic return. Orthop Trans 8:159, 1984
5. Denis F: The three column spine and its significance in the classification of acute thoracolumbar spinal injuries. Spine 8:817, 1983
6. Drummond D: The Wisconsin segmental spinal instrumentation system. Scoliosis Research Society Meeting, Montreal, 1981
7. Drummond D, Guadagni JS, Keene JS, Breed A, Narechania R: Interspinous process segmental spinal instrumentation. J Pediatr Orthop 4:397, 1984
8. Dunn HK, Goble EM, McBride GG, Daniels AU: An implant system for anterior stabilization. Orthop Trans 5:433, 1981
9. Dwyer AF: Experience of anterior correction of scoliosis. Clin Orthop 93:191, 1973
10. Dwyer AF, Newton NC, Sherwood AA: An anterior approach to scoliosis. Clin Orthop 62:192, 1969
11. Flesch JR, Leider LL, Erickson DL, Chou SN, Bradford DS: Harrington instrumentation and spine fusion for thoracic and lumbar spine fractures. J Bone Joint Surg 59A:143, 1977
12. Gaines RW: Stabilization of thoracic and thoracolumbar fracture dislocations with Harrington rods and sublaminar wires. Scoliosis Research Society Meeting, Denver, 1982

13. Harrington PR: Treatment of scoliosis correction. J Bone Joint Surg 44A:591, 1962
14. Harrington PR: Technical details in relation to the successful use of instrumentation in scoliosis. Orthop Clin North Am 3:49, 1972
15. Hibbs RA: An operation for progressive spinal deformities. NY Med J 93:1013, 1911
16. Kaneda K, Abumi K, Fujiya M: Birth fractures of the thoracolumbar and lumbar spine with neurologic involvement—Anterior decompression and fusion with instrumentation. Orthop Trans 7:16, 1983
17. Kaufer H: The Thoracolumbar Spine. In Rockwood CA, Green DP: Fractures, vol 2. Philadelphia, J.B. Lippincott, 1975, p. 861
18. Luque ER: The anatomic basis and development of segmental spinal instrumentation. Spine 7:256, 1982
19. Luque ER: The correction of postural curves of the spine. Spine 7:270, 1982
20. Luque ER: Cordosa A: Segmental of scoliosis with a rigid internal fixation. Scoliosis Research Society Meeting. Ottawa, 1976
21. McCarthy RE, Dwyer AP, Harrison BH: Comparison of Luque segmental fixation with three types of posterior spinal fixation using the spinous process. Scoliosis Research Society Meeting, New Orleans, 1983
22. Moe JH, Winter RB, Bradford DS, Lonstein JE: Scoliosis and Other Spinal Deformities. Philadelphia, W.B. Saunders, 1978, pp. 485–499
23. Murphy W, Southwick W: Treatment of the unstable spine with combination Harrington distraction and compression rods. Scoliosis Research Society meeting, Montreal, 1981
24. Nachemson A, Gosta Elfstrom M: Intravital wireless telemetry of axial forces in Harrington distraction rods in patients with idiopathic scoliosis. J Bone Joint Surg 53A:445, 1971
25. Nasca RJ, Hollis JM, Lamons JE: Cyclic

axioloading of spinal implants. Orthop Trans 8:167, 1984

26. Shufflebarger HL, Kahn A, Rinsky LA, Shank M: Segmental spinal instrumentation in idiopathic scoliosis: A retrospective analysis of 234 cases. Scoliosis Research Society Meeting, Orlando, FL, 1984

27. Simmons E: Biomechanical studies with scoliotic stimulator. Scoliosis Research Society Meeting, Toronto, 1970

28. Waugh TR: Intravital measurements during instrumental correction of idiopathic scoliosis. Acta Orthop Scand (Suppl) 93:1-87, 1966

29. Wenger DR, Carrollo JJ: Biomechanics of scoliosis—correction of segmental spinal instrumentation. Spine 7:260, 1982

30. Wenger DR, Carrollo JJ: Laboratory testing of segmental spinal instrumentation versus traditional Harrington instrumentation for scoliosis treatment. Spine 7:265, 1982

31. White AA, Panjabi MM: The clinical biomechanics of kyphotic deformities. Clin Orthop 12B:8, 1977

32. White AA, Panjabi MM (eds): Clinical Biomechanics of the Spine. Philadelphia, J.B. Lippincott, 1978, pp 434–438

33. Winter RB: Posterior spinal arthrodesis with instrumentation and sublaminar wiring: 10 consecutive personal cases. Scoliosis Research Society Meeting, Orlando, FL, 1984

34. Yocum TD, Leatherman KD, Brower TD: The early rod fixation in the treatment of fracture dislocations of the spine. J Bone Joint Surg 52A:1257, 1970 (abstr)

Keith Bridwell
Thomas G. Saul

5

Upper Thoracic Spinal Instability

There are a number of obstacles to surgically stabilizing the upper thoracic spine that are not encountered in stabilizing the lower thoracic and lumbar spine. Most of these stem from the anatomy of the upper thoracic spine. It is quite difficult to achieve a wide anterior exposure from T1 to T3 because of the change in sagittal spinal alignment at the cervicothoracic junction and because of the location of the subclavian vessels. Posterior exposure is also slightly more difficult because of the presence of the shoulders and the change in sagittal spinal alignment. Posterior exposure often necessitates and is facilitated by tong or halo traction. Instrumentation of the upper thoracic spine is somewhat limited by the change in the posterior elements between C7 and T1. The posterior elements are much smaller in the cervical spine. Harrington rod instrumentation cannot be safely carried above T1. The upper thoracic spine cannot be immobilized externally with an underarm cast or orthosis. Radiographic assessment of the upper thoracic spine is more difficult because of the radiographic interference produced by the shoulders. All of these factors must be considered in assessing and achieving spinal stability in this portion of the spine and will be discussed in detail in this chapter.

For the purposes of the discussion, the upper thoracic spine is defined as the first six thoracic vertebrae. Because some stabilization procedures involve one to two vertebral levels above and below the level of instability, we will include the sixth and seventh cervical vertebrae in our anatomic discussions.

NEUROANATOMY

The intraspinal contents can be divided between the epidural and intradural spaces. The epidural space contains veins, arteries, and epidural fat. Under normal conditions, there is an abundant amount of epidural fat over the posterior surface of the dural tube and virtually none posteriorly. The components of the spinal nerve can also be considered contents of the epidural space. Dorsal and ventral roots at this level exit the dural tube separately and unite to form the spinal nerve root in the intervertebral foramen. In the upper thoracic spine, the vertebral column levels do not coincide with the spinal cord levels. For example, the third thoracic vertebra is at the same level as the fifth spinal cord segment.

The T2–T6 spinal nerve roots innervate intercostal muscles and provide sensory innervation for the respective dermatomes. The ventral ramus of the T1 spinal nerve root becomes part of the brachial plexus and innervates intrinsic hand muscles. The C8 spinal nerve root exits between C7 and T1 and enters the brachial plexus. It also innervates the intrinsic hand muscles and supplies some innervation for finger extension and flexion. The C7 nerve root exits between the sixth and seventh cervical vertebrae and innervates the triceps and the extensors and flexors of the hand. The C7 and C8 nerve roots supply sensory innervation to specific dermatomes of the hand. These nerve roots are mentioned because instrumentation and stabilization procedures of the upper thoracic spine often must include the lower cervical spine. This information therefore is necessary for proper preoperative planning as well as for instructing the patient about the possible risks of any given procedure.

In addition to understanding the functions of the nerve roots in this area, a knowledge of the relationships of the cervicothoracic (stellate) ganglion of the sympathetic chain is also important. This ganglion sends gray rami communicantes to the seventh and eighth cervical and first thoracic nerves.[25] Disease processes in this area of the spinal column often produce a Horner's syndrome because of disruption of the sympathetic fibers at these levels. Furthermore, when instrumentation or operative procedures are planned to include these levels or the nerve roots at these levels, patients should be warned preoperatively of the risk of developing a Horner's syndrome.

The spinal cord in the upper thoracic region is round in configuration and is smaller than the cervical and lumbar portions of the cord. In addition, the sagittal diameter of the canal at this level is also smaller than in other areas. In the midthoracic region the transverse diameter of the spinal cord is approximately 10 mm and the sagittal diameter is approximately 8 mm. Structurally the spinal cord at this level has relatively less gray matter than is seen in the cervical or lumbar areas because the latter areas innervate the large muscles of the extremities. In the thoracic area only the smaller intercostal and abdominal muscles are innervated.

The vasculature in this area of the cord is particularly important. In general, the anterior two thirds of the spinal cord receives its arterial supply from the anterior spinal artery, which runs along the ventral aspect of the spinal cord in the median sulcus. This midline artery or arterial network receives contributions from the spinal radicular arteries, which enter the spinal canal through the neural foramen.[12] These spinal radicular arteries are not present at each level of the spinal column and they are not symmetrical. The number of cervical radicular arteries that contribute to the anterior spinal artery may vary from one to six. The thoracic region may receive two to four spinal radicular arteries and the lumbosacral region may receive several of these contributory arteries.[12] It is this variation in the anterior spinal artery network that accounts for the variability in the blood supply to the spinal cord throughout it length. It is believed that the thoracic spinal cord (approximately T3 to T9) has a relative paucity of spinal radicular arteries entering the neural foramen.[4,12] Gillilan maintains that there are only two or three spinal radicular arteries that enter the spinal canal in the thoracic region.[12] Domisse maintains that there are several important clinical observations related to this matter.[4] It is interesting that the spinal cord is narrowest from T4 to T9 and this corresponds with the part of the cord that has the smallest arterial supply.

Domisse and Enslin reported four cases of paraplegia complicating 68 spinal operations.[5] Three of the four cases occurred between T5 and T9, while only 18 of the 68 procedures were done in this region. Because of these facts, they emphasized that the area from T4 to T9 is the "critical zone of the spinal cord." Truex and Carpenter[25] maintained that the area of diminished blood supply to the thoracic cord actually begins at T1 and is least profuse at the T4-5 level. Because of the small numbers of these spinal radicular arteries and because of the subsequent great length between these major contributing arteries, a blockage or disruption of any of them, either by disease or by surgical intervention, could have devastating results on cord function. This tenuous supply to the anterior portion of the thoracic spinal cord might have direct implications for both the preoperative and postoperative care of these patients, for we believe that poor perfusion states may worsen neurologic deficits.

The arterial supply to the posterior one third of the spinal cord is much more abundant and less variable than the anterior circulation. This region of the cord is supplied by the paired posterior spinal arteries, which begin as branches from the vertebral arteries and course caudally. They are located just medial to the posterior roots (dorsal root entry zone). These posterior arterial networks receive a more abundant supply throughout the course of the spinal cord from the posterior spinal radicular arteries. In addition, there are more anastomotic channels on this aspect of the spinal cord.

Because many of the conditions that cause instability in the upper thoracic region affect the ventral aspect of the vertebral column, the anterior spinal cord and the anterior spinal artery are often compressed. Many of these patients therefore have the anterior spinal artery syndrome described by Schneider.[28] Classically, this consists of preservation of the posterior column functions of proprioception and touch combined with a loss of pyramidal tract motor function and spinothalamic function.

SUPPORTING STRUCTURES OF THE UPPER THORACIC SPINE

The anterior, middle, and posterior columns of the upper thoracic spine derive support from both primary and secondary supporting structures (Table 5-1). The yellow ligament is very strong in the thoracic area and the capsular ligaments are comparatively weak. Therefore, multiple midline laminectomies coupled with a physiologic kyphosis may create instability even when the facet articulations are spared *if* there is loss of some of the anterior supporting structures of the spine as well. The interspinous and supraspinous ligaments are not as thick in the thoracic spine as in the lumbar spine and do not provide a major stabilizing force. The radiate ligaments and the various costotransverse ligaments provide stability by binding the adjacent vertebra to the interconnecting ribs. The anterior and posterior longitudinal ligaments and the annulus are major factors in clinical stability of the spine anteriorly.

The ribs, both by their connection to the rib cage and by their coupling to the vertebrae of the spine, increase the stability of the thoracic spine. The transverse

Table 5-1.
Supporting structures of the upper thoracic spine

Important Supporting Structures
Anterior:
Anterior longitudinal ligament
Posterior longitudinal ligament
Anulus
Disc
Vertebral body
Posterior:
Ligamentum flavum
Facet joints
Middle:
Pedicles
Costovertebral-transverse process Complex
Lesser Supporting Structures
Spinous proceses and neural arch
Supraspinous ligaments
Interspinous ligaments
Facet capsular ligaments

processes and ribs (except T1 and T2) are larger in the upper thoracic spine than the lower thoracic spine. White and Panjabi[26] have shown that even when all the posterior elements are cut, the spine remains stable in flexion until the costovertebral articulation is destroyed. The facets in the upper thoracic spine provide stability against anterior displacement. The facet joints in the upper thoracic spine have more of a sagittal orientation than the joints of the lower thoracic spine. The facet orientation resists rotatory injuries. Therefore, a considerable amount of force is required to create an unstable fracture of the upper thoracic spine. When such a fracture does occur, it is usually associated with neurologic injury. Most instabilities secondary to fracture are associated with disruption of the posterior longitudinal ligament and at least two of the important posterior structures: the ligamentum flavum, the facet joints, or the costovertebral joints.

The vertebral bodies and discs in the thoracic spine get progressively larger rostrally to caudally. The upper thoracic discs are smaller than the lower thoracic, cervical, and lumbar spine discs in vertical dimensions; however, the thoracic discs are larger in cross-sectional area than the discs in the cervical spine.

The thoracic spinal canal has a relatively constant size and contour throughout its length. The small size of the canal at this level also contributes to the very high incidence of severe spinal cord injuries when an unstable fracture occurs. The spinal canal is smaller in the upper and middle portions of the thoracic spine than in any other area from T1 caudally. The canal is round with equal transverse and sagittal diameters. However, at T1 and T2 the canal becomes more elliptical and flattens in the sagittal plane, similar to the canal in the cervical spine.

At the cervicothoracic junction there is a sharp reversal from cervical lordosis to thoracic kyphosis. The usual apex of physiologic thoracic kyphosis is between T6 and T9; the apex of cervical lordosis is between C5 and T2.

PRINCIPLES AND CAUSES OF INSTABILITY

Spinal instability can be defined as either abnormally increased mobility at a certain level or a tendency toward loss of normal contour in the coronal or sagittal planes. The most common form of instability in the upper thoracic spine is in the sagittal plane, creating kyphosis. In adults, a kyphosis can be created by significant injury to the anterior and posterior columns of the spine such as an anterior fracture and a posterior ligamentous injury. Tumors or infections that lead to destruction of the vertebral body may lead to kyphosis, especially if involvement of the pedicles exists as well. The upper part of the thoracic spine is often difficult to visualize on plain films because the vertebral bodies are smaller and the anatomy of the sagittal plane is obscured by the shoulder girdle. This roentgenographic obscuration makes evaluation of stability difficult (Figure 5-1). Tomograms and CT scans of the upper thoracic spine in these cases are helpful.

If there is any doubt about the stability of the upper thoracic spine, it is best to stabilize it. With fusion there is minimal if any noticeable loss of motion because the upper thoracic spine contributes only a small percentage to total spine motion. Also, fusing this part of the spine in a young patient is less apt to cause noticeable loss of trunk height than fusion of the lumbar spine at an early age[6] because the vertebral bodies in the upper thoracic spine are relatively small and contribute less to the longitudinal growth of the trunk than do the larger lower thoracic and lumbar vertebrae. However, stopping a fusion or instrumentation at the transitional zone of C7-T1 may create late instability at this level.[6]

The upper thoracic spine is a relatively uncommon location for unstable spinal fractures.[1,3] The lower end of the cervical spine, the thoracolumbar junction, and the lumbar spine are the more common areas of fractures. Whereas pure burst fractures are commonly seen in the lower thoracic and lumbar spine, they are uncommon in the upper thoracic spine. When they do occur, they are often associated with a significant spinal cord injury because of the large amounts of force required to fracture this part of the spine and the small size of the spinal canal at this level.

Harrington or Moe distraction rod instrumentation will stabilize most deformities in the upper thoracic spine created by fractures (Figure 5-2). This instrumentation can be used from T1 distally in the thoracic spine. Because the laminae become thinner and the sagittal alignment changes at the cervicothoracic junction, it is difficult to place a Harrington hook above T1. Luque instrumentation is useful in stabilizing fractures of the flexion-shear variety but does not provide resistance to axial compression (Figure 5-3).

Tumors and Infection

As with fractures, the upper thoracic spine is a relatively uncommon location for osteomyelitis and tumor.[10,15,27] With both tumor and infection, the area of vertebral involvement is usually anterior and is accompanied by vertebral body collapse. In cases of collapse and kyphosis, anterior decompression can often be performed with costotransversectomy. More complete removal of an anteriorly situated tumor can be performed through a high transthoracic approach.[11,17] Decompression can be performed through a costotransversectomy, but it is more difficult to graft bone to the spine anteriorly after decompression. Grafting can be accomplished more easily

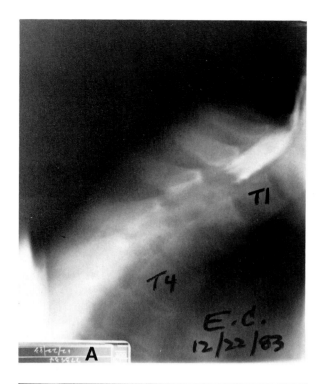

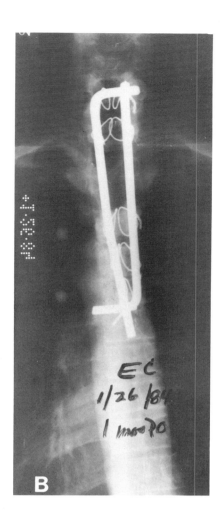

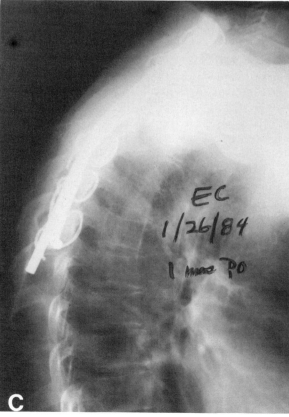

Figure 5-1. (A) A tomogram shows that this 58-year-old man has metastatic cancer to T2-3 and an extradural defect and block on a myelogram. He had pain and loss of proprioception and long track signs in both extremities. (B,C) He was treated with a posterolateral anterior decompression at T2 and T3 on the left side and instrumented with bilateral 1/4-inch Luque rods and methylmethacrylate from C7 to T6. Perhaps the instrumentation here should have been longer above and below. The patient was given radiotherapy after the wound healed.

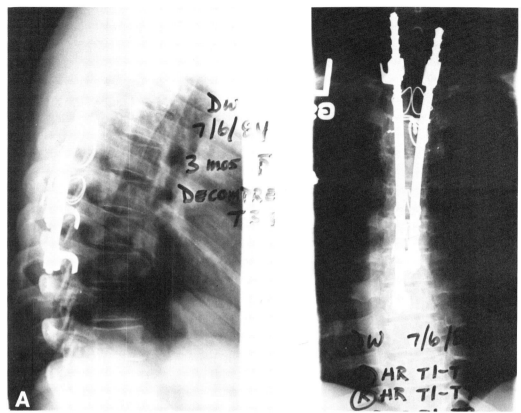

Figure 5-2. (A,B) This 22-year-old man sustained a gunshot wound to the posterior portions of the T3 and T4 vertebral bodies and through the pedicles of T3 and T4 on the left side. In addition, bone was retropulsed into the patient's spinal canal on the left side. He developed a Brown-Sequard syndrome. He was treated surgically with anterior decompression through posterolateral approaches on the left side. Because of the instability created by both the gunshot wound and the surgical removal of two pedicles and parts of two ribs as well as parts of the posterior portions of the T3 and T4 vertebral bodies on the left side, the spine was rendered unstable. Harrington rods were placed from T1 to T7 on the right side and from T1 to T8 on the left side. Posterolateral spine fusion was performed from T1 to T8, including facet fusions and transverse process fusions. Sublaminar wires were used at each level where the laminae were intact. Zielke bifid hooks were placed straddling the pedicles of T1 superiorly. The use of sublaminar wiring and the use of the bifid hooks straddling the pedicles increased the stability of the system. The distal hooks were square hooks to control rotation of the rods.

through a transthoracic approach. For access to levels higher than C6 as well as the upper thoracic spine, we prefer either a sternal splitting approach or a simultaneous anterior cervical and high transthoracic approach. With tumor destruction anteriorly and laminectomy posteriorly, kyphosis may worsen and enhance the possibility of recurrent spinal cord compression.[17]

For benign tumors and tubercular osteomyelitis, it is necessary to insert a strut graft in the spine anteriorly after anterior debridement and decompression. For certain

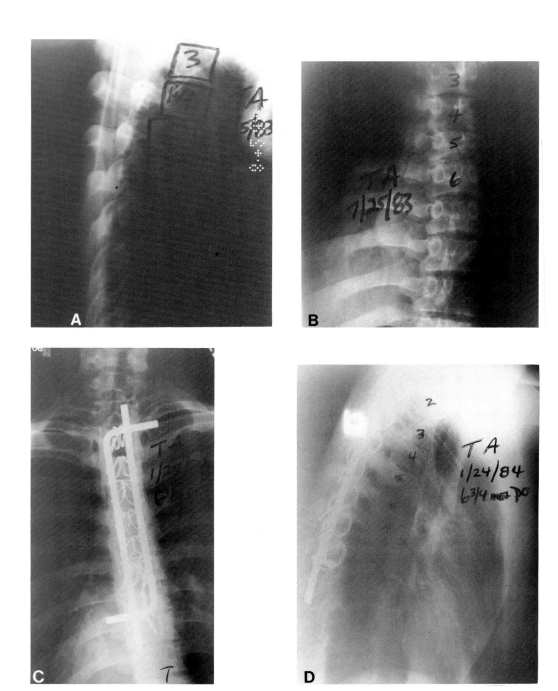

Figure 5-3. (A,B) Preoperative lateral x-ray films of this 20-year-old man demonstrate a fracture dislocation at T4-5 with anterior subluxation of T4 on T5, a posterior fracture, and ligamentous injury. He suffered a complete spinal cord injury at this level. (C,D) He was treated with bilateral Luque rods from T2 to T8 and a posterior spinal fusion with an autogenous fibular bone graft. This fracture could also have been treated with bilateral Harrington or Moe rods and SSI.

Table 5-2.
Method of spinal reconstruction for malignant tumor

Technique	Advantages	Disadvantages
1. Methylmethacrylate vertebral body reconstruction anteriorly.	1. Tumor resection complete as possible and decompression Good resistance to compression forces.	1. Difficult if disease is not limited to one or two adjacent levels with sparing of levels above and below.
2. Methylmethacrylate anteriorly plus Steinmann pin reinforcement.	2. Resistance to shear stresses as well as above.	
3. Harrington rods plus SSI plus methylmethacrylate posteriorly two levels above and below last levels of instability.	3. Useful for (1) multilevel tumor involvement, (2) loss of anterior plus posterior stabilizing structures.	3. Difficult to place instruments above T1.
4. Luque rods plus SSI plus methylmethacrylate more than 3 levels above and below last levels of instability.	4. Useful when instrumentation into the cervical spine is needed to provide stability.	4. Kyphosis at the top of instrumentation. Less resistance to axial compression.
5. Halo cast.	5. Provides stability for 6 to 12 weeks without morbidity of surgery.	5. Will last only as long as the Halo pins (6–12 weeks). External cast/ orthosis often tolerated poorly.

cases of pyogenic osteomyelitis a spontaneous interbody fusion may occur.[16] The likelihood of spontaneous interbody fusion is enhanced by resting and stabilizing the spine through bedrest, plaster immobilization, or instrumentation.

Stabilization is required after removal of a metastatic tumor anteriorly (Table 5-2). If instability is limited to one or two levels and to the anterior column, then anterior stabilization with methylmethacrylate coupled with pins or a spacer may suffice. If more than two vertebral levels are involved or if the middle or posterior columns are involved, segmental spinal instrumentation two or three levels above and below the level of pathologic or traumatic involvement may be necessary. Reinforcement of the posterior construct with methylmethacrylate may increase its stability. See Table 5-3 for further guidelines.

Iatrogenic Instability

Adult

In adults, performing a midline laminectomy in the upper thoracic spine usually will not create instability unless it is coupled with a destructive process in the anterior portion of the spine. Any disruption of the rib cage or the pedicles (costotransversectomy) will increase the incidence of instability. The rib cage is an important stabilizing

Table 5-3.
Spinal tumors

Indications for Anterior Reconstruction
Benign process involving the vertebral body.
Single level metastatic tumor involvement with sparing of pedicles and posterior elements.
Indication for Posterior Reconstruction
Multi-level spinal involvement anteriorly.
Loss of anterior and posterior supporting structures.
Destructive process limited to posterior structures.

astructure in the thoracic spine. Therefore, a costotransversectomy coupled with a laminectomy may create instability with minimal anterior involvement. Removal of an appreciable portion of the vertebral body (greater than 50 percent) may lead to kyphosis even with totally unaffected posterior structures. The various treatments for iatrogenic instability and the patterns of instability are listed in Tables 5-4 and 5-5.

Pediatric

In the pediatric population, laminectomy alone may lead to instability.[19] Kyphosis will occur in at least 50 percent of the pediatric patients who undergo laminectomy for astrocytoma, neuroblastoma, or neurofibroma. If the facet joints are left intact, the kyphosis will be a gentle rounded one; if the facet joints are removed, it will more likely be a sharp angular kyphosis that may stretch the spinal cord and produce paralysis.

APPROACHES TO THE UPPER THORACIC SPINE

Several approaches can be used to gain access to the upper thoracic spine (Table 5-6). These are the midline posterior approach, costotransversectomy, the high transthoracic approach, and a combined low cervical and high transthoracic approach or a sternal splitting approach.

Midline Posterior Approach

The midline posterior approach to the upper thoracic spine should be used whenever direct exposure of the spinous processes, laminae, and facet joints is desired or when one intends to explore the posterior spinal canal and its contents. A variety of instrumentation procedures for the correction of spinal deformities can be performed through this approach.

A direct midline posterior approach to the spine can be used for posterolateral decompression of the spinal canal.[1] This procedure is particularly tailored to lesions that are primarily unilateral and located in the lateral or anterolateral aspect of the canal. Whereas midline laminectomy provides access to the posterior and the posterolateral aspects of the canal, posterolateral decompression allows entry into the lateral and anterolateral compartment of the spinal canal.

This operation is performed by removing the lateralmost aspect of the lamina and,

Table 5-4.
Treatment of iatrogenic instability (No deformity—all other supporting
structures intact)

Cause	Treatment
Resection of 50 percent or more of vertebral body	Anterior strut fusion
Laminectomy without facetectomy	Adult—no treatment Pediatric—facet and transverse process fusion
Laminectomy with facetectomy	Transverse process or anterior fusion or both
Unilateral hemilaminectomy plus costotransversectomy	Contralateral facet and transverse process fusion or anterior fusion or both

using high-speed instruments, drilling into and removing the pedicle at the appropriate level. By drilling through the pedicle at that level, the posterior and lateral part of the vertebral body can be removed (Figure 5-4). This procedure has been particularly applicable in treating fractures of a vertebral body with asymmetric retropulsion of bone into one side of the spinal canal and in treating patients with unilateral metastatic tumors in the lateral area of the canal.

Although posterolateral decompression provides adequate exposure of the lateral aspects of the canal, medially situated masses will be very difficult to remove in the upper thoracic spine via this approach. In our judgment, posterolateral decompression usually should be accompanied by an appropriate stabilization procedure. Often instrumentation can be performed before formal decompression in treating upper thoracic fractures that require posterolateral decompression. If the anterior longitudinal ligament is intact, the instrumentation procedure itself may decompress the spinal canal. This can be ascertained by putting one of the rods into position initially, performing a limited laminectomy, exploring the lateral gutter of the spinal canal to determine whether this has adequately decompressed the spinal canal, and continuing with the posterolateral decompression if this has not occurred.

Table 5-5.
Patterns of instability

Destruction of a vertebral body totaling 50 percent or more

Destruction of a vertebral body totaling 35 percent or more plus destruction of a pedicle or costovertebral articulation

Laminectomy plus destruction of 35 percent or more of a vertebral body

Collapse into kyphosis
   Single level
   Multiple adjacent levels

Pediatric patient
   Laminectomy
   Laminectomy plus facetectomy

Table 5-6.
Approaches to the upper thoracic spine

Posterior/posterolateral
Costotransversectomy
Sternal splitting
High transthoracic
Low cervical anterior
Combined high transthoracic plus low cervical anterior

Costotransversectomy

Using an exposure that combines removal of a transverse process and the rib articulating at that level, the pedicle at that level and the posterior portion of the vertebral body can be removed. This provides wider access to the anterior aspects of the spinal canal than the posterolateral approach just described (Figure 5-5). A costotransversectomy in the upper thoracic spine can be accomplished through one of two incisions.[21] A curvilinear incision that begins just lateral to the midline and is carried directly over the course of the rib to be removed can be used. The other incision that can be used is a midline longitudinal incision with lateral stripping of the paraspinal muscles out to the ribs.

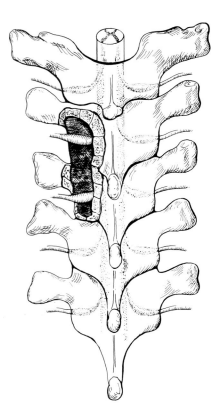

Figure 5-4. The bony exposure accomplished by a posterior lateral decompressive procedure.

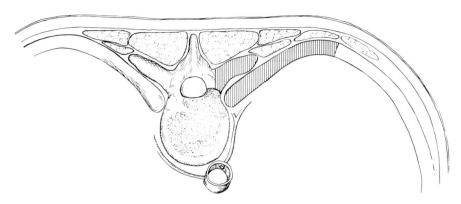

Figure 5-5. The bony structures removed in a costotransversectomy. The cross-hatched areas show the transverse process and rib articulation that are removed. The stippled area is the portion of the vertebral body accessible through this procedure.

Anterior decompression through this approach is easier to accomplish if there is a significant kyphosis. It is certainly a destabilizing procedure, since the pedicle and part of the link to the rib cage on one side are removed. If there is significant destruction of the anterior vertebral body by tumor or infection, the spine should be stabilized after a costotransversectomy. Costotransversectomy can be done over several adjacent levels or even at two widely separate locations if needed.

High Transthoracic Approach

A kyphotic deformity tends to force the cervical spine into the chest, in which case the high transthoracic approach can give access to levels as high as C6.[14] Without significant kyphosis, exposure up to T1 is possible. The incision for the approach is the upper thoracoplasty J incision, followed by division of the inferior periscapular muscles and forward mobilization of the scapula (Figure 5-6). One or several of the ribs (3 to 5) are then removed to gain entry into the chest. Fusion of the vertebral bodies and insertion of a bone graft is technically difficult because of the small vertebral bodies and the narrowing thoracic inlet, which reduces the working space. The innominate vessels usually limit the exposure superiorly. This exposure is best for total anterior vertebrectomy and bilateral anterior spinal cord transposition/decompression.

Low Cervical Approach Plus High Transthoracic Approach
or Sternal Splitting Approach

The low cervical approach can provide access to levels as low as T1 or T2 depending upon the height of the clavicle.[21] This can be judged on lateral spine films. For exposure from C4 to T4, a combination of the low cervical approach and the high transthoracic approach may be used[20] (Figure 5-7). A sternal splitting approach may also be used[9] (Figure 5-8). These approaches require careful work on both sides of the innominate vessels and, at times, mobilization of the vessels. Ligation of the innominate vein often is required. The combined low cervical, high transthoracic approach produces a wider exposure than the sternal splitting approach.

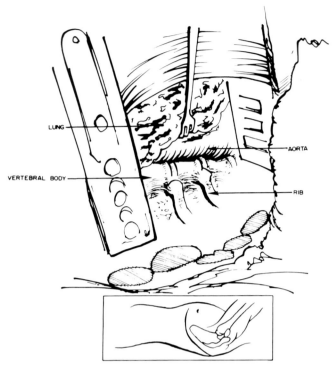

Figure 5-6.   Periscapular approach. Removal of the third rib will allow exposure up to T1 if there is no deformity. If kyphosis exists, exposure up to C6 may be possible. (Reprinted from Pierce DS, Nickel VH: The Total Care of Spinal Cord Injuries. Boston, Little, Brown, 1977, pp. 64. With permission.)

METHODS OF STABILIZATION

Harrington distraction instrumentation provides resistance to axial compression and is useful in the reduction of flexion-shear fractures.[1] The square distraction Moe rods allow the sagittal plane to be contoured. Additional stability may be provided by adding Luque sublaminar wires. To adequately support a one-level instability, the Harrington instrumentation needs to be placed two levels above and below the unstable segment. The instruments must also be contoured in order to apply three-point fixation to the spine at the apex of the deformity. The principle limitation of Harrington instrumentation is that it is impossible to securely place the hooks any higher than the T1 lamina. In order to get maximal purchase rostrally, it is advisable to use Zielke bifid hooks and to place them around the pedicle (Figure 5-9). This is especially important at T1 and T2, where the laminae are smaller. Placing the collar-end hooks in the middle or lower thoracic spine necessitates using smaller hooks. An alternative is to instrument on down to L1 where large hooks can be used.

Luque instrumentation has a distinct advantage in that it can be used all the way up to the occiput. It may be quite helpful in cases where both anterior and posterior destruction is present at several levels of the upper thoracic spine (Figure 5-10). Sublaminar passage of the wires in the cervical and upper thoracic spine is safe if the

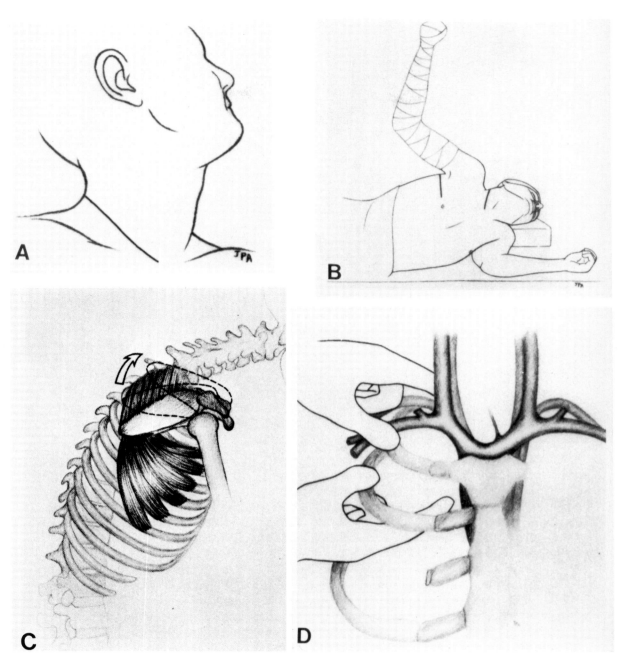

Figure 5-7. (A) The patient is positioned in the lateral decubitus attitude with the side of the convexity of the scoliosis uppermost and the upper extremity draped free and included in the operative field. The thoracic and cervical incisions are shown. (B) An oblique supraclavicular incision is used for the cervical portion of the procedure. (C) Mobilization and superior displacement of the scapula are accomplished by releasing the portions of the serratus anterior and rhomboid muscles attached to its lower margins (heavy broken line and arrows). (D) The combined cervical and thoracic approach exposes the spine and provides ready access to the great vessels for hemostatic control if needed. (Reprinted from Micheli LJ, Hood RW: Anterior exposure of the cervicothoracic spine using a combined cervical and thoracic approach. J Bone Joint Surg 65A:992, 1983. With permission.)

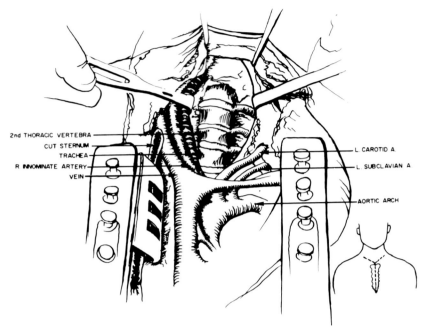

2nd THORACIC VERTEBRA
CUT STERNUM
TRACHEA
R INNOMINATE ARTERY
VEIN

L CAROTID A
L SUBCLAVIAN A

AORTIC ARCH

Figure 5-8. Sternal splitting anterior exposure to visualize C6 to T4. (Reprinted from Pierce DS, Nickel VH: The Total Care of Spinal Cord Injuries. Boston, Little, Brown, 1977, pp. 64. With permission.)

canal is patent. The Luque system does not provide the resistance to axial compression that the Harrington distraction system does. However, the application of methylmethacrylate to the construct does provide some additional resistance. To adequately stabilize the spine with Luque instrumentation it is best to instrument three levels above and below the level of instability. Therefore, if T2, T3, and T4 are void of posterior elements and there is destruction anteriorly, it is recommended that the spine be instrumented from at least C6 to T7. Also, it is quite easy to contour Luque rods to whatever sagittal conformation is desirable. For rather significant deformity in the sagittal plane, it is more desirable to use the thicker 1/4-inch rods.

A disadvantage of Luque instrumentation is that up to T2 it necessitates removal of the ligamentum flavum at T1-2 or up to C7 it necessitates removal of the ligamentum flavum at C6-7. The removal of these posterior ligamentous supporting structures coupled with the transfer of stresses to this upper level will often produce a kyphosis at the level just above the instrumentation.

Compression rods are useful in correcting kyphosis by shortening the posterior column. With a burst fracture, tumor, or infection, however, they encourage further retropulsion of material into the canal. Compression rods provide no resistance to axial compression and they cannot be used above T1. The indication for compression rods is the correction of longstanding kyphosis after the appropriate anterior releases. They are of little benefit for acute fractures since pure distraction or Chance fractures are exceedingly rare in this part of the spine. The role of the newer Cotrel-Dubousset rods, which allow multiple hook fixation, application of compression and distraction forces,

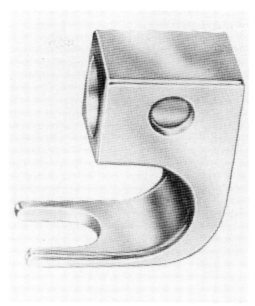

Figure 5-9. A Zielke bifid hook. The bifid shoe fits around
the thoracic pedicle.

and more rigid transverse linkage of bilateral rods to control rotation, is yet to be
determined.

Roy-Camille plates have been used for stabilization of the spine after tumor
resection. These plates are quite rigid, and it may be more difficult to make them
conform to the sagittal alignment of the upper thoracic spine than to the rest of the
thoracic and lumbar spine. The technique consists of placing screws through the intact
pedicles (from a posterior approach) into the vertebral bodies. The plates are placed
bilaterally at least two levels above and below the level of tumor or deformity.

The indications for a posterior approach and instrumentation are:

1. A one-level instability created by a flexion-shear fracture where there is destruction
    of the posterior longitudinal ligament, possible damage to the vertebral body
    anteriorly, and posterior ligamentous disruption including the ligamentum flavum
    and the interspinous and supraspinous ligaments. Usually such an injury is
    treatable by Harrington rod instrumentation two levels above and below the injury
    provided the anterior longitudinal ligament is intact.
2. Single or multiple level instability caused by a metastatic tumor. In cases of tumor
    with multiple level instability, it is possible to decompress the spine anteriorly
    through a costotransversectomy, which is easier to perform when there is kyphosis
    present. The spine may then be instrumented and stabilized with Luque or
    Harrington rods several levels above and below the unstable segment (see Figure
    5-10). If the tumor process is benign, then a high transthoracic anterior approach
    with more complete removal of the tumor and bone grafting anteriorly will be
    desirable as well. For palliation in a metastatic tumor, simultaneous posterior

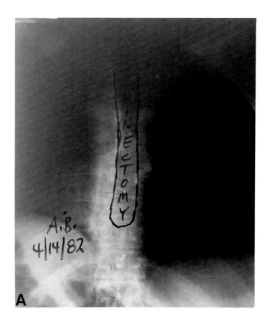

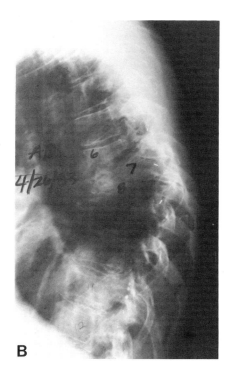

B

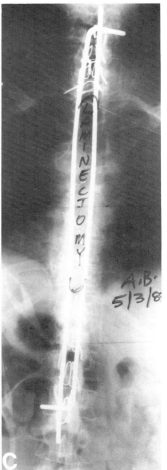

Figure 5-10. A 38-year-old man with metastatic pheochromocytoma to all vertebral bodies (T1–T10). (A) His status preoperatively as demonstrated by this anteroposterior film is one failed anterior fusion and multiple laminectomies and costotransversectomies from T1 to T10. (B) This preoperative lateral film shows that he is devoid of most of his supporting structures from T1 to T10 anteriorly and posteriorly and that he has developed a fracture-dislocation at T7-8. (C) He was stabilized with bilateral contoured Luque rods and methylmethacrylate from C4 to L2 as shown in this anteroposterior film. Probably thicker 1/4-inch rods should have been used.

instrumentation and anterior decompression through costotransversectomy is often sufficient.[2]

3. With metastatic tumor involvement at T1 or T2, anterior debridement and stabilization is often technically difficult. It is often feasible to debride through a costotransversectomy (bilaterally if necessary) and to stabilize with segmental instrumentation or to combine "anterior transthoracic" decompression (or "low cervical" depending on patient anatomy) with posterior instrumentation.

Anterior Instrumentation

The following bone grafts are available. Bicortical iliac crest will incorporate fairly rapidly and provide reasonable strength. The strength of rib bone is not as good but the ribs are quite accessible. Vascularized rib potentially will incorporate more rapidly than avascular rib. Autogenous fibula is quite strong but probably incorporates somewhat slower than bone from the rib and iliac crest, since less of its density is cancellous bone.

Nonbiologic materials such as Steinmann pins or fiber-metal struts or ceramic spacers with methylmethacrylate may be used when a tumor with spinal cord compression is present at a single level such as T4. A transthoracic procedure can then be performed with removal of the T4 vertebra and spanning of the area with methylmethacrylate and a Steinmann pin for palliation. Because methylmethacrylate is a nonbiologic material, it will ultimately fail from shear forces. In cases of metastatic disease, however, it usually has an adequate life span.

Anterior distraction devices such as the Dunn device, Kaneda instruments, the Bradford distraction device, or AO plates are designed to provide resistance to axial compression. These instrumentation systems are somewhat bulky, however, and therefore are harder to use in this part of the spine, where space is more limited because of the narrowing rib cage and closely applied great vessels.

The indications for an anterior approach and stabilization are:

1. Single level malignant spine disease with preservation of the pedicles and posterior elements. This may be stabilized by tumor resection and methylmethacrylate body replacement (with or without Steinmann pins, fiber-metal implants, or ceramic spacers). If there is significant posterior destruction (the pedicles, costovertebral articulation, facets, and so forth), this may not provide sufficient stabilization.
2. Benign tumor. Any benign tumor should be completely removed through a transthoracic approach and bone grafts placed anteriorly.
3. Osteomyelitis. Bone grafts should be placed anteriorly for any tubercular vertebral osteomyelitis requiring anterior debridement to prevent further collapse and recurrent neurologic deficits.

Halo Vest or Halo Cast Immobilization

In contrast to the lumbar spine, semirigid deformities of the upper thoracic spine are often amenable to traction and reduction through the use of halo traction. Certain cranial nerve, brachial plexus, and long track signs must be carefully monitored while the traction is applied. Semirigid deformities or kyphosis resulting from tumor or infection can often be reduced by halo gravity traction if reduction by posterior instrumentation alone is deemed unsafe or inadvisable.

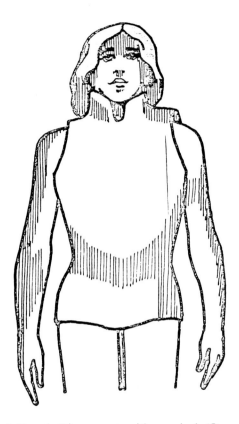

Figure 5-11. A Risser cast with cervical (Queen Anne) collar, which allows better control of the upper thoracic spine.

Unlike the midthoracic spine, it is quite difficult to immobilize the upper thoracic spine from T1 to T6 with the use of an underarm Risser cast or underarm orthosis. For rigid immobilization of the upper thoracic spine, it is necessary either to incorporate a Queen Anne collar (Figure 5-11) into the underarm cast or to place the patient in a halo vest or a halo cast. The halo cast provides the most rigid external immobilization of the upper thoracic spine. Operative procedures may even be performed with a halo cast or halo vest in place. For osteotomies of the upper thoracic spine or the cervical thoracic spine, such as Simmons osteotomy, halo cast immobilization is ideal to achieve reduction and maintain position.

A halo cast can be used to stabilize metastatic deformities of the cervical and upper thoracic spine. The lifetime of a halo cast is usually limited by the problem of maintaining sterile halo pin tracks (about 12 weeks). Also, the bulky halo cast if often poorly tolerated by terminally ill patients.

SUMMARY

Operations in the upper thoracic region require caution and meticulous care because of the tenuous vascular supply to the area of the spinal cord and because of the pathophysiologic changes that occur during spinal cord compression. When the spinal cord is injured, either by trauma or by some other compressive phenomenon, hemodynamic changes in the microcirculation of the cord and biochemical changes take place that make the cord especially vulnerable to alterations in systemic physiology.[7,8,24]

Animal experiments have confirmed that there is an additive detrimental effect when a compressive injury is combined with an ischemic one.[13]

Because of the small size of the upper thoracic spinal canal, almost any retraction of a compressed spinal cord can lead to worsening of neurologic function, and retraction of the cord should therefore be avoided.

Intraoperative spinal evoked or somatosensory responses are used as a monitor of spinal cord function. These electrophysiologic studies are very helpful in the various procedures discussed in this chapter, but it should be noted that these only monitor the posterior columns of the cord. They provide only indirect information about motor function or about the anterior tracts. Therefore maintaining normal somatosensory responses during an operation will not guarantee that spinal paralysis will not occur. There have been some preliminary reports on monitoring the motor tracts of the spinal cord during operative procedures. In the future, this, in addition to the use of somatosensory responses may be extremely helpful during these types of surgical procedures.[18]

Because of the complicated anatomy and relative paucity of disease in the upper thoracic spine, there is less experience and less agreement among spine surgeons about how to approach and stabilize this area of the spine. Only the occipital-cervical and lumbosacral junctions are equal to the cervicothoracic junction in surgical controversy. This chapter hopefully expresses certain principles, although further understanding and sophistication in stabilization of the upper thoracic spine is certain to evolve in the next few years.

ACKNOWLEDGMENT

The authors wish to extend special thanks to Gregory B. Krivchenia, II, M.D., Resident III, Department of Orthopedic Surgery, University of Cincinnati, for his assistance.

REFERENCES

1. Bradford DS, Akbarnia BA, Winter RB, Seljeksog EL: Surgical stabilization of fracture and fracture dislocations of the thoracic spine. Spine 2:185, 1977

2. Bridwell KH, DeWald RL, Prodramas C: Reconstructive spine surgery as palliation for primary and metastatic malignancies. Presented at the Fiftieth Annual Meeting of the AAOS, Anaheim, CA, 1983

3. Burke DC, Murray DD: The management of thoracic and thoracolumbar injuries of the spine with neurologic involvement. J Bone Joint Surg 58B:72, 1976

4. Domisse GF: The blood supply of the spinal cord. J Bone Joint Surg 56B:225, 1974

5. Domisse GF, Enslin TB: Hodgson's circumferential osteotomy in the correction of spinal deformity. J Bone Joint Surg 52B:778, 1970

6. Drennan JC, King EW: Cervical dislocation following fusion of the upper thoracic spine for scoliosis: A case report. J Bone Joint Surg 60A:1003, 1978

7. Ducker TB, Kindt GW: The effect of trauma on the vasomotor control of spinal cord blood flow. Curr Top Surg Res 3:163, 1971

8. Ducker TB, Salcman M, Perot PL, et al: Experimental spinal cord trauma. I. Correlation of blood flow, tissue, oxygen, and neurologic status in the dog. Surg Neurol 10:60, 1978

9. Fang HSY, Ong GB, Hodgson AR: Anterior spinal fusion. Clin Orthop Rel Res 35:16, 1964

10. Garcia A, Grantham SA: Hematogenous pyogenic vertebral osteomyelitis. J Bone Joint Surg 42A:429, 1960

11. Gertzbein SD, Cruickshank B, Hoffman H, Taylor GA, Cooper PW: Recurrent benign osteoblastoma of the second thoracic vertebra: A case report. J Bone Joint Surg 55B:841, 1973

12. Gillilan LA: Vascular supply of the spinal cord. In Chov SN, Seljeksog EL (eds): Spinal Deformities and Neurological Dysfunction. New York, Raven Press, 1978

13. Gooding MR, Wilson CB, Hoff JT: Experimental cervical myelopathy. Effects of ischemia and compression of the canine cervical spinal cord. J Neurosurg 43:9, 1975

14. Hall JE: The anterior approach to spinal deformities. Orthop Clin North Am 3:81, 1972

15. Harrington KD: The use of methylmethacrylate for vertebral body replacement and anterior stabilization of pathologic fracture dislocations of the spine due to metastatic malignant disease. J Bone Joint Surg 63A:36, 1981

16. Kulowski J: Pyogenic osteomyelitis of the spine: An analysis and discussion of 102 cases. J Bone Joint Surg 18:343, 1936

17. Larsson SE: Removal of the third thoracic vertebra and partial lung resection for a radioresistant giant cell tumor of the spine. J Bone Joint Surg 61B:489, 1979

18. Levy WJ, York DH: Evoked potentials from the motor tracts in humans. Neurosurgery 12:422, 1983

19. Lonstein JE: Post-laminectomy kyphosis. Clin Orthop Rel Res 128:93, 1977

20. Michelli LJ, Hood RW: Anterior exposure of the cervicothoracic spine using a combined cervical and thoracic approach. J Bone Joint Surg 65A:992, 1983

21. Rothman RH, Simeone FA: The Spine. Philadelphia, W.B. Saunders, 1982

22. Schneider RG: The syndrome of acute anterior spinal injury. J Neurosurg 12:95, 1955

23. Simmons EH: Kyphotic deformity of the spine in ankylosing spondylitis. Clin Orthop Rel Res 128:65, 1977

24. Smith AL, McCreery DB, Bloedel JR, et al: Hyperemia, CO2 responsiveness, and autoregulation in the white matter following experimental spinal cord injury. J Neurosurg 48:239, 1970

25. Truex RC, Carpenter MB: Human Neuroanatomy, 6th ed. Baltimore, Williams & Wilkins, 1969

26. White AW, Panjabi MM: Clinical Biomechanics of the Spine. Philadelphia, J.B. Lippincott, 1978

27. Yau ACMC, Hsu LCS, O'Brien JP, Hodgson AR: Tuberculous kyphosis. J Bone Joint Surg. 56A:1419, 1974

Michael L.J. Apuzzo
Robert G. Watkins
William R. Dobkin

6

Therapeutic Considerations in the Surgical Management of Lesions Affecting the Midthoracic Spine

The biomechanics of the spine depend upon the interaction of its various supporting structures. An understanding of the role of these supporting tissues therefore is requisite before biomechanical principles can be applied to the treatment of disorders of the thoracic spine.

In this chapter we will expound the two-column principle of spinal stability as distinct from the three-column concept described in Chapter 1. The spine may be roughly divided into two parallel columns. The anterior column comprises the disc, the vertebral bodies, and the longitudinal ligaments; the posterior column is formed by the pedicles, the facet joints, the spinous processes, and their associated ligaments. The basic functions of these columns differ. The anterior column must resist compression. The posterior column must resist tensile or distracting forces. Most movements, however, produce complex stresses that must be resisted by both columns simultaneously. These include combinations of shear, lateral bending, tension, compression, and rotation. These complex mechanical stresses have both mechanical and biologic effects on the spine. The mechanical effects may result in disruption of the supporting structures of the spine, while the biologic effects may result in remodeling of bone, loss of calcium from the bony matrix, or the induction of differentiation of multipotential reticuloendothelial cells.

Because of the natural curvature of the spine in the sagittal plane, the center of gravity in the midthoracic region is anterior to the spine. Consequently, structural diseases affecting this portion of the vertebral column may result in the development of a progressive kyphotic deformity that exceeds the normal range of 20 to 40 degrees. When the forces produced by such a deformity exceed the adaptive abilities of the neural and vascular elements, progressive radiculomyelopathy will develop.

Clinical experience and scientific data have produced guidelines for the amount of deformity that can be resisted by an average spine. For most spines, a kyphotic angle

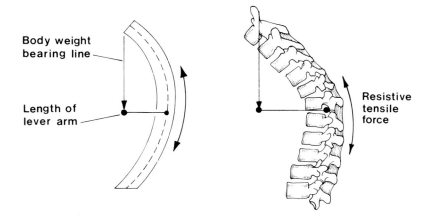

Figure 6-1. A lever arm is the distance between the weight-bearing line of body weight and the axis of rotation at the spine. An increase in the lever arm or an increase in body weight results in an increase in the resistive tensile forces. Without adequate resistive extensile force, the kyphotic angle will increase.

of 60 degrees or greater requires tremendous amounts of force to prevent increasing kyphotic deformity (Figure 6-1).

Another important stabilizing structure in the region of the thoracic spine is the thoracic cavity, i.e., the ribs and their articulations with the spine (Figure 6-2). The thoracic cavity may be responsible for up to 40 percent of midthoracic spinal stability. There are two anatomic mechanisms by which the ribs enhance stability in this region: (1) the actual articulations of the costotransverse and costovertebral joints and their accompanying ligaments provide a significant amount of articular strength. Each rib articulates with the cephalad half of its appropriate vertebral body and the disc space above that vertebral body. The strong costovertebral ligaments attach to the vertebral bodies, the longitudinal ligaments, and, very importantly, to the annulus of the intervertebral disc. (2) The cross-sectional diameter of the thoracic cavity effectively increases the bending strength of the column. For example, it is harder to bend a steel tube that is 20 inches in diameter than a steel tube that is 1 inch in diameter. This has important implications in the treatment of fractures of the thoracic spine. A spinal fracture occurring in conjunction with a major disruption of the thoracic cavity such as multiple rib fractures or a transverse sternal fracture is an unstable thoracic spinal fracture.

BIOLOGIC EFFECTS OF STRESS

The biomechanical effects of stress will produce biologic effects. The multipotential cells respond to their bioelectric environment by differentiation into cells of different ultimate functions (Figure 6-3). Compression produces osteoblasts from the same multipotential reticuloendothelial cells that in distraction evolve into fibroblasts.

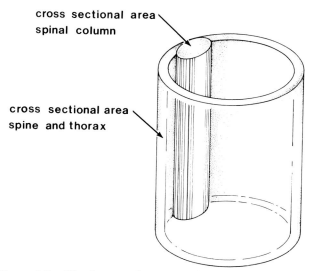

cross sectional area
spinal column

cross sectional area
spine and thorax

Figure 6-2. The increased cross-sectional area of the spine and the thoracic cavity combined increases the resistance of the spinal column to bending. The rib cage accounts for approximately 40 percent of the bending strength and stability of the thoracic spine.

Accordingly, a bone graft will reabsorb in an area of distraction and be replaced by fibrous tissue. These concepts have clinical application in the treatment of injuries or disease of the midthoracic spine. Placing bone grafts on the posterior column of the thoracic spine with a significant amount of kyphotic deformity, such as 70 to 80 degrees, will not produce a solid union. By avoiding the tension on the posterior side of a kyphotic spine and placing a strut graft on the compressed anterior side, bony healing can be produced through compression even at 80 degrees of kyphosis.

GENERAL DIAGNOSTIC PRINCIPLES

The following approach to diagnosis should be considered in cases of possible lesions of the midthoracic spine: (1) Strictly define the neurologic and physiologic level, (2) define the precise structural alterations, and (3) define the exact etiologic factors. Considerations related to obtaining a history and the physical and neurologic examination are obviously rudimentary; however, important steps in this method involve the proper use of radiographic adjuvants. In considering plain films, the greatest pitfall is the initial improper assessment of the anteroposterior thoracic spine films. A systematic method of progressing from posterior to anterior structures, identifying each bony element and the appropriate distance between them is recommended. Ligamentous injury can often be diagnosed by identifying displacement of the bony elements. By assessing the spinous processes first, the distance between these processes and the degree of rotation may be determined. Proceeding on, the lamina should be examined for vertical or horizontal fractures. Next, the facet joints should be examined for dislocation, displacement, or fracture. The transverse processes are inspected next for

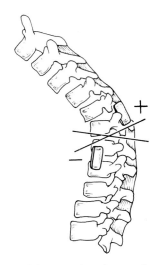

Figure 6-3. The negative charge of compression stimulates differentiation of multipotential cells into osteoblasts and stimulates bone formation. The plus charge of distraction stimulates multipotential cells to differentiate into fibroblasts and impairs formation of bone structure.

elements of fracture. The costotransverse ligaments may be damaged or separated. The pedicles may be spread or fractured transversely. The posterior body wall may be fractured vertically or transversely. The anterior column may demonstrate damage to the intervertebral disc, the longitudinal ligaments, or the costovertebral articulation.

Judicious use of high-resolution computed tomography with and without metrizamide myelography is an invaluable diagnostic adjunct in assessing bony alterations and compromise of the spinal canal at this level. The use of these techniques of imaging will refine the appreciation of structural alterations and develop a comprehension of the three-dimensional architecture that serves as a basis for management strategy.

Needle aspiration under fluoroscopic or computerized tomographic monitoring should be considered as a diagnostic adjunct in the treatment of patients with neoplasms or infections. The discrete use of needle aspiration with any number of devices, including a Craig needle or a long spinal needle, is helpful in establishing preoperatively a more exact diagnosis in many cases of tumor or infection.

GENERAL MANAGEMENT PRINCIPLES

The goals of treatment should include (1) prevention of the occurrence of or the progression of a neurologic deficit; (2) reduction of spinal deformity; (3) decompression of the spinal cord; (4) restoration of the structural integrity and stability of the spine; and (5) prevention of future pain.

The critical issues of treatment are decisions concerning decompression, reduction, stabilization, and fusion. As for decompression, it is important to define specifically the nature and extent of the neurologic deficit, the factors related to such a deficit, and the precise structural components related to the etiologic factors. The compressing structure should be removed. For example, in patients with incomplete neurologic lesions, removal of a mass lesion that has compromised the neural canal should either improve neurologic function or arrest the progression of deterioration. However, attempts to do this may occasionally produce a loss of neurologic function.

In general, if there is an anterior column lesion producing a mass effect with neural compromise, it should be properly removed from an anterior approach. If there is a fractured lamina compromising the spinal canal, it should be excised posteriorly. In the midthoracic spine, manipulation of the spinal cord is not advisable because of biomechanical factors and vascular anatomic conditions that raise a risk of exacerbating existing deficits. Although not widely practiced, we believe spinal angiography should be employed as an essential step in the selection and planning of operative procedures intended to treat middle and lower thoracic spinal lesions, especially procedures where sacrifice or injury to a predominant radiculomedullary vessel is a possibility.

When possible, the surgical approach should be through the area of greatest ligamentous damage. In the event that there is marked ligamentous disruption of the posterior bony column, approaching the anterior column by destroying an intact anterior or posterior longitudinal ligament is undesirable. There are, however, times when the previously described principles of treatment are in contradiction. For example, there may be ligamentous disruption of the posterior column combined with a fragment of bone from the anterior column producing a neurologic deficit. Anterior decompression may then be combined with simultaneous or subsequent stabilization.

Stability must be restored in the face of instability. Instability is present when the structural integrity of the spinal column is insufficient to prevent a neurologic deficit or progressive deformity and pain. The decision to surgically stabilize a spine is tempered by other decision-making factors. For example, many unstable spinal lesions will become stable with nonoperative care. Therefore, it is important to identify a spine at risk of developing chronic instability, such as a spine with ligamentous injuries that are less likely to heal.

Reduction or realignment of the spine may be needed to correct deformities. Isolated deformities of 40 degrees or more and generalized deformities of 60 degrees or more should be corrected. Operative stabilization and reduction may require metal fixation to achieve the reduction, to enhance healing of a fusion, and to provide spinal stability until the fusion heals. Metal fixation is only as effective as the fusion. Failure to obtain a solid fusion within the fatigue life of the metal instrumentation will result in metal failure. It is important to realize that a malaligned spine is less likely to fuse and become stable and is more likely to prevent neurologic recovery.

TECHNIQUES OF DECOMPRESSING THE MIDTHORACIC SPINAL CANAL

A number of operative techniques are available for decompressing the midthoracic spine and may be applied under appropriate pathologic circumstances. These include (1) laminectomy, (2) costotransversectomy, (3) transthoracic anterior decompression, and (4) transpedicular decompression.

Laminectomy

When indicated and the option is available, we prefer to undertake laminectomy in the lateral position (left lateral decubitus) with rotation of the thorax to the right 20 degrees. Radiographically defined marking of the operative level is beneficial. Before the incision is made, the paraspinal musculature and supraspinous midline are infiltrated with 0.5-percent Xylocaine with epinephrine. After a subperiosteal dissection and exposure of the appropriate lamina, laminectomy is undertaken with a combination of high-speed drills, rongeurs, curettes, and narrow foot-plated bone punches. Care is taken to minimize contact and transient deformity of the dural tube. Somatosensory evoked responses may be monitored during positioning and decompression. Appropriate decompression can be accomplished without disruption of the facet joints.

Costotransversectomy, Lateral Rhachotomy, and the Anterior Decompression of Dott and Alexander

As has been noted, a combination of factors contribute to the neurologic sequela produced by masses impinging on the ventral surface of the spinal cord. These are both mechanical and vascular. In animals, failure of a decompression laminectomy to restore normal spinal cord hemodynamics in the presence of an anterior epidural mass has been documented angiographically. In addition to direct vascular compromise, an anterior mass produces axial tension that may stretch the cord. This may reach a critical degree over the convex posterior surface of the cord, leading either to ischemia or to increased intramedullary pressure, which may then result in further neural injury. Posterior decompression may be inadequate to relieve this tension. These experimental studies suggest why the extent of the spinal cord injury is often out of proportion to the size of the offending mass and also why laminectomy may be without benefit and may be potentially hazardous. The potential effects of these mechanisms may be greatly magnified in the watershed region.

Conventional laminectomy not only carries an unacceptable risk when used to deal with ventrally placed thoracic spine lesions, but also posterior decompression alone may fail to reduce the impact of the lesion on the spinal cord. Clinical observations have tended to corroborate the experimental conditions suggested above. In reviewing a number of series, Patterson and Arbit[7] found 45 percent of patients with anterior spinal lesions to either deteriorate or fail to improve after laminectomy. Consequently, posterolateral and anterolateral approaches to the spine have been developed to facilitate treatment of these lesions.[4]

Current practice employs several variations of costotransversectomy, the selected approach being dependent on the nature of the existing pathologic condition.[10] Either a prone or a modified lateral decubitus position with the patient's body rotated slightly anteriorly is used. Optimum exposure for an extensive procedure encompassing the resection of two intervertebral discs and the intervening vertebral body is through the semilateral decubitus position. When the entire vertebral body is to be resected, an anterior interbody fusion is contemplated, or resection of a lesion extending into the center of the body or its contralateral side is considered, a paraspinous curvilinear incision with a corresponding fascial incision offers optimal surgical exposure. For decompression after rod stabilization, it is necessary to have a sufficiently long midline incision to permit lateral retraction beyond the costotransverse joint and onto the rib. Alternately, adequate exposure may be obtained by extending a "T" limb from the midline incision over the rib at the involved level. This allows for resection of the transverse process, resection of the pedicle, and decompression of the spinal canal. This approach is appropriate for biopsy of an intervertebral disc or vertebral body.

When a paraspinous incision is used, the incision straddles the lateral border of the paraspinous musculature. The underlying fascia is divided laterally and the paraspinous muscle mass is elevated medially. With a combination of sharp periosteal elevation and judicious electrocautery, the periosteum overlying the dorsal surface of the rib, the capsule of the costotransverse joint and the fascia, and periosteum of the transverse process are removed. Either sharp dissection or electrocautery is then used to incise the costotransverse joint, which is then removed with rongeurs back to its confluence with the lamina, the pedicle, and the superior articular process. Isolation of the neurovascular bundle should be done at this point to avoid its unintentional injury. This structure courses slightly cephalad from the base of the transverse process and comes to reside in its recess in the rib within several centimeters. Periosteal elevators are used to circumferentially remove the periosteum from the rib, with care being taken not to injure the underlying endothoracic fascia and pleura. Rib cutters are then used to remove a section of the rib extending from the region of the resected costotransverse joint to the angle of the rib, approximately 4–5 cm. The remainder of the proximal rib is now resected with rongeurs and the cut surfaces smoothed and waxed. A combination of sharp and blunt dissection is directed along the pedicle to expose the vertebral body and adjacent intervertebral disc. If necessary, the pedicle may be removed with rongeurs and a high-speed drill. Once this is accomplished, the adjacent lamina may be resected. If further resection of the posterior spinal elements is not essential, the anterior dural surface may be identified and dissected free from the underlying ligamentous and bony structures. This may be facilitated by gentle posterior traction on the intercostal nerve. Kerrison rongeurs may be used to enlarge the intervertebral foramen. As in any approach, caution should be exercised when dealing with rigid elements protruding into the spinal canal. Under these circumstances, a trough may be drilled in the vertebral body and the impinging lesion delivered from the dura into the defect. The procedure may be facilitated by the use of an operating microscope during the final stages of decompression. Rib strut grafts may be interposed between the vertebral bodies when conditions dictate.

Because this procedure not only disrupts the costovertebral articulations but may also damage or destroy the zygapophyseal joint, intervertebral disc and posterior longitudinal ligament, an unstable spine may easily be produced. As mentioned, an anterior strut graft may be interposed between adjacent vertebral bodies. If Harrington rod stabilization has been used, a posterior or posterolateral spinal fusion may be accomplished.

Anterolateral Transthoracic Approach

Tuberculous abscess of the spine with its potential for producing skeletal deformity and myelopathy inspired the transthoracic anterolateral spinal approach. Successful application of this procedure, however, had to await the evolution of surgical and anesthetic techniques that would allow for acceptable morbidity and mortality. This approach has been applied to a variety of lesions affecting the second through the twelfth thoracic vertebrae. It has been found useful in resecting tumors of vertebral bodies that require extensive replacement with bone grafts.[8,11] It has found application in treating severe kyphotic deformities where anterior osteotomy and bone grafting are superior to posterior fixation because the compressive forces produce a greater probability of satisfactory fusion. Of major importance, however, has been its application to lesions compressing the spinal cord from the ventral surface. These have included infections of the vertebral bodies, disc spaces, and epidural tissues as well as tumors, herniated discs, and fractures that have a significant intraspinal component.

In general, the right lateral decubitus position is preferred. It avoids the significant obstacle presented by the liver and eliminates potentially disastrous manipulation of the delicate vena cava. After a standard thoracotomy skin incision over the rib to be resected, the subcutaneous tissue is opened from the lateral border of the paraspinous musculature to the sternocostal junction. If there is any doubt about which is the appropriate rib, it is better to err toward selection of the more rostral one, since it is easier to approach a lesion from above than from below. The periosteum from the rib to be resected is incised with electrocautery and elevated circumferentially, with care taken not to injure the underlying pleura. The rib is then cut from its costochondral articulation anteriorly to the angle of the rib posteriorly. The rib is gently elevated; the endothoracic fascia and pleura are left intact. The parietal pleura underlying the rib bed is incised and opened in line with the rib after blunt dissection has freed any pleural adhesions. The lung is manually deflated and retracted medially. It is important to ensure that the cut ends of the rib do not present any unusually sharp edges. The cut bone edges may be waxed for hemostasis. The rib is saved for possible bone grafting. In cases of infectious processes, spinal neoplasms, or trauma, identification of the level of the pathologic condition usually presents no challenge. However, it occasionally is necessary to identify the rib level with absolute accuracy at this juncture. Although this can usually be done by palpation either within the thoracic cavity or after the serratus anterior muscle has been reflected, localization through x-ray films is preferable. Once the appropriate level is identified, an incision is made into the parietal pleura overlying the posterior rib and extended over the vertebral body. This exposure is advantageous for lesions at or adjacent to one interspace. Alternately, the pleura may be opened in a vertical fashion over the anterolateral surface of the vertebral bodies when surgery is directed toward an extensive lesion. The pleura is bluntly elevated, preserving both the sympathetic chain and the segmental vessels that cross the midportion of each vertebral body. For a restricted lesion, especially at the level of the interspace, it may be possible to retract the vessels from the operative field. In extensive operative procedures, however, it is usually necessary to ligate and divide these segmental vessels. Although the possibility of ischemic infarction of the spinal cord theoretically exists, especially in the poorly supplied midthoracic region, ligation of these vessels has not proved to be a significant problem when proper identification of the primary radiculomedullary vessel has been realized.

Resection of the rib head will allow access to the posterolateral disc and the spinal canal. Furthermore, identification of the pedicle will allow improved localization of the spinal canal. Removal of the discs above and below an affected vertebral body will allow the level of the anterior wall of the spinal canal to be anticipated if the goal is the complete removal of the vertebral body. When there has been destruction of the vertebral bodies or of the posterior longitudinal ligament, the main dural tube may be identified by following the intercostal nerve to its origin. Gentle traction on the intercostal nerve will facilitate its dissection from the overlying structures. Lesions affecting the bodies, disc spaces, and adjacent costal articulations can be removed with a combination of high-speed air drill, rongeurs, and curettes. Since the costovertebral articulations afford considerable stability to the spine in this region, attempts should be made to preserve this articulation if possible.

In order to limit potential complications, it is preferable to close the parietal pleura over the spine. The ribs are approximated with woven Dacron sutures and the overlying muscular layers reapposed with absorbable sutures. Closed chest drainage is instituted for 48 to 72 hours. The incidence of CSF fistulas or complications from thoracotomy is relatively low. This approach offers maximum exposure and relative ease of decompression of the spinal canal over as many as eight segments.[10]

Transpedicular Approach to the Thoracic Spine

Because posterolateral and anterolateral approaches are often extensive, complex procedures that carry additional risks to the patient, a posterior approach through the pedicle has been advocated.[7] One of the limitations of this procedure, however, is that it has limited surgical exposure. Furthermore, since the pedicle joins the vertebral body at its cephalic end, it is primarily useful for lesions limited to the disc space and the immediately adjacent vertebral body and that tend to lateralize to one side of the vertebra.

After a midline incision, electrocautery is used to extend the incision to the level of the spinous processes. Subperiosteal dissection of the paravertebral muscles from the spinous processes and the lamina is then performed bilaterally. On the side harboring the lesion, exposure continues laterally beyond the facet joint. The facet joint and underlying pedicle are then removed with a high-speed air drill. A cutting burr is appropriate except when the dura is approached, at which time a diamond-tipped burr is used. This creates a cavity as deep as the diameter of the spinal canal, approximately 1.5 to 1.0 cm. Once the pedicle has been resected to the vertebral body, there is good exposure of the rostral aspect of the vertebral body as well as the adjacent intervertebral disc. Soft lesions may now be removed with careful curettage. However, firm or bony lesions should be delivered from the dura and spinal cord into a cavity made in the posterior aspect of the body with a high-speed drill. Only with this technique can the possibility of producing cord injury be minimized.

After the cord is decompressed anteriorly, a laminectomy can be safely accomplished, starting laterally and moving medially across the midline to the opposite side. Usually the dura need not be opened. If an intradural or intramedullary component to the lesion is suspected, however, the dura should be opened after laminectomy and the cord gently displaced so that the anterior surface of the dura and cord can be inspected. Although this maneuver carries some risk, such risk is minimized by the previous steps taken to allow lateral exposure and ventral decompression.

This procedure obviously causes impairment or destruction of both the zygapophyseal joint and the ligamentous complex formed by the intervertebral disc and the posterior longitudinal ligament. It does not, however, affect the costovertebral articulation, which affords significant stability to the thoracic spine. Depending upon the degree of resection of the ligamentous structures and facet joint, a posterolateral fusion may be indicated.

Because the surgical exposure is quite varied, lesions that are totally ventral or extend a significant distance into the vertebral body may be better approached posterolaterally or anterolaterally. Also, lesions that are too extensive to be easily dealt with at one level probably are best dealt with by one of the alternate approaches.

SPECIFIC PROBLEMS IN MANAGEMENT

Spinal Infection

Infectious diseases generally affect the spine through blood-borne metastasis. The initial complaints are usually pain and associated systemic manifestations of infection, which may vary from malaise to septic shock. Spine films are often revealing. In general, tuberculosis and fungal diseases involve the vertebral body and pyogenic diseases predominantly involves the disc space. The most common early roentgenographic finding in any type of infection is endplate disruption and disc space narrowing. Pyogenic diseases do not involve the disc space directly, but begin at the vertebral endplate. Plain films often disclose pathologic fractures, absent pedicles, or soft tissue abscesses.

Diagnostic Management

Important steps in the diagnostic definition of infections of the spine include:

1. History and physical examination. The history should detail exposure to infection such as intravenous drug abuse and symptoms of infectious disease such as unrelenting spinal pain at night, fever, or chills. The physical examination will often be highlighted by the finding of localized spinal tenderness. Palpation may indicate warmth and evidence of a paravertebral abscess. The precise neurologic status must be defined from the moment the patient is evaluated and any change well documented. Too often, decisions regarding treatment are made on the basis of changing neurologic status, and frequently the initial examination and subsequent examinations are inadequate baselines.
2. Roentgenographic assessment. It is important to evaluate the anterior column. This will help to localize the disease process as well as to identify the origin or site of neurologic dysfunction. It should be determined whether there is an abscess attendant to the process. A paravertebral abscess in the thoracic spine can be well visualized on plain films. Appreciation of such a process has been greatly refined by the introduction of contrast-enhanced computerized tomography. Metrizamide myelography can further refine the structural substrate.
3. Agent definition. Every effort should be made to identify the infectious agent before any surgical intervention. This provides a basis for appropriate antibiotic coverage, thus protecting the patient from generalized sepsis. Pretreatment of tuberculous patients, even those with Pott's paraplegia, has been effective in walling off an abscess, thus allowing a safer, more definitive surgical approach. This regimen usually improves the neurologic deficit before surgery. The time required for needle biopsy or aspiration in this region is minimal and such procedures may be carried out quite effectively. Evaluation of specimens with Gram's stain or Ziehl-Neelsen stain permits the adequate treatment to be initiated, even in the face of emergency surgery.

Techniques of Surgical Aspiration

After the patient has been placed in the prone position on the image intensifier table, anteroposterior and lateral roentgenograms are obtained. A centimeter ruler should be included in the films. The ruler can be used to calculate the number of centimeters from the tip of the spinous process of the involved vertebra to the middle and anterior column. The presence of the ruler in the roentgenograms also eliminates the possibility of magnification errors.

The point of entry for the needle is determined by taking the distance from the spinous process to the middle or anterior column on the films and measuring this same distance directly the skin laterally from the spinous process. Once the insertion point is determined, the needle is positioned at this point at an angle of 45 degrees lateral in the transverse plane and 20 degrees cephalad in the parasagittal plane. The needle is advanced with frequent checks in both planes on the image intensifier. The needle must never enter the spinal canal in either plane. When a Craig needle is used, a small-bore long needle or blunt-tipped obturator should be used first. Good quality x-ray films should be obtained before the Craig cutting core is inserted and again when the biopsy or aspiration needle is at its maximum depth. If the angle of insertion in the transverse plane is changed, then trigonometric functions must be used to calculate the depth of insertion. This is done by knowing the length of one side and two angles of a triangle. The use of a greater angle of insertion, such as 55 or 60 degrees, is felt by some to be safer, but the distance of the insertion point from the spinous process must then be calculated rather than directly measured. As an alternative technique, CT-monitored biopsy and aspiration may be considered. Formal CT-guided systems are currently under development (Trent Wells, Inc., Southgate, California).

Treatment Initiatives

Antibiotic or antitubercular therapy is begun as soon as possible after aspiration. The presence of a pyogenic agent does not eliminate tuberculosis or a fungus as a concomitant infectious agent. Skin tests, complement-fixation titers and total body cultures should be done initially. If there is any suspicion of tuberculosis, antituberculosis agents should be used until the cultures assessment is completed.

For apparent tuberculosis, every attempt should be made to treat the patient for a period of 6 weeks before surgical intervention. In some patients the spine will fuse and not require surgery. In others, the abscess will be better localized and encapsulated and there will be better systemic control. In bacterial processes, antibiotics should be employed at the onset. It is advisable to drain paravertebral abscesses of unacceptable size. The precise volume of acceptability is not well defined; however, such variables as the location of the abscess, the condition of the patient, and the etiologic agent should be considered. In general, abscesses over 6 cm in diameter should be drained. The administration of high-potency glucocorticoids should be initiated in patients with neurologic deficits concurrently with measures to define the etiologic agent.

As noted, decompression should be undertaken from the direction of the compressing structure, which in most instances dictates an anterior approach. An approach through the area of greatest ligamentous damage should be planned and destruction of normal ligamentous structures should be avoided.

Structural stability should be evaluated. Before surgery an estimate should be made of the amount of destruction caused by the disease and the anticipated amount of iatrogenic structural alteration attendant to the decompression procedure. An important consideration in the performance of grafting at the time of decompression is the virulence of the organism. In the case of tuberculous processes and most fungal infections bone grafting may be done at the time of decompression. Instability caused by most pyogenic bacteria, especially *Staphylococcus aureus* and various aggressive Gram-negative organisms, should be treated by primary decompression only and insertion of irrigation tubes when applicable. All infected debris exclusive of neurologic tissues and such vital structures such as the aorta should be removed during the decompression procedure. Bone grafting should be undertaken as a secondary procedure.

It is important to stress that there are difficulties involved in performing a laminectomy for osteomyelitis of the anterior column of the thoracic spine with or without an epidural extension of the abscess. These include (1) the expansile anterior column mass produces an increased amount of displacement of the spinal cord after laminectomy; (2) normal portions of the spine, namely the posterior ligamentous structures, are removed, thus producing two unstable columns rather than one; (3) a structural substrate is established that results in an increased kyphotic deformity because the resistive tensile forces of the posterior column are removed, which often increases a neurologic deficit by increasing the mass effect of the anterior infected debris and abscess; (4) there is an increased possibility of meningitis from dural penetration; (5) this method of decompression creates bacterial contamination and precludes the possibility of fusing the posterior column to stabilize the spine. There are cases in which a second-stage posterior instrumentation and fusion after anterior decompression and control of the infection may provide protection of neurologic elements and early mobilization.

Spinal Tumors

Certain tumors have a predilection for either the anterior or the posterior column. Common posterior column tumors include osteoblastomas, osteoid osteomas, aneurysmal bone cysts, and giant cell tumors. Such tumors may involve the entire spinal column and may be associated with instability. Giant cell tumors and aneurysmal bone cysts may involve the entire spinal column. Vascular tumors of various kinds, osteoblastomas, and giant cell tumors often grow until they produce a neurologic compromise. Anterior column tumors include metastatic processes, multiple myelomas, hemangiomas, and sarcomas (visceral tumors with direct penetration) and are commonly associated with instability.

There are four major considerations in the evaluation and treatment of spinal tumors: (1) diagnosis of tumor type in conjunction with definition of the extent of structural alteration and neurologic deficit; (2) adequate decompression of all neural elements with maintenance of appropriate patency and structure of the spinal and root canals; (3) specific treatment of the tumor; and (4) maintenance of the stability of the spinal column.

Diagnosis begins with a complete history and physical examination. Patients generally have midline or radicular thoracic pain that is unrelenting and problematic at night or on standing and occasionally associated with malaise, generalized weakness, and weight loss. The evaluation should proceed from baseline immunologic and serum enzyme assays and progress to plain films of the region in question. Naturally, appropriate investigation should be undertaken regarding the possibility of metastatic neoplasms concomitantly with the evaluations of the focal spinal disease. Computed tomography with and without contrast media or associated metrizamide myelography is an important step in determining the structural alterations present. Spinal angiography is a critical consideration in the event that surgical strategies require potential manipulation or sacrifice of regional radicular arteries.

In the event that these measures do not specifically lead to a diagnosis of a tumor, a spinal biopsy may be considered. For posterior column tumors, an open biopsy technique is preferred and for the majority of those an excisional biopsy is undertaken. Biopsy of laterally placed lesions involving both the anterior and posterior columns is easily accomplished through a costotransversectomy approach, which allows easy access to the vertebral body by following the rib to the costovertebral articulation. It is possible to do a needle biopsy through a partial costotransversectomy approach. Additionally, access to the vertebral body may be obtained down the tube of the pedicle by following the pedicle to the vertebral body via the posterior approach.

After the tissue diagnosis has been established, appropriate treatment of the tumor may be undertaken. This step may or may not require surgery, depending upon the neurologic and histologic indications for such an approach. It is important to consider and to assess the structural integrity of the spine, however, and prophylactic fusion before treatment of a tumor is an important option. In cases of severe instability of the skeletal column, Harrington rods or Luque instrumentation reinforced with either bone grafts or methylmethacrylate can provide excellent protection during tumor treatment. Luque instrumentation provides excellent fixation with multiple levels available for fixation, and it allows safe, early ambulation of the patient. Methylmethacrylate reinforcement for the Harrington system in distraction provides good stabilization. Most anterior column instabilities are not adequately supported by a compression system. Great care must be taken when stabilizing a patient with a neurologic deficit or canal obstruction. Any change in spinal alignment produces the risk of neurologic loss. Fixation in situ is safer. Decompression of neural elements should be undertaken with appropriate operative technique and adjuvants including the operating microscope, laser instrumentation, and monitoring of evoked potentials.

Stabilization in the Face of Tumor

Posterior element tumors. Any tumor that involves the neural arch potentially decreases the stability of the entire spinal column if the neural arch is removed. The lamina serves as the insertion of the ligamentum flavum. Removal of the ligamentum flavum at one level of the thoracic spine in itself does not destabilize that segment, but if done in conjunction with resection of the costovertebral articulation bilaterally or in conjunction with major structural changes to the anterior column, it can be a destabilizing procedure. Removal of an articular facet in conjunction with other structures is a major destabilizing process for the thoracic spine. While the thoracic facet joint capsules are not as strong as those in other regions, the orientation of the articular surfaces of the facet are a significant restraint to forward subluxation. Pedicular involvement essentially removes bony support from one half of the posterior column.

Anterior element tumors. Neoplasms involving the anterior column frequently weaken the bone and bony endplate. This process may destroy or negate the stabilizing restraints of the longitudinal ligaments. Anterior column instability will usually exist with major destruction to one or more of the vertebral bodies. Because of the destruction and shortening of the anterior column, the ligaments loose their restraining ability in the shortened condition and a significant amount of subluxation is possible. Lytic tumors can be quite deceptive in terms of their appearance of instability. A large lytic lesion may spare a reasonable amount of soft tissue support. There is no appreciable way to judge the mechanical integrity of this pathologic condition. Blastic tumors are considered more stable, but bone with blastic metastasis is weak and very susceptible to pathologic fracture.

Maintenance of stability.   It is important to consider the possibility of instability of the spine and subsequent spinal cord injury in the face of operative or nonoperative treatment of the neoplasm in question. In the midthoracic spine, the use of Luque instrumentation is our preferred technique for stabilizing an unstable anterior column. Harrington rods reinforced with methylmethacrylate, special hooks, or wire fixation may be employed. The use of methylmethacrylate in the posterior elements where it is essentially subjected to distraction forces is not ideal. Prophylactic fusion also may be of benefit with metal fixation. Luque instrumentation allows stabilization and early mobilization of the patient during the treatment period. This circumvents the complications of bed rest, which an unstable and generally symptomatically painful tumor of the spine usually requires. Prophylactic surgical stabilization is often indicated for patients with static and incomplete neurologic deficits resulting from an unstable large lytic lesion of the anterior column.

Posterior Column Curative Resection

Resection of tumors in the posterior elements essentially involves removal of the tumor and involved bone with preservation of neural elements. The intercostal nerve may be sacrificed, however, enblock resection involving the spinal cord is rarely indicated. There is no absolute need for internal fixation or fusion after total removal of the posterior elements of one level of the midthoracic spine if the anterior column is intact. Close observation of the problem for potential instability should be undertaken in the postoperative period. Removal of one hemipedicle, transverse process, and facet joint or bilateral removal of all structures to the pedicles at one level with a costovertebral articulation is not an absolute indication for fusion or internal fixation. Disruption of a costovertebral articulation and all the posterior elements at one level is a relative indication for fusion and internal fixation. Destabilization of the posterior column and removal of both costovertebral articulations is usually an indication for internal fixation and fusion.

Anterior Column Curative Resection

Strict attention should be given to defining the limits of the tumor. There frequently are soft tissue extensions that are difficult to delineate on any study. In anterior column tumors in which resection is frequently contemplated, such as in an apparent isolated metastasis, localized intrinsic sarcoma, or benign local tumor, the following approach may be considered: (1) assess the stability of the posterior column; (2) perform appropriate angiographic studies to define the extent of the vascularity of the lesion, the spinal axis, and the neural axis, since preoperative embolization may be one option; (3) assess the levels above and below the region of apparent tumor carefully for evidence of tumor extension, since any resection procedure will require normal adjacent bone to provide firm fixation for the replacement device or graft. Soft tissue erosion, drainage fistulas, vascular fistulas, bowel fistulas, and so forth, should be carefully assessed before any anterior surgery.

Methods of Anterior Fixation

The Dunn device has some potential for stabilization in thoracic tumors. This device provides distraction or compression, ease in fitting bone grafts, and good visualization of articular surfaces; however, the presence of soft bone precludes satisfactory use of this unit.

Other constructs for anterior tumor replacement consist of methylmethacrylate and metal composite structures. Use of Knodt rods hooked into the vertebrae above and below or Steinmann pins driven vertically into the center of the body and reinforced with methylmethacrylate give a composite structure similar to reinforced concrete. Tumors of the anterior column treated by resection of the entire tumor should be reinforced posteriorly unless the resection areas are small and stable.

Spinal Trauma

Mechanisms of Injury

There are four potential mechanisms of injury in the midthoracic spine: (1) flexion, (2) compression, (3) shear, and (4) flexion rotation. There may be any number of combinations of these four mechanisms in any given traumatic event.[3]

Management of Spinal Fractures

With midthoracic fractures a number of considerations are imperative: (1) protecting the patient against increased neurologic injury; (2) establishing a basis for maximal neurologic recovery; (3) obtaining a stable reduction of the deformity; (4) restoring the structural integrity of the spinal column; (5) allowing the patient to return to active function as soon as possible; (6) preventing the emergence of spinal related pain; and (7) protecting the patient's life. Decision-making in the management of spinal fractures is based on consideration of all of these factors. There is often one that seems of paramount importance, but failure to consider all of these factors in each case may be to the great detriment of the patient.

Preventing a neurologic deficit from increasing and establishing a substrate for maximal neurologic recovery are the most critical factors in the management of patients with injuries to the spinal column. The amount and type of neurologic deficit is usually the overriding factor and must take precedence over structural stability when the two are in contradiction.

As a general rule, patients with no neurologic deficit whose spines will fuse within 6 to 12 weeks of bedrest with ancillary orthoses are treated nonoperatively. Patients with ligamentous injuries and a probable substrate for chronic instability are treated by operative reduction and stabilization. It is rarely necessary to decompress the spinal cord of a neurologically intact patient.

Patients with an incomplete cord lesion usually show some neurologic improvement with nonoperative treatment. Treatment decisions are made with due consideration of the extent of the lesion, the rapidity of return of neurologic function, the condition of the patient, and the potential for chronic spinal instability. Decompression is usually accomplished at the time of reduction and stabilization and may be done by one of several methods. Reduction with Harrington rods may totally decompress the spinal cord. Vertebrectomy may be needed if the space-occupying lesion is located anteriorly. Laminectomy may be used with reduction and stabilization if the cord compression can be relieved anteriorly.

Patients with a complete thoracic cord lesion may need reduction and stabilization to enhance restabilization or prevent chronic instability and deformity. Decompression is not indicated.

Midthoracic deformities may be reduced without surgery. An effort should be made to retunr the spine to a configuration as close as possible to the natural anatomic condition, whether this is 0 degrees or whether it is simply less than 40 degrees. The amount of kyphotic deformity in the thoracic spine can be up to 40 degrees, however, an angle of 40 degrees at one vertebra is unacceptable.

Reduction of the thoracic spine can be obtained by a number of techniques:

1. Halo femoral traction. Halo femoral traction requires the insertion of Gardner-Wells tongs or a halo device and femoral pins. The patient should be observed very carefully for the many possible complications of this technique, including increased myelopathy and cranial nerve palsies, as well as peripheral neuropathies in the region of the knee.
2. Halo pelvic traction. Halo pelvic traction is another technique with potential applications in the thoracic region but with elements of risk in inexperienced hands.
3. Positioning. This technique can reduce a kyphotic deformity in the thoracic region and is accomplished by positioning the patient over pillows. This method gently reestablishes alignment when the pillows are positioned at the apex of the kyphotic deformity. Reduction may be obtained and in the event that healing proceeds appropriately it may be maintained. Positioning the patient on the operating table in the prone position may often significantly reduce a kyphotic deformity before surgery. Consideration must be given to the maintaining the reduction. Any reduction of a kyphotic deformity that is obtained by the application of an orthosis such as a hyperextension jacket will not be maintained. Frequently the orthosis will prevent further deformity, but it should not be relied upon to maintain a closed manipulative type of reduction. Axial loading increases kyphotic deformity and axial loading in inherent in the upright position and cannot be negated by an orthosis.

Spinal stability is the state of structural integrity of the spinal column that prevents neurologic damage, increasing deformity, or spinal pain. A spine may be acutely unstable at the time of injury but heal and stabilize without surgery within 6 to 12 weeks or a spine may fail to heal, resulting in permanent instability that requires special operative intervention.

Bony injuries to the thoracic spine, especially those of a compressive nature involving the anterior column will, in general, heal within 6 to 12 weeks. In cases of ligamentous injuries, a determination must be made whether or not the extent of ligamentous damage is such that it carries a risk of increasing neurologic deficit even after a prolonged period of bedrest. In such cases, earlier operative intervention and surgical stabilization are indicated.

A treatment initiative that allows the patient to be ambulated early decreases the hazards of bedrest, and in patients with pronounced neurologic deficits operative intervention to treat an unstable fracture is preferable because it allows the patient to be mobilized early without the emotional and physical impact of long periods of bedrest. For the patient who is neurologically intact, the circumstances may be different. Operative intervention does not carry a specific risk of increased neurologic deficit.

The prevention of spinal pain is a complex and multifaceted issue. Operating to prevent future pain is not an intellectually honest endeavor in the majority of cases. The realigned spine in an patient without neurologic deficit is certainly less likely to produce a chronic benign pain syndrome than a deformed unstable spine in a neurologically impaired patient, but it had been difficult to prove on a statistical basis.

Patients with an unstable thoracic spine caused by trauma have usually suffered a high-velocity thoracic impact injury. A ruptured thoracic aorta, pneumohemothorax, ruptured diaphragm, ruptured viscus, and cardiac contusion are common concomitant injuries. Emergency surgery to restore spinal stability must take this into consideration; the life of the patient must be protected.

Management Related to Mechanism of Injury

The mechanism of injury is an indicator of spinal instability, and management of spinal instability may be derived from a knowledge of the pathomechanisms. Using the two-column concept, injury mechanisms can be described as flexion, compression, shear, flexion-rotation, and combined. These injury mechanisms guide treatment.

Flexion. As a result of flexion, there is most often bony or ligamentous instability to the posterior column and an intact anterior longitudinal ligament. Therefore, Harrington distraction rods can distract against the anterior longitudinal ligament and produce a reduction of a kyphotic deformity by three-point pressure. There will be instances in which distraction rods fail to reduce the horizontal cleavage gap of the posterior column, but if the kyphotic deformity is reduced and grafting is carried out in the area of the fracture, the gap will not be of major consequence. An additional method of treatment of this injury is a compression apparatus applied to the posterior column. In this technique a Harrington compression apparatus is applied over four levels or a Knodt rod compression over two levels. The compression apparatus substitutes for the distracted damaged ligamentous structures. It is imperative to undertake careful preoperative evaluation of the spinal canal before employing compression in the management of spinal fractures. The integrity of the posterior body wall, posterior annulus, and intervertebral disc must be determined before institution of compression to prevent displacement of anterior column fragments of disc or bone into the spinal canal.

As a general rule, 2 cm of posterior distraction should be reduced, but in the majority of instances, it is the overall kyphotic deformity that is the important factor, not the amount of distraction between the bone of the posterior column. A majority of Chance fractures that are entirely bony in nature can be treated nonoperatively within the variables of acceptable reduction. Such patients seldom require prolonged bedrest and can be ambulated within 7 to 10 days in a hyperextension jacket, which usually prevents progression of the deformity but does not produce reduction. Therefore, with flexion injuries it is advisable to reduce the deformity within safe limits and maintain that reduction in an orthosis when possible. If reduction must be obtained operatively, compression or distraction apparatuses are available and compression techniques are probably more reliable.

Compression. Simple compression-type injuries in which there is no major structural damage are, in general, stable lesions. With an intact thoracic cage and no evidence of posterior column distraction or rotation, there is no amount of anterior compression per se that requires an operation. A totally collapsed, crushed vertebral body, such as is seen in a pathologic fracture, is a stable lesion. An isolated anterior wedge fracture, even with greater than 50 percent of anterior wedging, requires no operative intervention. A major axial loading injury with disruption of the posterior body wall is more dangerous in the acute phase but is a bone injury that will heal with bedrest. A vertical laminar fracture is a stable lesion, emphasizing that not all posterior element fractures are unstable. Horizontal cleavage and distraction rotation of the posterior column are unstable and may indicate the need for operative intervention to provide stability.

Because of the vascular supply and the anatomic relationships in this region, most midthoracic lesions produce an immediate and complete paraplegia. Occasionally, operative intervention is indicated for either progressive or stable incomplete neurologic deficits accompnaying these fractures. In these instances, the patient undergoes a decompression procedure after a period of neurologic observation to enhance the climate for recovery within the spinal canal. There are two basic methods of approaching this problem: (1) posterior distraction instrumentation to reduce any kyphotic deformity using a posterior element for three-point fixation distraction and realignment of the canal. This method rarely produces a reduction in the amount of bone in the canal although it is possible to decrease the anterior mass effect from the fracture and produce neurologic improvement. (2) Anterior decompression and removal of all anterior column bone encroaching into the spinal canal with reduction of the deformity anteriorly and bone grafting to reestablish the stability of the anterior column. The advantages of the anterior approach are that the posterior column, which is generally intact, is not disrupted.

A deformity may be reduced by the newer anterior fixation devices such as the Dunn device. Bone grafting anteriorly is usually superior to bone grafting posteriorly because of the large surface area in compression between the vertebrae. Anterior grafting becomes more and more effective with any degree of kyphotic deformity. The available instrumentation includes the Dunn device and the bottle-jack devices. The bottle-jack devices do obstruct a portion of the potential graft area in the anterior body but provide good reduction forces and will usually leave adequate exposure for stable grafting. Strut grafting techniques also may be employed in which the spine is manually reduced and the strut graft placed under tension to maintain the reduction.

A combination of the two approaches is very commonly employed, especially in treating older fixed deformities. A total reduction of the spine can be obtained by performing a combined approach with the patient in the lateral position and 45 degrees from vertical posteriorly for anterior release and then being side-tilted 45 degrees anteriorly for reduction of the spine with either a compression or a distraction device, then returning to the anterior approach for grafting or supplemental internal fixation. We prefer the combined approach and thoracotomy to the costotransversectomy approach, which provides limited exposure.

Shear. Shear injuries produce an unstable posterior and anterior column. Distraction rods are seldom indicated in that there are no resisting ligamentous structures. Decompression is frequently required because of the neurologic deficit. The fixation devices available for this unstable type of lesion are usually of the compression type, but a combined compression-distraction system at times may be of benefit.

In shear fractures with total ligamentous disruption, as in flexion-rotation injuries with a disrupted thoracic cage, Luque instrumentation does provide stable fixation without a cast. It is our preferred treatment at this time for unstable fractures that do not require distraction for neurologic improvement of a gross deformity.

Plate fixation in the midthoracic spine provides the same static fixation as the Luque system. The location of the screws is critical. Placement of the screws through the spinous processes is very tenuous and is not considered effective. Screws directed down the pedicle and into the vertebral body provide optimal fixation for the thoracic plates. However, this requires expertise in order to avoid encroachment into the spinal or root canals.

Flexion-rotation. Flexion-rotation injuries without associated thoracic cage disruption are stable; however, with thoracic disruption they may become unstable. Plating of the sternum has been employed, obviously with short screws, and this has restored stability to transverse sternal fractures and thereby the overall stability of the spine.

Flexion-rotation injuries do have the potential for producing total ligamentous disruption. In spite of this potential risk, however, distraction rods are the preferred method of treatment because of their advantage in restoring alignment. When using any distraction apparatus, very careful study of intraoperative x-ray films must be done to assess the potential for overdistraction. With kyphotic deformity and the use of three-point fixation and Harrington rod distraction, the tips of the spinous processes should move toward each other rather than apart. Monitoring and visual observation during distraction will often detect alterations of somatosensory evoked responses or increasing distance between the spinous processes, both signs of overdistraction and indications for immediate x-ray evaluation. Overdistraction is a cause of increased neurologic deficit after Harrington distraction fixation. Combined distraction-compression systems are therefore employed when evidence of axial instability is present. Under these circumstances, the compression devices are initially applied over the unstable segment and loosened with caution as the distraction system produces the required reduction.

Combined injuries. In the midthoracic spine, the most commonly observed injury is anterior compression-distraction. In this mechanism the anterior column is compressed and flexed, producing a wedge-type injury, and the posterior column has a distraction dislocation of the facets. In this case, the injured longitudinal ligament is usually intact and reduction can usually be obtained with distraction rod three point fixation. Combining compression with this distraction may be necessary to produce adequate bony reduction of the facet. Facet dislocations in this area should be preceded by removal of the cephalad half of the caudad facet involved in the dislocation. This makes the reduction easier and prevents possible neurologic compromise by those facets. The true danger of the wedged subluxation fracture is that its importance is missed at the time of initial evaluation. This fracture should be treated operatively because of the severe ligamentous disruption of the posterior column. This is a fracture that, after 3 months of bed rest, may progress and operative stabilization and fusion are therefore indicated to prevent severe late deformity. Again, the clinical implications of this fracture are worse in the thoracolumbar junction than in the midthoracic spine because of the important stabilizing effect of the thoracic cavity. This fracture, when seen in conjunction with an unstable thoracic cavity, is the classic example in which, at a later date, the transverse sternal fracture jumps and shortens and the spine annulates 100 degrees in a reasonably short period of time.

REFERENCES

1. Breig A: Adverse Mechanical Tension in the Central Nervous System. New York, John Wiley & Sons, 1978
2. Capener N: The evolution of lateral rhachotomy. J Bone Joint Surg 36B:173, 1954
3. Dorr LD, Harvey JF, Nickel VL: Clinical review of the early stability of spine injuries. Spine 76:545, 1982
4. Hulme A: The surgical approach to thoracic intervertebral disc protrusions. J Neurol Neurosurg Psychiatry 23:133, 1960
5. Lazorthes G, Gouaze A, Zadeh JO, Santini JJ, Lazorthes Y, Burdin P: Arterial vascularization of the spinal cord. J Neurosurg 35:252, 1971
6. Macon JB, Poletti CE, Sweet WH, Ojemann RG, Zervas NT: Conducted somatosensory evoked potentials during spinal surgery: Clinical applications. J Neurosurg 57:354, 1982
7. Patterson RH Jr, Arbit E: A surgical approach through the pedicle to protruded thoracic discs. J Neurosurg 48:760, 1978
8. Ransohoff J, Spencer F, Siew F, Gage L Jr: Transthoracic removal of thoracic discs: Case reports and technical notes. J Neurosurg 31:459, 1969   2
9. Turnbull IM: Microvasculature of the human spinal cord. J Neurosurg 35:141, 1971
10. Watkins RG: Surgical Approaches to the Spine. New York, Springer Verlag, 1983
11. Weiss MH, Heiden JS, Apuzzo MLJ, Kurze T: Anterior decompression of the thoracic and thoracolumbar spine. Bull LA Neurol Soc 40:112, 1978
12. White AA, Panjabi MD: Clinical Biomechanics of The Spine. Philadelphia, J.B. Lippincott, 1978

Sanford J. Larson

7

The Thoracolumbar Junction

Most fractures of the thoracic and lumbar vertebrae occur between T10 and L2. This area, the thoracolumbar junction, is a zone of structural and functional transition, and it is helpful to understand the anatomic and biomechanical features that are unique to this area.

ANATOMY AND BIOMECHANICS OF THE THORACOLUMBAR JUNCTION

The configuration of the tenth, eleventh, and twelfth thoracic vertebrae is similar to that of the first and second lumbar vertebrae. The tenth, eleventh, and twelfth ribs are attached to the bodies of the tenth, eleventh, and twelfth vertebrae, while the second through the ninth ribs each are attached to two vertebral bodies, straddling the interspace. The eleventh and twelfth thoracic vertebrae lack a costotransverse articulation. When viewed from the side (see, for example, Figure 7-8A), the articular processes of the thoracic vertebrae are nearly horizontal, that is, they are parallel to the long axis of the vertebral column, which is a configuration that inhibits flexion. Flexion is also restricted by the costovertebral and costotransverse articulations and related ligaments, as is lateral movement. Extension is severely restricted by contact between the inferior articular processes and the subjacent laminae. The superior articular processes from T1 to T11 are directed dorsally and laterally, while the inferior articular processes from T1 to T10 are directed medially and ventrally. Consequently, the articular surfaces lie on the circumference of a circle, the center of which is located in the midventral region of the vertebral body. This configuration permits rotation, which is the predominant direction of motion in the thoracic spinal column.

In contrast to the thoracic articular processes, the lumbar facets have a more vertical orientation, paralleling the sagittal plane of the vertebral column. This

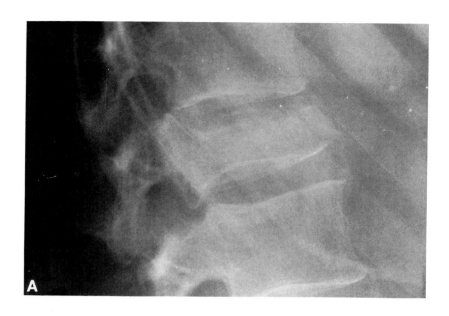

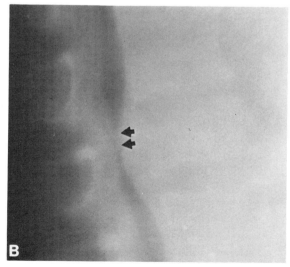

128

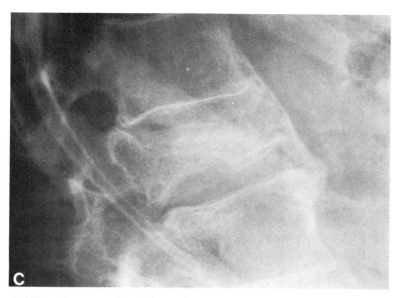

Figure 7-1. (A) Burst fracture of L1. The patient had a mild neurologic deficit that cleared within a few days. (B) Gas myelogram done 1 week later. The spinal cord is not deformed (arrows) and the posterior elements are intact. After his back pain subsided, he was allowed out of bed in a rigid orthosis. (C) The same patient 3 years later. He was neurologically normal and without symptoms.

configuration permits flexion, extension, and lateral movement but little rotation. One of the lower thoracic vertebra, usually the eleventh but sometimes the twelfth, is transitional, with superior processes of the thoracic type and inferior processes of the lumbar type. While the vertebrae of the thoracolumbar junction have lumbar characteristics, they are not as stout as the third through the fifth lumbar vertebrae.

The thoracolumbar junction therefore is an area where the long lever arm of the thoracic spine, which is rigid with regard to flexion and extension, joins a portion of the vertebral column that permits flexion and extension but lacks the support of the ribs and the strength of the lower lumbar elements. It is also an area where the rotational movement of the thoracic spine is abruptly impeded by the vertically oriented articular processes of the transitional and lumbar vertebrae.

Although the transitional nature of the thoracolumbar junction makes this area vulnerable to fracture, the type of deformity produced depends upon the direction of the force applied. A strictly axial load is absorbed by the vertebral bodies and a burst fracture is produced. Flexion produces anterior wedging and, if sufficiently severe, disruption of the posterior elements. Rotational stresses cause disruption of the posterior elements followed by injury to the vertebral body.[9] Each of these stresses can occur alone or in combination. Distraction with flexion produces a splitting injury beginning posteriorly and then proceeding anteriorly through the vertebral body. Extension injuries and translational injuries secondary to shear forces are rare in the thoracolumbar region.

STABLE AND UNSTABLE FRACTURES OF THE
THORACOLUMBAR JUNCTION

Regardless of the mechanisms of injury, the primary problem is actual or potential injury to the spinal cord or cauda equina, and the major concern is the measures that must be taken to prevent or reverse neurologic deficit. In this regard, it is important to determine whether a fracture is stable or unstable. A stable fracture is one in which the vertebral body is damaged without disruption of the posterior elements (Figure 7-1). For additional deformity to occur, a force exceeding that which caused the original injury must be applied.[9,14] Consequently, in stable fractures surgical treatment is not required unless there is an associated neurologic deficit. On the other hand, an unstable fracture is one in which progressive deformity in the direction of the originally deforming force can be anticipated under physiologic loads.[3,13] In the thoracolumbar region, this is almost invariably flexion, which produces increased axial tension in the spinal cord with a corresponding adverse effect on neurologic function.[4]

Various criteria have been proposed to define an unstable fracture. These have included such variables as angulation greater than 30 degrees or a decrease in the height of the anterior surface of the vertebral body to less than 50 percent of the height of the posterior surface.[3] However, a wedge fracture with these characteristics may be stable and heal if the posterior elements are intact (Figure 7-2). Patients with this type of fracture consequently could be immobilized in a rigid orthosis; surgical treatment would be reserved for those patients who develop a progressive deformity or who have persistent and disabling pain. If both anterior and posterior elements are disrupted, either by injury or by a surgical procedure such as laminectomy, the fracture should be considered unstable.[5,9,11,14] While the deformity produced by such fractures can be expected to increase under physiologic loads, the rate of progression can be variable, taking place rapidly (Figure 7-3) or gradually.[11]

MANAGEMENT OF UNSTABLE FRACTURES OF THE
THORACOLUMBAR JUNCTION

The management of an unstable thoracolumbar fracture usually includes fusion. Although healing may occur with nonsurgical methods,[1,7] these postural techniques require an undesirably long period of recumbency, and the overall results are not as good as those obtained with surgical treatment.[10] Fusion with external splinting by a rigid orthosis is acceptable but cannot be expected to restore and maintain a more normal vertebral alignment and may not be tolerated by patients whose skin is anesthetic. The most efficient technique is fusion of the involved segment and internal splinting with metallic instrumentation and external splinting with a removable rigid orthosis that is worn when the patient is not recumbent. This allows mobilization 1 to 2 weeks after surgery within limits determined by neurologic function and by associated injuries.[6]

Several surgical approaches are available, including a posterior approach with costotransversectomy,[15] a retroperitoneal sympathectomy-type approach,[16] a transthoracic and transabdominal thoracolumbar approach,[17] and a lateral extracavitary approach.[10] Each has advantages and disadvantages. The thoracolumbar and the lateral approaches provide the best exposure for reconstructing the spinal canal. With the

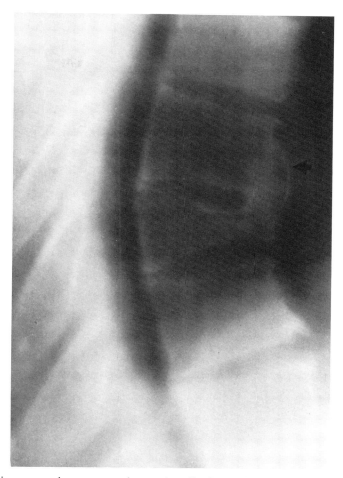

Figure 7-2. This gas myelogram was done primarily for evaluation of a cervical myelopathy. The patient gave a history of transient back pain after an automobile accident several years earlier.

thoracolumbar approach, the patient is in the lateral decubitus position for the reconstruction of the spinal canal, and therefore blood loss from the epidural veins will be less than with the extracavitary approach, which is done with the patient prone. The lateral extracavitary approach, however, permits a single-stage, single-incision operation for reconstruction of the spinal canal, interbody fusion, and instrumentation without the risks associated with thoracotomy and laparotomy. The details of the lateral approach are given later in this chapter.

The type of internal splint that is selected depends upon the direction in which the vertebral column has been deformed and the extent of bony and ligamentous disruption. Although a variety of fixation devices have been developed, those that are applied posteriorly are superior to those that are fixed to the vertebral bodies, such as the Dwyer and Zielke devices. The latter resist the forces that produce lateral deformity but cannot effectively control flexion and extension. The Dunn device for anterior fixation

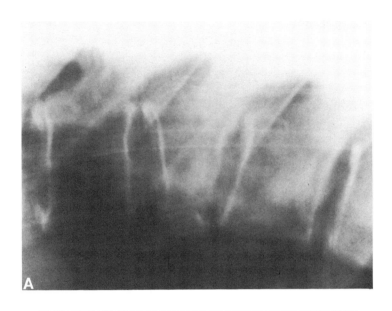

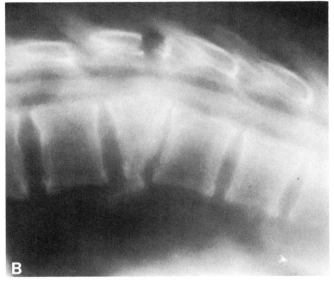

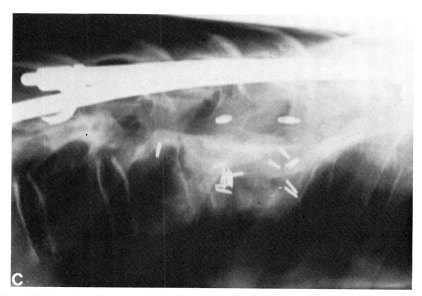

Figure 7-3. (A) A wedge fracture with reduction in the height of the vertebral body anteriorly of approximately 50 percent. The neurologic examination was normal. (B) The patient became paraparetic within two days after he was allowed out of bed. The gas myelogram demonstrates posterior disruption, deformity of the spinal cord, and increased angulation of the vertebral column. (C) A postoperative film of the same patient. The displaced bone has been resected, Harrington rods have been applied, and interbody fusion has been performed.

appears to provide satisfactory fixation but has not been used long enough or extensively enough to allow adequate evaluation. A number of techniques have been tried for posterior fixation. Recently, such devices as the Steffes or Roy-Camille screw plates have been advocated. These require placing screws through the pedicles into the vertebral bodies. While these devices may prove to be effective, they, like the Dunn device for anterior fixation, have not been used long enough or extensively enough to permit adequate evaluation. At present, three basic types of posteriorly applied devices are available. These are Harrington distraction rods, modified Weiss springs, and Luque rods. Each has a satisfactory resistance to loads applied axially and with three-point and four-point fixation. With the Harrington and Luque rods, failure is abrupt and irreversible, while with the modified Weiss springs failure is more gradual and recovery occurs when the load is released.[12] Each has advantages and disadvantages and particularly suitable applications.

In flexion injuries with anterior and posterior disruption, either rods or modified Weiss springs can be used. Each device produces an anteriorly directed force at the apex of the deformity (Figure 7-4). Harrington rods exert a force on the laminae and articular processes that has a posteriorly directed component, while the Weiss springs exert a force that is more parallel to the lamina. While each system will tend to straighten the vertebral column, neither can be relied upon to reconstruct the spinal canal.[11,15]

In addition to straightening the spinal column, Harrington distraction rods will also lengthen it. This increases the tension in the anterior and posterior longitudinal

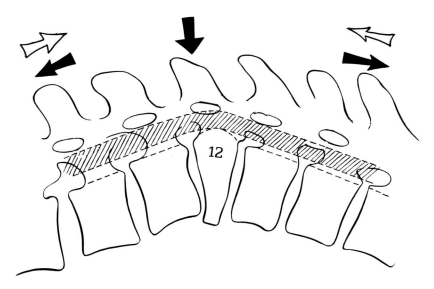

Figure 7-4. Harrington rods produce axial distraction (horizontal solid arrows) and the modified springs a compressive force (open arrows). Both devices exert an anteriorly directed force (vertical arrow) at the apex of the kyphus.

ligaments, developing forces that tend to restore the deformed vertebral body to a more normal configuration. The posterior longitudinal ligament, however, frequently is not strong enough to do this effectively, and the spinal cord may not only remain deformed but with sufficient vertebral distraction may be subjected to increased axial tension.[4] Depending upon the location of the axis of rotation, the application of modified Weiss springs may increase the height of the vertebral body anteriorly but may further compress the vertebral body posteriorly. Regardless of whether rods or springs are used, it is more prudent to surgically reconstruct the spinal canal before proceeding with instrumentation. A neurologic deficit cannot be correlated with the extent of angulation of the vertebral column or compromise of the spinal canal. Therefore, neither substantial improvement in alignment nor in the dimensions of the spinal canal can be considered as end points for treatment unless they are followed by satisfactory recovery of neurologic function or by radiographically demonstrable restoration of normal relationships between the spinal cord and the spinal canal.

Preoperative radiographic assessment should include myelography to demonstrate the spinal cord and its relationship to the spinal canal. This information is very helpful in planning the appropriate surgical procedure. For example, the patients whose x-ray films are shown in Figures 7-5 and 7-6 had unstable fractures. Each was functionally normal, but one required a more extensive operation than the other. Postoperative demonstration of the spinal cord is also necessary when anticipated recovery of function does not follow what appears to be satisfactory restoration of vertebral anatomy.

Although CT scans are valuable because they provide excellent demonstration of the bony elements, the spinal cord is never adequately demonstrated even by scanners with the highest resolution. For myelographic studies, CT scans enhanced by intrathe-

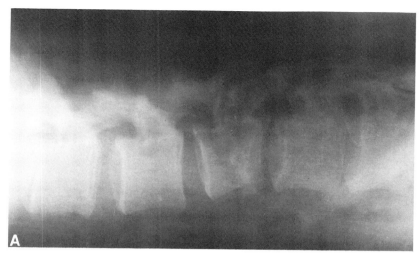

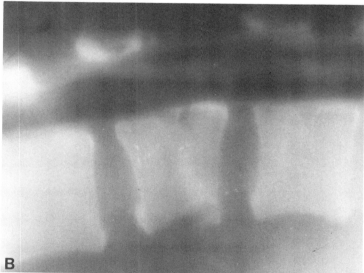

Figure 7-5. Lateral spine film (A) and gas myelogram (B) of a patient with an unstable fracture of L2. Although the lamina, pedicle, and body are fractured, the cord is not deformed and the subarachnoid space is patent anterior and posterior to the cord.

cal contrast or gas myelograms are satisfactory, although gas myelography is not available at many institutions. Contrast-enhanced CT scans are done with the patient supine, which is an advantage over gas myelography, where the patient is placed in the lateral decubitus position. This additional movement of the patient, however, has not been a source of problems.[8] Headache can be a complication of each procedure; however, gas myelography does not have adverse effects other than headache, whereas, in addition to headache, intrathecal metrizamide has a low but nevertheless significant incidence of complications including convulsions. Also, since gas myelog-

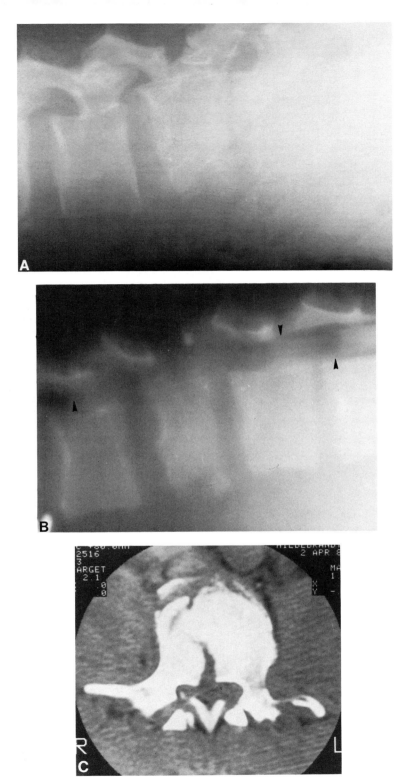

Figure 7-6. This fracture is similar to that shown in Figure 7-5. (B) The gas myelogram shows considerable involvement of the spinal cord with occlusion of the subarachnoid space from L1 to the lower portion of L3 (arrows). Although CT scans demonstrate the fracture very well, the spinal cord is not visible in the standard cuts (C) nor in the sagittal reconstruction

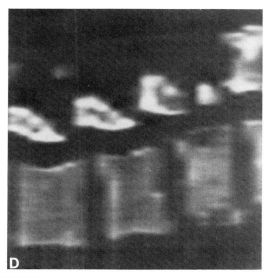

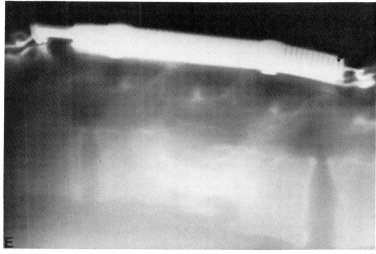

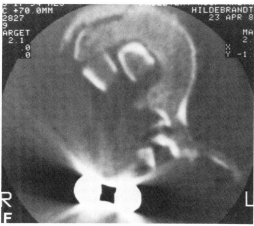

Figure 7-6. *(Continued)* (D). Postoperative polytomography (E) and CT scans (F) show that adequate bony resection was accomplished and that the position of the bone grafts was satisfactory.

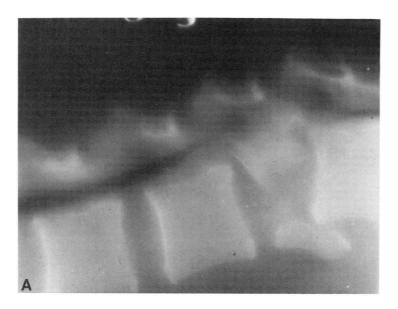

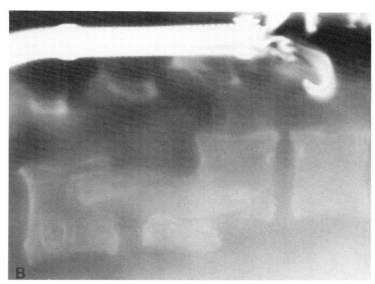

Figure 7-7. (A) A preoperative gas myelogram of a patient with severe paraparesis. (B) Postoperative polytomography demonstrates adequate resection of bone and satisfactory vertebral alignment. The patient made good neurologic recovery and was walking without assistance. He continued to have defective control of micturition.

raphy requires hypocycloidal polytomography in the sagittal planes (Figure 7-7), additional information about bony disruption is provided to supplement that obtained from CT scans. The development of nuclear magnetic resonance imaging (NMRI) can be expected to greatly reduce the need for contrast media.

An unstable fracture produced by flexion and compression can be satisfactorily treated with Harrington rods (Figure 7-3). The area immobilized is extensive, since the hooks must be applied at least two levels above and two levels below the level of instability. For thoracolumbar injuries, the superior hooks are placed beneath the inferior articular processes of a thoracic vertebra and the inferior hooks beneath the leading edge of a lumbar lamina. Consequently, flexion and extension will be restricted at the lumbar end and rotation will be restricted at the thoracic end. Since the fusion usually extends for only the length of the unstable segment, the portion of the vertebral column fixed by the rods is considerably longer than that fixed by bony union. Tension developed at the hook–bone interface subsequent to flexion, extension, and rotational movement may eventually cause symptoms and in some cases result in dislocation of the hooks. Therefore, some surgeons who use Harrington rods remove them electively after the fusion has become solid.[2]

Fractures produced by flexion and compression can also be managed with modified Weiss springs. Although plain Weiss springs provide no support against rotational or lateral stresses, modified Weiss springs, which contain stainless steel rods, provide excellent resistance against such stresses,[12] particularly when the rodded portion of the spring is fixed to the spinous processes by Parham bands (Figure 7-8B). It is necessary for the portion of the spring containing the rod to rest upon one lamina above and one below the area of instability. This amount of fixation is essential; if it is not achieved initial correction of alignment may not be maintained. Since the springs adapt partially to rotational movement at the thoracic end and flexion-extension movement at the lumbar end (Figure 7-8), the region of restricted spinal motion is less than with Harrington rods. Because some motion is possible at the hook–spring interface, the modified Weiss springs are better tolerated over the long term. Of 127 patients with thoracic and lumbar fracture in whom modified Weiss springs were placed at the Medical College of Wisconsin Affiliated Hospitals, the springs had to be removed in 4 patients because of pain that developed after the springs broke. Although the possibility of battery action produced by dissimilar metals exists, corrosion of the hooks, bands, or springs was not observed despite intervals between placement and removal of 1 to 4 years. While the Weiss springs do not tend to restore the normal length of the spinal canal and may even shorten it, this is an advantage rather than a drawback, since axial tension in the spinal cord will be decreased rather than increased as may be the case with Harrington rods.*

If rotation is added to flexion and compression, a slice fracture is produced.[9] If, for example, rotation is such that the spinous process of the rotating vertebra moves to the left, the left inferior articular process of the rotating vertebra hits the left superior process of the subjacent vertebra. The joint is disrupted and the pedicle and transverse process are avulsed and displaced laterally. On the opposite side, the facet joint is also disrupted, allowing medial movement of the inferior process of the rotating vertebra. The body of the subjacent vertebra is also disrupted. usually in a circumferential manner with a portion remaining attached to the rotating vertebral body (Figure 7-9). Because bony and ligamentous disruption is complete, this fracture is very unstable. If malalignment is not severe, a compressive device combined with interbody fusion can be used (Figure 7-10). However, with substantial lateral deformity, while fusion may be

---

* Editors' Note: Although most spinal surgeons have not used the Weiss springs because the metal has fatigued early, Dr. Larson has demonstrated how they can be used successfully. He uses a modified variety that contain a steel rod in the center of the spring's helix. These rods impart greater resistance to flexion forces than the unmodified springs. The Parham bands that Dr. Larson uses resist rotational forces.

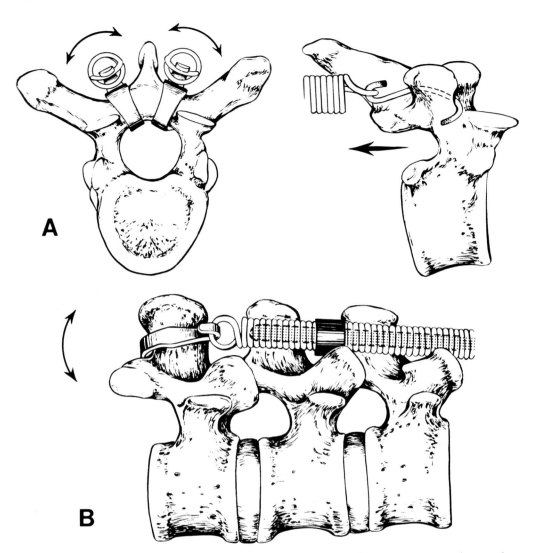

Figure 7-8. (A) At the thoracic end, the modified Weiss spring can accommodate at least partially to rotation (left) and the force exerted is parallel to the lamina (right). (B) Some flexion and extension is possible at the lumbar end of the modified springs. The Parham bands fix the rodded portion of the springs to the spinous processes, providing good resistance to lateral and rotational forces exerted across the fixed segment.

achieved, the deformity may not be corrected (Figure 7-11). Because disruption is circumferential, Harrington rods can produce excessive distraction. This may not be important in treating a patient with a complete transverse myelopathy (Figure 7-12), but it could produce further injury in a patient with an incomplete neurologic deficit.

Since both Harrington rods and Weiss springs require a resisting force to work against, neither is ideal for fractures with circumferential disruption and substantial dislocation (Figure 7-13). In this situation, Harrington rods could produce overdistrac-

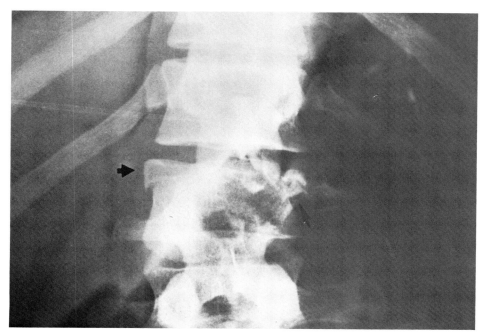

Figure 7-9. Anteroposterior projection in a patient with a slice fracture. A portion of the pedicle, superior articular process, and transverse process of L1 have been displaced laterally (small arrow). The superior portion of the body of L1 remains attached to T12 (broad arrow).

tion, while restoration of alignment would be difficult to achieve or control with modified Weiss springs. For this type of fracture, Luque rods provide the best means for obtaining accurately controlled realignment and stabilization. Luque rods are fixed to the spine by wiring the rods to the laminae for at least two levels above and two levels below the level of instability. The rods are bent to the configuration desired for the vertebral column, which is then brought into conformity with the rods by progressively tightening the wire loops. Because the Luque rods can be bent, they are particularly applicable for treating patients with flexion deformities who have had a laminectomy. The disadvantage of Luque rods is the length of time required for application and the possibility that the spinal cord could be injured as the wires are passed beneath the laminae. Luque rods also form a very rigid system, which is subjected to rotational stress at the upper end and flexion stress at the lower end when used for fixation of thoracolumbar fractures.

The optimal application for Harrington rods is a situation that requires correction of angulation and an increase in length of the vertebral column with subsequent strong vertical support. Since the rods can be bent, they can be used even if a laminectomy has been done. When combined with segmental wiring, the rods are also well suited for use in patients who are unable to tolerate a rigid orthosis because of cutaneous anesthesia.

The optimal application for Weiss springs is in treating a lap belt fracture produced by flexion and distraction (Figure 7-14). In this situation, the action of the springs, which is directly opposite to the forces that produced the injury, restores a normal

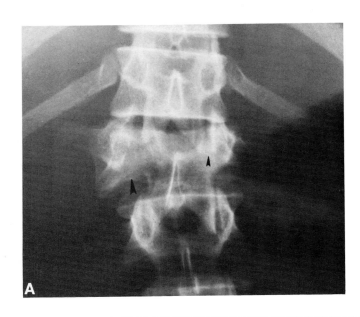

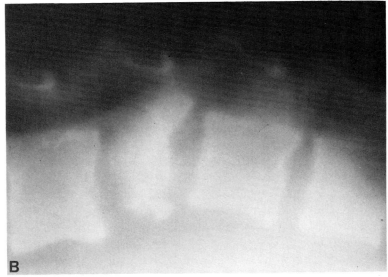

142

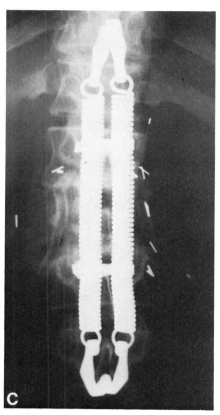

Figure 7-10. (A) Slice fracture in a patient with incomplete myelopathy. The laterally displaced fragment is unusually large (large arrow). The opposite facet joint is also disrupted (small arrow). (B) A gas myelogram of the same patient. Bone is displaced into the canal, and although the angulation is not severe, the cord is deformed. (C) Anteroposterior view 1 year after surgical reconstruction of the canal, interbody fusion, and application of modified Weiss springs. A bilateral approach was used. The patient regained normal neurologic function.

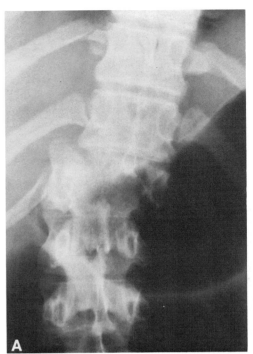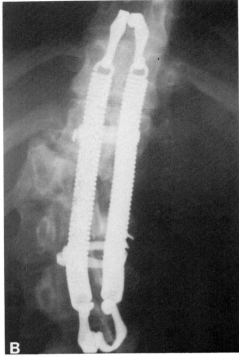

Figure 7-11. Anteroposterior view of a slice fracture with substantial lateral diplacement. The patient had a complete myelopathy. (B) The same patient 2 years later. Solid fusion has occurred and alignment, while unchanged, is not satisfactory. Luque rods would probably have provided better correction but were not available when this patient was treated.

configuration to the vertebral column. The springs usually cannot be used in patients with flexion deformities who have had a laminectomy.

The objectives of treatment in unstable thoracolumbar fractures are prevention of progressive deformity and pain in patients with complete myelopathy, improvement in neurologic function in patients with incomplete myelopathy, and preservation of function in patients who are neurologically normal. The overriding consideration is protection of the spinal cord. Treatment therefore must be directed at restoring a normal anatomic relationship between the spinal cord and the spinal canal and maintaining this relationship by making an unstable vertebral column stable. For these purposes, the posteriorly applied metallic fixation devices are very useful in correcting spinal deformity and in providing sufficient stability to permit early mobilization of the patient. It must be emphasized, however, that they serve principally as an internal splint. Long-term stability depends on solid bony union achieved either by the healing of the fracture or by bone grafts. Although relatively normal vertebral alignment may be obtained with these devices, the spinal cord may remain deformed by displaced fragments of bone or disc. Consequently, in most cases it is advisable to surgically reconstruct the spinal canal before proceeding with instrumentation.

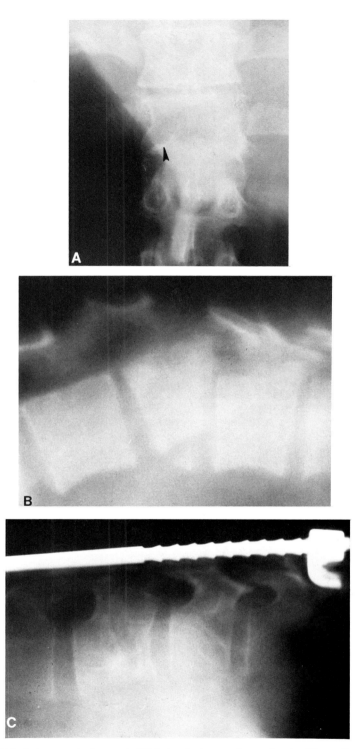

Figure 7-12. (A) Anteroposterior and (B) lateral views of a patient with a slice fracture and complete myelopathy. Harrington rods provided good fixation and correction of alignment but produced over distraction (C).

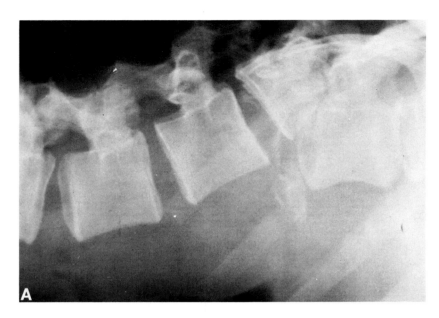

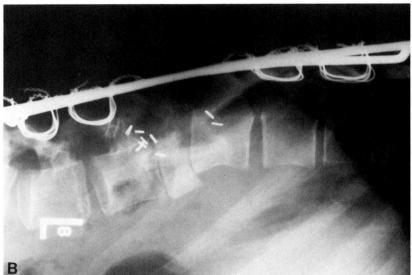

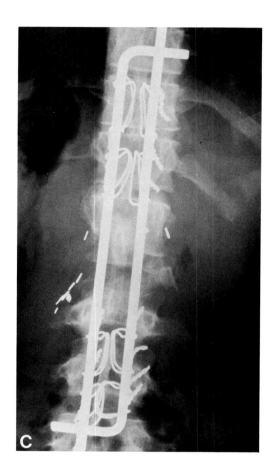

Figure 7-13. (A) The patient with this fracture dislocation at L1-2 was only-able to flex the toes and had reduced sensory perception below L2. (B) A lateral view after surgical reconstruction of the spinal canal, application of Luque rods, and interbody fusion. The appearance of residual deformity of the spinal canal is misleading and is produced by the unresected lateral portion of the body of L1. Lateral tomograms demonstrated that satisfactory reconstruction of the spinal canal has been achieved. (C) Anteroposterior projection. The patient regained normal neurologic function.

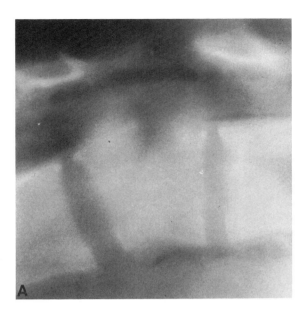

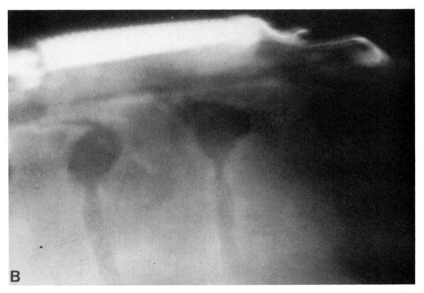

Figure 7-14. (A) A flexion distraction fracture in a patient with severe neurologic deficit. (B) The same patient after reconstruction of the canal and application of modified Weiss springs. The polytomographic cut was made through the pedicle on the side opposite the surgical approach. Neurologic function returned to normal.

THE LATERAL APPROACH TO THE THORACIC AND
LUMBAR VERTEBRAL BODIES

A skin incision is made in the midline and curved laterally at the lower end for about 10 to 12 cm or longer if necessary (Figure 7-15A). The lumbodorsal fascia is incised transversely at the level of the fracture and the incision is extended superiorly and inferiorly to separate the fascia from the spinous processes. In the thoracic area, it is usually necessary to include the trapezius muscle. After the fascial flaps are reflected, the lateral edge of the erector spinae muscle is identified, and dissection is carried out medially in the plane between the erector spinae and the quadratus lumborum. If the erector spinae is bulky, it is sometimes advantageous to split it. In the thoracic area, the longissimus, iliocostalis, and latissimus dorsi muscles are split and dissected from the ribs. The ribs are divided about 8 cm from the costotransverse joints and the medial portion is removed. The transverse processes are resected (Figure 7-15B). The spinal nerves are identified and separated from the surrounding tissue. In the thoracic area the nerve is divided about 3 cm lateral to the dorsal root ganglion and a ligature is placed on the central end of the root for retraction. The pleura, diaphragm, and retroperitoneal tissues are separated from the vertebral bodies. During this stage of the procedure, the segmental arteries are dissected from the vertebral bodies, ligated, and divided. The nerves above and below the fractured vertebral body are traced to their root foramina, and the intervening pedicle and facet joint are resected. A brace and bit is used to drill out the intervertebral disc about three fourths of the way across the vertebral body (Figure 7-15C). The intervening bone is removed with rongeurs and then curettes are used to remove the bone remaining in the posterior portion of the vertebral body beneath the floor of the spinal canal. When the floor of the canal becomes thin enough that it can be bent downward with modest pressure from a curette, upward-angled curettes are used to fracture the floor of the canal into the defect that has been created in the vertebral body. It is essential to have the floor of the canal very thin because this portion of the procedure must sometimes be done rapidly to prevent excessive blood loss from the epidural veins. Additional bone is removed to create slots in the vertebral bodies above and below the area of resection to provide a seat for the bone grafts and prevent posterior migration of the bone grafts into the spinal canal (Figure 7-15D). The self-retaining retractors are withdrawn and the spinous processes and laminae of the appropriate number of vertebrae are exposed. When this is completed, the dura is visible through the defect produced by resection of the pedicle and facet joint. After the metallic devices have been applied (Figure 7-15E), the erector spinae and other medial muscles are again retracted medially. Bone grafts are cut to a length slightly greater than the distance to be spanned. They are put into position (Figure 7-15F) and impacted. The site is inspected with a dental mirror before and after introduction of the grafts to make sure that the resection has been adequate and that the dural sac and its contents are not deformed.

A Hemovac drain is usually left in the paravertebral region for about 12 hours after surgery. If the pleura has been opened a chest tube is placed and connected to underwater drainage to prevent accumulation of blood in the thoracic cavity.

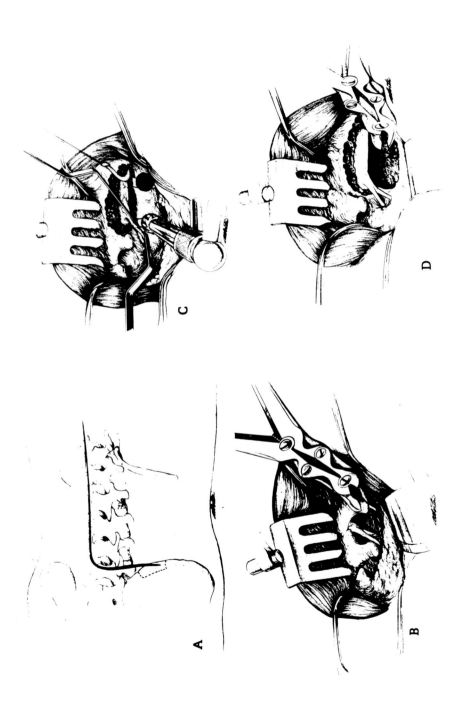

Figure 7-15. (A) This operation was done on a patient who had an unstable fracture of the second lumbar vertebra. A skin incision was begun in the lower thoracic area and curved laterally across the iliac crest. The twelfth rib, which will be resected to provide adequate exposure, and the iliac crest are available for use as bone grafts. If a bilateral approach is necessary, the lower limb of the incision can be extended across to the other side. (B) The erector spinae muscles have been separated from the quadratus lumborum and are retracted medially. The transverse process of L1 is being resected and the second lumbar nerve is visible between the first and second lumbar transverse processes. (C) The first lumbar root has been divided and is being retracted. The pedicle of L2 and the L1-2 facet joint have been resected. The L1-L2 intervertebral disc has been drilled out and the bit is being introduced into the L2-3 interspace. The diaphragm and retroperitoneal tissues have been dissected from the vertebral bodies nearly to the anterior surfaces. (D) A substantial part of the second lumbar body has been resected and the floor of the spinal canal has been removed by breaking it down into the bony defect. The bed for the bone graft is being prepared. (E) Modified Weiss springs have been applied with the portions of the springs containing the rods placed on the laminae of L1, L2, and L3. Parham bands have been used to bind the portion of the springs containing rods to the spinous processes to prevent lateral and rotational movement. The dura and second lumbar root are visible through the defect created by removal of the pedicle and facet joint. (F) The erector spinae muscle is again retracted medially and the bone graft is introduced. In this case ribs were used. Depending on the configuration of the ribs, at least two and usually three pieces can be put into the defect.

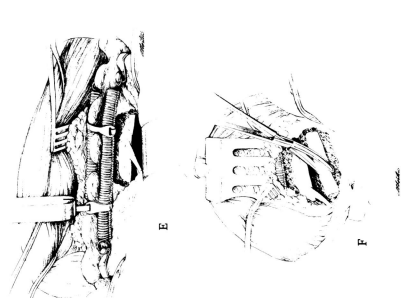

E

F

REFERENCES

1. Bedbrook GM: Spinal injuries with tetraplegia and paraplegia. J Bone Joint Surg 61B:267, 1979

2. Benzel EC, Larson SJ: Operative stabilization of the post-traumatic thoracic and lumbar spine. Surg Forum 33:507, 1982

3. Bohlman HH, Ducker TB, Lucas JT: Spine and spinal cord injuries. In Rothman RH, Simeone FA (eds): The Spine. Philadelphia, W.B. Saunders, 1982, pp 661–757

4. Breig A: Biomechanics of the central nervous system. Some basic normal and pathologic phenomena. Stockholm, Almquist and Wiksell, 1960

5. Dickson JH, Harrington PR, Erwin WD: Results of reduction and stabilization of the severely fractured thoracic and lumbar spine. J Bone Joint Surg 60A:799, 1978

6. Flesch JR, Leider LL, Erickson DL, Chou SN, Bradford DS: Harrington instrumentation and spine fusion for unstable fractures and fracture dislocations of the thoracic and lumbar spine. J Bone Joint Surg 59A:143, 1977

7. Frankel HL, Hancock DO, Hyslop G: The value of postural reduction in the initial management of closed injuries of the spine with paraplegia and tetraplegia. Paraplegia 7:179, 1969

8. Hemmy DC, Larson SJ: Gas myelography in spinal cord injury. J Trauma 19:145, 1979

9. Holdsworth FW: Fractures, dislocations and fracture-dislocations of the spine. J Bone Joint Surg 45B:6, 1963

10. Larson SJ, Holst RA, Hemmy DC, Sances A Jr: Lateral extracavitary approach to traumatic lesions of the thoracic and lumbar spine. J Neurosurg 45:628, 1976

11. Maiman DJ, Larson SJ, Benzel BC: Neurological improvement associated with late decompression of the thoracolumbar spinal cord. Neurosurgery 14:302, 1984

12. Maiman DJ, Sances A Jr, Myklebust J, Larson SJ, Flatley T, Neseman S: Comparison of the failure biomechanics of spinal fixation devices. Neurosurgery 17:574, 1985

13. Malcolm BW, Bradford DS, Winter RB, Chou SN: Post-traumatic kyphosis: A review of forty-eight surgically treated patients. J Bone Joint Surg 63A:891, 1981

14. Nicoll EA: Fractures of the dorso-lumbar spine. J Bone Joint Surg 31B:376, 1949

15. Schmidek HH, Gomes FB, Seligson D, McSherry JW: Management of acute unstable thoracolumbar fracture (T11-L1) with and without neurological deficit. Neurosurgery 7:30, 1980

16. Southwick WO, Robinson RA: Surgical approaches to the vertebral bodies in the cervical and lumbar regions. J Bone Joint Surg 39A:631, 1957

17. Whitesides TE Jr, Shaw SGA: On the management of unstable fractures of the thoracolumbar spine: Rationale for use of anterior decompression and fusion and posterior stabilization. Spine 1:99, 1976

Frank J. Eismont
Barth A. Green

8

Technical Considerations in the Management of the Unstable Lumbar Spine

Contemporary spinal surgeons have developed an approach to the unstable spine that combines the principles of adequate neural decompression with those of providing stability. In this context, it is timely to discuss the appropriate indications for lumbar spinal decompression or stabilization, what determines the appropriate degree of decompression of the neurologic elements, and the relative advantages of the available surgical techniques for stabilization of the lumbar spine and their potential complications.

THERAPEUTIC PATHWAYS

Patients with significant lumbar fractures who do not have a neurologic deficit are kept immobilized on a Roto Rest Kinetic Treatment Table[16,17] until they can be scheduled for elective decompression and stabilization. During this period, their neurologic condition is repeatedly monitored. If a patient develops evidence of a progressive deficit, he or she undergoes emergency surgery if indicated. In most cases, even those of severe fractures, the use of the kinetic bed allows us to perform the operative procedures on an elective basis.[27,28] Patients who have a significant neurologic deficit and evidence of impingement of the spinal canal on CT scans are treated by immediate decompression and stabilization. It is our belief that lumbar dislocations with minimal bony disruption are best treated with Harrington distraction or compression rod or Luque rod instrumentation,[1–5,12,15,18,20] since these are predominantly posterior ligamentous injuries and the reduction itself should accomplish the desired degree of bony realignment. Burst fractures of the vertebral body can be treated either with Harrington distraction rods or Harrington distraction rods combined with a simultaneous posterolateral decompression[10] or alternatively by anterior corpectomy and stabilization using strut bone grafts. Luque instrumentation is not appropriate in the treatment of burst fractures because the spine may telescope along the rods, resulting in further retropulsion of vertebral body fragments into the spinal canal. We are inclined to use anterior decompression and fusion for injuries involving the vertebral bodies of L3 and L4 because of our reluctance to immobilize and fuse the entire lower lumbar spine or lumbar spine and sacrum.[8] The anterior approach, however, cannot be used by itself if there is significant disruption of the posterior elements.[10] Injuries at the level of L5 present unique surgical problems because of the difficulties of attaching instrumentation to the pelvis or sacrum, and at present Luque instrumentation offers the best solution. There is no role for lumbar laminectomy in the primary treatment of the vast majority of closed injuries to the lumbar spine. Laminectomy results in further spinal instability, a potentially greater deformity (Figure 8-1), and, possibly, progressive neurologic deficit.[23,25]

There are three different surgical approaches to the unstable lumbar spine. The midline posterior approach performed with either a bilateral transverse process fusion,[24] or with rods and wires and bony fusion[4,7,14,15,18,20] (these procedures may be combined with posterolateral decompressions[12]); anterior decompressions and fusions of the spine performed by a retroperitoneal transabdominal or a transthoracic approach[3,5,22]; or by combined anterior and posterior approaches to the lumbar spine.[13]

POSTERIOR APPROACH TO THE LUMBAR SPINE

Because of the instability of the spine and the potential for worsening a neurologic deficit, patients with spinal instability resulting from disruption of anterior and posterior elements should be intubated while awake, turned to the prone position, checked neurologically, and then anesthetized. In these cases an appropriate frame is used to support the patient. Once the patient has been log-rolled to the prone position and anesthetized, baseline somatosensory evoked potential recordings are checked to monitor for neurologic deterioration. These recordings can be continued throughout the remainder of the operative procedure if specific anesthetics such as nitrous/narcotic or light fluothane are used.

Posterolateral Fusion In Situ

For patients with a minor degree of spinal instability, a bilateral lateral transverse process fusion is performed. This operation is preferable to the various posterior midline fusions because these may result in fusion mass overgrowth[21,24], which may produce a secondary stenosis of the lumbar canal. The technique is performed through a posterior midline incision with exposure of the spinous processes, lamina, facet joints, and transverse processes at each level to be fused. The posterior cortical surface of the transverse processes is then removed either with a high-speed burr or with a sharp curette. Decortication is carried out medially onto the lateral surface of the facet of the same numbered vertebra, which increases the surface area of exposed bone for fusion. The facet joints to be fused are prepared by first removing the posterior joint capsule and the joint cartilage from both the medial and lateral aspects of each facet joint. Corticocancellous strips of bone are placed over the transverse processes to be fused and cancellous bone is impacted into each of the facet joints with a bone tamp and mallet.

Lumbar lordosis should be preserved whenever possible when the Harrington distraction system is used. To accomplish this, square-ended Moe rods should be used with a 1201-50 hook on the inferior end of the rod to prevent rotation of the rod and to allow lordosis to be bent into the rod for injuries below L1. If a standard round-ended Harrington rod and 1254 hook were to be used and lordosis was bent into the rod, the rod would eventually rotate 180 degrees and would result in a lumbar kyphosis being held in place with the rods rather than the desired lordosis.

A major difference between the thoracic spine and the lumbar spine is that the length of fusion in the thoracic or thoracolumbar spine does not have a major effect on the patient's subsequent mobility or predispose him or her to significant future degenerative problems. In the lumbar spine it is important whether there are one or two mobile segments below a fusion. As the number of unfused segments is diminished, the concentration of stress within the joints is increased and the propensity for degenerative changes and future back pain are increased. When it is necessary to fuse to the pelvis, adequate lordosis should be maintained to prevent an abnormal stance and gait.

The two problems of having a small number of mobile segments below a fusion and of obtaining proper posture when the lumbar spine is fused to the pelvis can be managed partially by the concept of "rodding long and fusing short," with elective removal of the Harrington rods approximately 1 year later.

Technical considerations in the positioning of the Harrington rods include placing the upper 1253 Harrington rod hooks or Edwards hooks under the medial part of the lamina to decrease the chances of the hooks fracturing through the facet joints or the inferior aspect of the lamina as the patient flexes forward.* The inferior hooks can be placed on the lamina as far caudally as the fifth lumbar vertebra. The hook should not be placed on the first sacral lamina because of the thinness of this structure. When fixation to the sacrum is necessary, it should always be accomplished with sacral alar hooks and used in conjunction with square-ended Moe rods. These hooks should be secured into the alar processes of the sacrum bilaterally. Using the specifically designated hooks and creating an angle with the rod allows the lateral degree of placement. The Harrington rods should extend three levels above and two levels below an unstable segment. This construct is mechanically stable and reduces the incidence of hook cut-out.[26] Before the insertion of the Harrington rods, the intervening facet joint capsules and facet joint cartilages are removed and each of these joints is packed with autogenous iliac cancellous bone. The transverse processes are prepared as described previously.

When Harrington rods are used to reduce fractures of the lumbar spine, it may be necessary to use a straight Harrington rod on one side, then insert a slightly lordotic Harrington rod on the opposite side, after which the straight Harrington rod is replaced with a rod having a lordotic curve. This maneuver may have to be repeated until the desired degree of lordosis is achieved. To reduce the incidence of rod dislodgement, double-thickness 18-gauge stainless steel wires are passed beneath the laminae and around the Harrington rod at the level below the upper hooks and at the level above the lower hooks.[4] Care must be taken that when the hooks are placed under the lamina there is not excessive anterior-to-posterior movement of the rods. This is occasionally seen in patients with thin laminae. If excessive movement is present and the segmental wires are tightened, the hooks may be forced into the spinal canal and produce a

---

* Editors' Note: Some authors believe that the superior hooks should be placed into the facet.

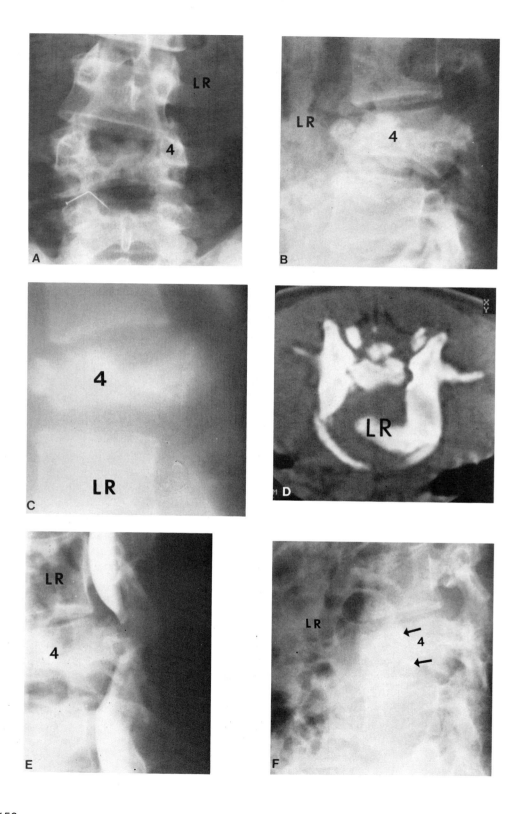

neurologic deficit. The wires are tightened in a clockwise direction with the rostral end of the loop medial to the rod and the caudal loop lateral to the rod in a "Christmas Tree" configuration proximally and in the appropriate manner distally. Additional bone grafts are applied around the rods on the segments to be fused. Copious amounts of antibiotic solution are used to irrigate the surgical field, and the deep fascia is closed with inverted simple sutures of a heavy monofilament to avoid wound dehiscence.

There are two situations in which the use of Harrington distraction rods can be disadvantageous. In patients with an extremely unstable spine, such as in cases of acute trauma in which there is disruption of all anterior and posterior ligaments, Harrington rods may overdistract the bony and neural elements and produce or aggravate a neurologic deficit. The other situation is one in which the patient has a fixed deformity, such as a fixed kyphosis, and there is a healed fracture with bone protruding into the spinal canal, or a tumor extending into the canal from the posterior aspect of the

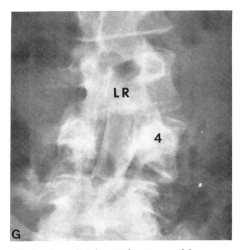

Figure 8-1. This patient sustained an L4 burst fracture with severe paralysis of the L4 nerve roots and all more distal nerve roots, with complete loss of bowel and bladder control. He was treated acutely with an L4 laminectomy but did not improve neurologically. (A) An anteroposterior roentgenogram shows moderate scoliosis. (B) A lateral roentgenogram suggests that there is a significant amount of bone that has been retropulsed into the spinal canal. (C) A midsagittal lateral tomogram confirms the extent of spinal canal impingement by the retropulsed bone. (D) A CT scan also reveals bone fragments protruding into the spinal canal. (E) A myleogram initially showed a complete blockage at the L4 level and this myelogram required an injection of metrizamide above and below the L4 level. A lateral roentgenogram of the myelography procedure shows severe impingement on the neural elements from anteriorly placed bone fragments. The neural compression has not been altered by the laminectomy. (F) The patient was treated with a posterolateral transverse process fusion followed the same day by an anterior transabdominal approach for resection of the L4 vertebral body and anterior fusion of L3 to L5 with an autogenous iliac graft. This shows the posterior aspect of the bone graft (see arrows). (G) The vertebral body resection can be seen on this anteroposterior roentgenogram. This extends from one L4 pedicle to the opposite side and the iliac bone graft can again be seen. The anterior decompression and fusion could also have been achieved via a retroperitoneal sympathectomy approach and this would now be the approach of choice. This patient's neurologic function improved significantly.

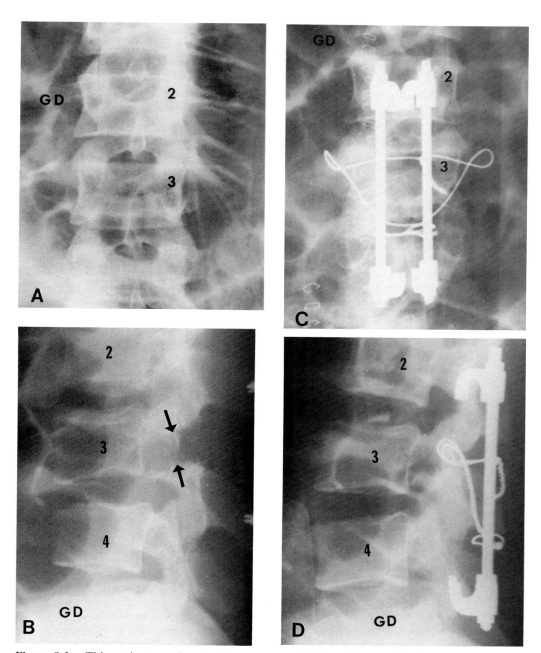

Figure 8-2. This patient was involved in a motor vehicle accident and had severe midlumbar spine pain and a severe paraparesis with diminished bowel and bladder control. (A) An anteroposterior roentgenogram reveals grossly normal alignment of the spine, and the distance between the spinous processes is approximately normal. The patient is most tender between the L2 and L3 spinous processes. (B) A lateral roentgenogram taken intraoperatively reveals abnormal angulation at the L3-4 interspace with this interspace being wider posteriorly than would normally be seen. A fracture at the pars interarticularlis (arrows) can also be seen. This x-ray film also shows an increased distance between the L2 and L3 spinous processes consistent

158

vertebral body. Distraction rods would cause the neural elements to be pulled more tightly across such a deformity which may produce or aggravate a neurologic deficit. The first situation can be recognized intraoperatively by palpating the dura, by obtaining intraoperative roentgenograms, or by using intraoperative real-time ultrasound. The second problem can be averted by recognizing when a patient has a point of fixed impingement in the canal and removing such an anteriorly situated pathologic condition before the distraction instrumentation is inserted.

Harrington Compression Rods for the Unstable Lumbar Spine

Harrington compression rods are threaded rods of either 1/8th- or 3/16th-inch diameter and are used with either 1259 or 1254 hooks. In the thoracolumbar and lumbar spine, these hooks are placed under the lamina and rigidly fix the spine. In laboratory testing, the strength provided by Harrington compression rods is greater than that provided by Harrington distraction rods (without added segmental wiring). The distraction rods can lose their purchase on the upper and lower lamina as a result of gradual stretching of the intervening soft tissue structures at each level. The Harrington compression system has less of a tendency to loosen with time. A compression system should not be used if the middle column of the spine is unstable, as in the case of a burst fracture, because it could cause further extrusion of bone into the canal. Harrington compression rods are best used when the posterior aspects of the vertebral bodies are intact and the major cause of the instability is posterior ligamentous disruption[18] (Figure 8-2). They are indicated for lumbar dislocations and for Chance fractures, both of which occur as a result of flexion and distraction. When Harrington compression rods are used the loss of lordosis is not as significant a consideration as when distraction rods are used because compression rods are usually placed only one segment above and one segment below the level of ligamentous disruption. The fusion is then short and the patient will be able to compensate with an adequate range of motion above and below the fusion. Also, as the Harrington compression rods are tightened, they produce a degree of lordosis by shortening the posterior column of the spine.

Harrington compression rods are inserted through the same exposure as is used for distraction rods. Laminotomies are performed at the interspace where the hooks will be placed under the lamina and in the spinal canal. No bone is removed from the lamina that will support the hooks. If any bone has to be removed in order to allow placement,

---

with a fracture of the pars. At surgery there was gross instability at the L3-4 interspace with complete disruption of the posterior longitudinal ligament as well as the annulus fibrosis. This was clinically suspected because of the patient's severe degree of paralysis with no evidence of bone retropulsed into the spinal canal. (C) A postoperative anteroposterior roentgenogram reveals Harrington compression rods extending from the L2 to the L4 lamina in order to bridge the lamina, which was free floating. The 18-gauge wire had been passed around the transverse processes of the L3 vertebra and was then looped under the loose L3 lamina in order to serve as a tension-band and reapproximate this fracture. (D) A postoperative lateral roentgenogram reveals the Harrington compression rods in place as well as the tension-band wire. The gap that was previously present at the pars interarticularis has been greatly diminished. At this time the spine is clinically stable. Postoperatively, the patient's neurologic deficit gradually improved. He was ambulated immediately after surgery in a total-contact body jacket.

it should be taken from the lamina proximal to the hook placement site in the case of the rostral hooks and from the lamina distal to the caudal hook. Just as with placing the hooks for Harrington distraction rods, the pars interarticularis should not be violated because it is the point of greatest weakness and where the system will frequently fail.[15] A simple way to tighten the nuts on the threaded rods and to tighten the lower hook is to place the rod holder on the caudal end of the rod and a hook holder on the lowest hook. The Harrington distractor is then used to spread between these and the nut can then be advanced easily up the threaded rod by simply spinning it with a Penfield dissector.

Harrington compression and distraction rods should always be used in pairs, one rod being located on each side of the central spinous processes. Scoliosis will develop if the rods are not used in pairs. Once the nuts have been tightened on both rods, the threads adjacent to the nut are stripped to prevent loosening and loss of reduction. Alternatively, the nut and the threaded rod can be covered with a small amount of methylmethacrylate to prevent the nut from loosening. If the Wisconsin system of slotted hooks and sleeves is used, then the methylmethacrylate can be placed over the sleeves and hook as well as the nut and threaded rod in order to prevent dislodgement of the hook from the sleeve. A small amount of methylmethacrylate is advisable because the cement does not provide additional strength.

Harrington compression rods can be used with Harrington distraction rods to prevent overdistraction at the site of instability and thereby decrease the chances of dislodgement of the upper hooks (Figure 8-3). To use this combination of rods, the Harrington distraction rods are inserted and a laminotomy is performed one level rostral to the laminotomy for the upper 1253 hooks. A similar laminotomy is then performed at a level caudal to the 1254 hook and a 1/8th-inch Harrington compression rod is used in combination with a 1259 hook above and below, which is placed under the lamina at the new laminotomy sites. By tightening this system, the lamina is prevented from moving up and over the upper 1253 hook when the patient flexes forward. Once the nuts have been tightened on both ends of the rod the threads adjacent to the nut are stripped or a small amount of methylmethacrylate is placed over the sleeves and hook as well as the nut and threaded rod to prevent loosening. This combination of rods is best suited for fractures that require a degree of distraction to achieve a reduction but that are extremely unstable and may be overdistracted. The transverse processes and the intervening facet joints are prepared for fusion exactly as previously described. Autogenous iliac bone grafts are used in addition to local bone graft to enhance the fusion rate.

Luque Rods for the Unstable Lumbar Spine

Luque instrumentation is an extremely rigid system but it cannot apply distraction or compression. Luque rods are bent to achieve lordosis in an unstable segment that is kyphotic or neutral. Luque rods control lateral translation extremely well. In cases of trauma, Luque rods can be used as an alternative to Harrington compression rods to treat dislocations (Figure 8-4). They should not be used to treat fractures with comminution of the posterior vertebral body because the spine may telescope along the course of the Luque rods and allow bone fragments to protrude further into the spinal canal. Two advantages of this system are (1) because of its great strength and rigidity, patients may often be mobilized without postoperative bracing; and (2) the L-rod system provides the most secure system of instrumentation for fixing the lumbar spine to the pelvis.[1] By incorporating lumbar lordosis into the rods and by carefully calculating the angle of fixation to the pelvis, a very normal posture may be achieved and a flat back and the "jumper's posture" can be avoided.

Use of this system in the treatment of instability requires instrumentation with fixation to at least two laminae above and below the unstable segment. The rigidity may be increased by adding a third segment above and below the unstable segment into the construct. A small central laminotomy is performed superior and inferior to the rod and at each intervening segment. Double-thickness 18-gauge stainless steel wire is passed under the lamina at the laminotomy sites.

When treating a spine deformity as in scoliosis, only one wire, which has been doubled, is passed beneath the lamina at each level. This is cut and one of the wires wrapped around each side of the lamina. In cases of instability resulting from tumor,[11] trauma, or infection, two doubled wires should be passed at each level to decrease the possibility of subsequent wire breakage. These wires should never be "fed" into the spinal canal; rather, they should be pulled through the spinal canal with a wire holder firmly attached to the tip while traction is simultaneously applied to the loose end of the wire. This will ensure that the wire is kept against the underside of the lamina as it is being passed through the spinal canal. The free ends of the wire are then secured with clamps having similar markings to facilitate correct pairing and to keep the wire ends out of the way of the surgeons.

The Luque L-shaped rods are then cut to length. In cases of significant spinal instability, the 1/4th-inch L-shaped rods are used. The 3/16th-inch L-rods often are used for fixation to the pelvis, since it is very difficult to contour the 1/4-inch rods. For the lumbar spine, the required amount of lordosis is bent into the rods and adequate lengths are left on the short segment of the "L" so that it may be overlapped by the long segment of the L-rod on the opposite side of the spinous process, thereby forming a rectangle.

To decrease the chances of cutting through the lamina, the cephalad end of the wire should be medial to the rod and the caudad end of the wire should be lateral to the rod. Wiring is begun at the central portion of the L-rod and proceeds toward the end of the rod with the bend in it. Once one half of the rod is in place, the L-rod for the opposite side is inserted so that the short end of the "L" from the opposite side is under the long end of the L-rod being wired. The wires should be twisted clockwise while traction is applied upward and until the wires lose the sheen on their surface or until they begin to twist abnormally at their base. Care should always be taken to have the rod snugly secured to the lamina at the base of the spinous process and to twist the wires tight enough to hold the rod in place. The surgeon should not try to pull the rod toward the lamina by the twisting process itself, since this will cause fatigue fracture of the wires. The segmental wires at the point where the L-rods overlap should pass over both rods so that they stay overlapped by securing the long end of the L-rod on one side firmly over the short end of the L-rod on the opposite side. The two wires around the most cephalad lamina should be placed around the rods in the opposite direction from all the lower wires so that the caudal portion of the wire is medial and the cephalad portion of the wire is lateral.

For fixation to the pelvis, a hole is made in the medial aspect of the iliac crest at the base of the posterior superior iliac spine just adjacent to the sacrum. A 3/16th-inch or 1/4th-inch drill is driven through this hole more than 6 cm and if possible more than

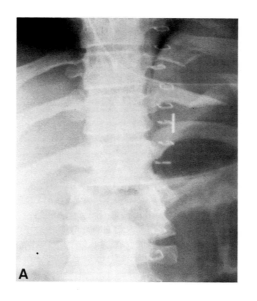

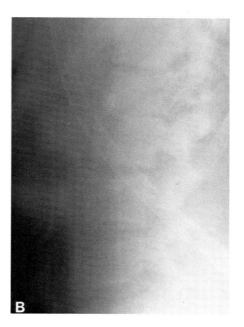

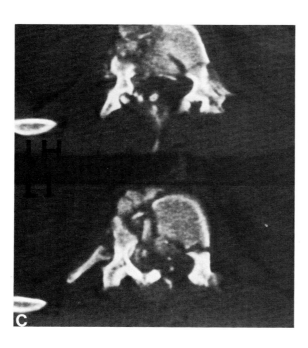

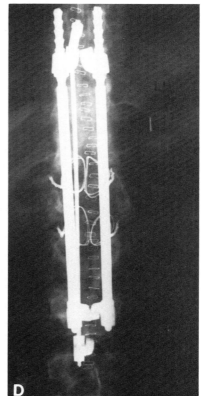

162

9 cm into the iliac crest. Before this is done, the lateral aspect of the ilium must be exposed so that the sciatic notch can be adequately identified by direct visualization. A Steinmann pin should be placed as close to the sciatic notch as possible without entering it and should definitely be less than 1.5 cm away from it. The Steinmann pin should course between the inner and outer tables of the pelvis. A 3/16th-inch or 1/4th-inch L-rod is then bent to allow it to be driven into the ilium along the course that

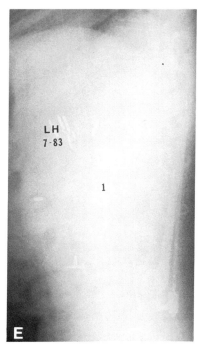

Figure 8-3. This patient sustained multiple injuries including an L1 fracture with incomplete paraplegia as a result of jumping from a building. (A) This anteroposterior roentgenogram demonstrates a fracture- dislocation at the L1 vertebral level with lateral listhesis. (B) A lateral roentgenogram again shows comminution of the L1 vertebral body but the degree of bony destruction is minimally evident on this view. (C) CT scans through the L1 vertebral body reveal multiple fracture lines with anterior and posterior disruption as well as significant encroachment on the spinal canal by bone fragments. At the time of surgery it was necessary for an assistant to stabilize the spine with clamps on the adjacent spinous processes to prevent displacment during the procedure. It was apparent that the anterior longitudinal ligament had also been disrupted in addition to the posterior elements. When Harrington distraction rods were initially positioned there was no resistance while the distraction was being accomplished. For this reason it was necessary to place a Harrington compression rod over this unstable segment once the proper vertebral height had been achieved. (D) The Harrington compression rod can be seen in this view spanning the entire length of the Harrington distraction rods and hence locking the hooks in place. Segmental wires were passed around the laminae to prevent side-to-side motion, which was still possible with the Harrington rods in place. (E) A lateral roentgenogram demonstrates the Harrington compression rod in place in addition to the Harrington distraction rods to prevent overdistraction. This patient later required an anterior corpectomy and fusion in order to fully obtain neural decompression.

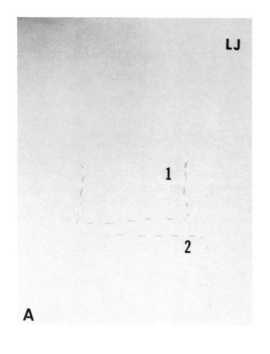

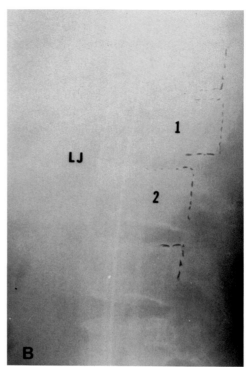

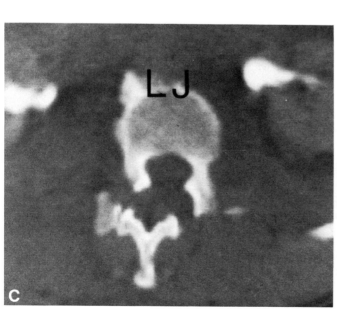

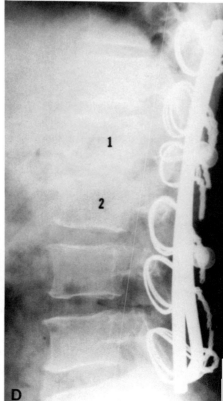

the Steinmann pin has traveled and then turn directly medial once exiting the pelvis so that it will lie directly on the sacrum. It should then be bent 90 degrees cephalad. The rods should have curvature bent into them to preserve lumbar lordosis. A high-speed burr is used to make a laminotomy at the inferior portion of the S1 lamina through the posterior roof of the sacrum, and a double-thickness segmental wire is then passed through this hole in the back of the sacrum and brought out through the L5-S1 interspace. This procedure is carried out bilaterally. After the L-rods are driven into the ilium, a sacral wire as well as the segmental wires at the other levels are tightened as the rod is approximated to the spine with direct manual pressure. This technique provides extremely rigid fixation to the pelvis and is the only system that allows adequate contouring of the rods to preserve normal lordosis (Figure 8-5). Bone grafts may still be obtained from the superior aspect of the lateral iliac crest as long as no supporting bone adjacent to the intrapelvic rod is removed. The ala of the sacrum is available for decortication and use as a site for placement of bone grafts. When this type of segmental spinal instrumentation with L-rods is used, the facet joints and the lamina are not decorticated since this would decrease the strength of the segmental wire fixation. The transverse processes are prepared simply by removing their posterior cortical surface and the lateral cortical surface from the superior facets. This provides an adequate bed to receive the bone grafts. Additional bone grafts are placed over the

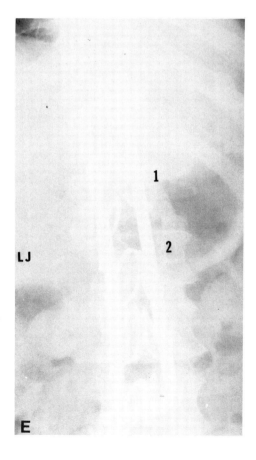

Figure 8-4. This patient sustained a spine injury and had a complete T12 level paraplegia. (A) An anteroposterior roentgenogram shows a 25 percent lateral listhesis at L1-2 with no apparent vertebral fractures. (B) A lateral roentgenogram demonstrates a 40-percent retrolisthesis of L1 on L2 with no obvious fractures. (C) A CT scan reveals a facet fracture on one side of L1-2 and a facet separation on the other side. This injury is predominantly ligamentous and the instability associated with these x-ray findings is unusually severe. (D) A postoperative lateral roentgenogram shows Luque rods in place with the subluxation decreased. Note the lordosis bent into these rods. The spine at surgery was extremely unstable with all ligaments disrupted both anteriorly and posteriorly. If Harrington distraction rods had been inserted in this case, the neural elements and spine would most likely have been severely overdistracted. (E) An anteroposterior roentgenogram shows the Luque rods and segmental wires in place. The patient was mobilized immediately after surgery in a total-contact body jacket. His neurologic condition has not improved significantly.

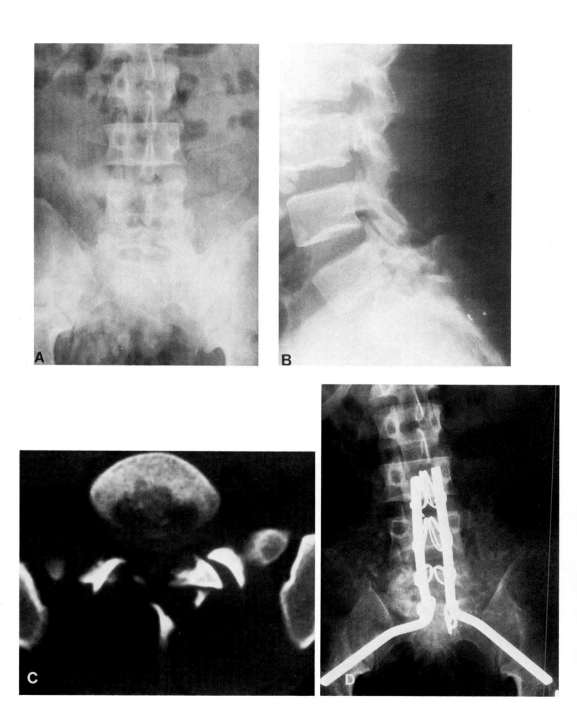

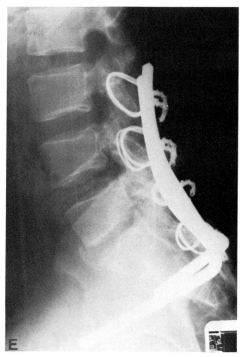

Figure 8-5. This patient had been involved in a motor vehicle accident and had severe low back pain as well as pain in the nerve root distribution of S1 and decreased perineal sensation. (A) An anteroposterior roentgenogram reveals fractures of the L3 and L4 transverse processes as well as a transverse fracture of the lamina of L5. (B) This lateral roentgenogram demonstrates a fracture of the spinous processes of L4 and L5 and is suggestive of a fracture at the level of the pars interarticularis of L5. (C) This CT scan at the L5-S1 level demonstrates the "empty facet" sign showing that the inferior facet of L5 is completely dislodged from its normal position adjacent to the S1 facet. Multiple fractures of the posterior elements are apparent. A large central disc extrusion is also visible at the L5-S1 level on this scan. The patient was taken to surgery for decompression of his neural elements and stabilization of his spine. At the time of surgery it was found that the L5 vertebra along with the upper lumbar spine could be easily dislocated from the sacrum with minimal force. It could be dislocated both anteriorly and posteriorly as well as from side to side. (D) The patient was treated with Luque rod fusion to the pelvis and up to L3 in order to adequately immobilize this area and allow ambulation in a total contact body orthosis. It should be noted that the Luque rod extends to within a centimeter of the sciatic notch joint on this anteroposterior view. At 6 months follow-up the extensive fusion from L3 to the pelvis is evident. At the time of surgery a large central disc extrusion was found and was removed before instrumentation. (E) This lateral roentgenogram demonstrates that adequate lordosis has been maintained with the use of the Luque rods. A spontaneous fusion has also occurred at the L5-S1 interspace as can be seen anteriorly and this again emphasizes the extent of trauma that was initially present.

bases of the spinous processes, which can be cut half-way down to the lamina and placed over the lamina, which has not been decorticated.

Posterolateral Decompression of the Spinal Canal

Posterolateral decompression of the spinal canal was described by Flesch et al.[12] and can be used for decompression of the anterior aspect of the spinal canal through a posterior exposure. It also can be used in combination with the various methods of fixation and fusion described previously. A CT scan is examined to determine the side of the canal that has the largest amount of anterior impingement so the side most affected can be approached through a laminotomy. Usually neural compression is caused by a burst fracture or by a tumor arising from the posterior portion of the vertebral body. The laminotomy provides access to the upper half of the vertebral body. Bone is removed to the pedicle, and the margins of the pedicle are defined. A high-speed drill is used to remove the medial one half to two thirds of the pedicle. The lateral one third of the pedicle should be left whenever possible to preserve the transverse process at that level and facilitate bone grafting and fusion. A gutter is fashioned in the posterolateral portion of the vertebral body with the high-speed drill. Reverse-angle curettes are used to remove the bone protruding into the spinal canal from the vertebral body by gently tapping it away from the neural elements and into the gutter. These pieces of bone can then be removed. Approximately three quarters of the width of the spinal canal may be decompressed from each side in this fashion. Often a pathologic condition on the opposite side cannot be eliminated unless a bilateral posterolateral exposure or a ventral exposure is used. In this circumstance, intraoperative ultrasound is particularly useful in verifying the degree of initial compression and in ensuring that adequate decompression has been accomplished (Figure 8-6).

With lumbar fracture-dislocations treated initially by reduction with Harrington rods, intraoperative ultrasonography can be used to repeatedly monitor the configuration of the spinal canal. This is done through a small laminotomy. If it is determined that the spinal canal has not been adequately reconstituted, the Harrington rod on the maximally affected side is cut out or maneuvered loose and a formal posterolateral decompression is performed, following which the Harrington rod is replaced. If residual compression remains on the opposite side as determined by ultrasonography, the procedure is repeated on that side.

ANTERIOR APPROACHES TO THE LUMBAR SPINE

The Retroperitoneal Approach to the Lumbar Spine

The retroperitoneal approach to the lumbar spine was described by Southwick and Robinson[29] and others[3] and provides excellent exposure from the first to the fifth lumbar vertebrae, allowing complete excision of the vertebral bodies and radical decompression of the spinal canal.

The patient is positioned in a straight lateral decubitus position so the back is perpendicular to the floor. The approach is usually from the patient's left flank and avoids the delicate inferior vena cava and allows easier exposure and palpation of the aorta. The incision is started directly over the midportion of the twelfth rib and extended anteriorly to the lateral edge of the rectus sheath, aiming at a point halfway between the umbilicus and the symphysis pubis. The skin, subcutaneous tissue, deep fascia, external abdominal oblique, internal abdominal oblique, and transversus abdominus muscles are incised. Posteriorly, the incision is extended through the anterior portion of the latissimus dorsi muscle before encountering the twelfth rib. The periosteum is incised in the midline along the length of the rib and then rolled cephalad and caudad to the edge of the rib. A Cobb elevator or a rib stripper then is used to elevate the periosteum off the inner aspect of the rib. The twelfth rib is cut at its midportion. The peritoneum is encountered just beneath the transversus abdominus muscle and the transversalis fascia. It is usually covered with a thin layer of fat. This fat can be rolled from the peritoneum with a sponge placed on the tip of the index finger. The dissection is continued posteriorly and medially so that the peritoneum and its contents fall away from the flank. The plane of the dissection is anterior to the iliopsoas muscle (if by error the dissection is carried posterior to the iliopsoas muscle a blind pouch will be entered). The spine can then be palpated and blunt dissection should be used to expose the anterior portion of the lumbar vertebral bodies. The crus of the diaphragm has fibers originating from the anterior surface of the first and second lumbar vertebrae that can be detached with electrocautery. There is a thin layer of fascia and areolar tissue overlying the lumbar spine at this point. If the surgeon is positioned at the anterior aspect of the incision a hand can be placed on the abdominal contents and the aorta and the segmental artery and vein can be cut. These vessels are located exactly in the middle position of each vertebral body coursing from the aorta and vena cava toward the neural forminae. These vessels should always be divided halfway between the aorta and the edge of the iliopsoas muscle. Bleeding can be controlled by placing a finger directly over the proximal end of the segmental vessels. An assistant can aid in obtaining hemostasis by placing pressure on the distal ends of the segmental vessels with a small sponge held in a clamp. The vessels are then cauterized. Hemostasis is tested by first withdrawing pressure on the distal ends of the vessels and then withdrawing pressure on the proximal ends of the vessels.

If exposure of the fourth and fifth lumbar vertebrae is required, the iliac artery and the iliac vein are visualized and protected to avoid injury (particularly the iliac vein). It must be remembered that as the peritoneal contents and the great vessels are rotated anteriorly, the aorta is anterior to the inferior vena cava and the iliac artery is anterior to the common iliac vein, making these structures more vulnerable to injury. The sympathetic chain lies immediately medial to the psoas muscle on the anterior surface of the vertebral bodies. This may be cut without adverse effects although the patient may subsequently complain of the opposite leg feeling cold.* Blunt dissection should be used to develop an extraperiosteal plane beneath the segmental vessels to expose the opposite side of the vertebral body and dissect the psoas muscle from the lateral aspect of the vertebral bodies to the level of the neural foramina.

A chest retractor is placed against the eleventh rib superiorly and the iliac crest inferiorly to maintain the exposure. The crossbar for the retractor is placed anteriorly and a 2-inch malleable retractor is placed on the opposite side of the lumbar spine from which the exposure has been developed and is attached to the crossbar of the retractor

---

* Editors' Note: Impotence may occur after division of the parasympathetic chain. The frequency of this complication can be reduced by avoiding use of electrocautery during dissection in the region of the body of L5.

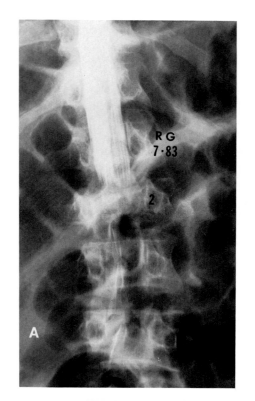

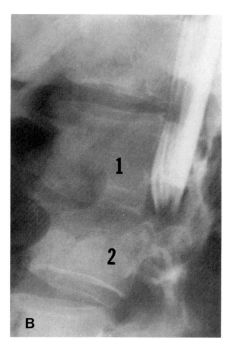

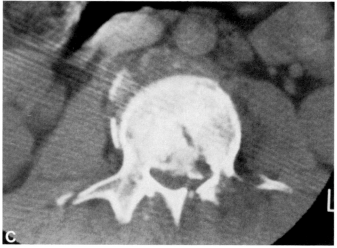

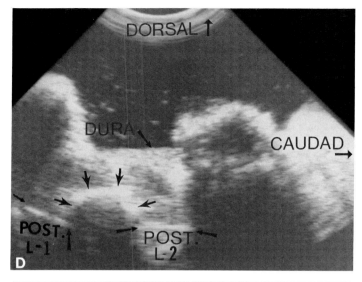

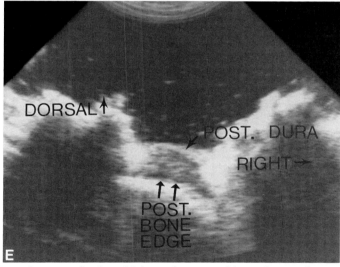

Figure 8-6. This patient sustained an L2 burst fracture with weakness of several lumbar nerve roots. He had normal bowel and bladder function. (A) An anteroposterior roentgenogram revealed a complete blockage of the myelographic dye at the L2 level. (B) A lateral roentgenogram shows the blockage at the superior portion of the L2 vertebral body resulting from retropulsed bone fragments. (C) A CT scan at the superior portion of L2 shows the bone fragments retropulsed from the vertebral body into the spinal canal. (D) The patient was taken to surgery for a posterolateral decompression and insertion of Harrington distraction rods. Intraoperative spinal sonography was used to document the extent of initial neural compression. This midsagittal sonogram shows a large bone fragment (arrows) protruding into the spinal canal and compressing the neural elements. (E) This is a corresponding transverse section of the spinal canal at the level of major compression. Note that no subarachnoid space is present at this level. The posterior aspect of the bone fragment is marked with arrows.

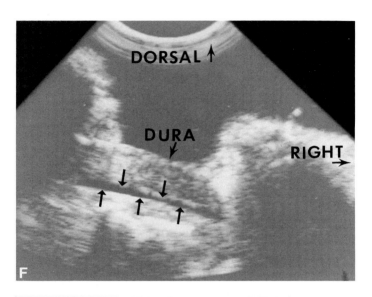

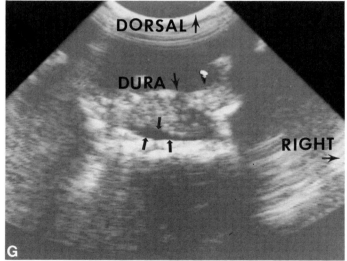

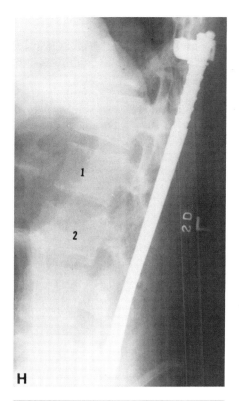

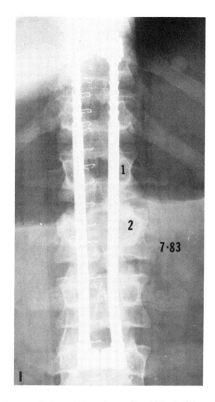

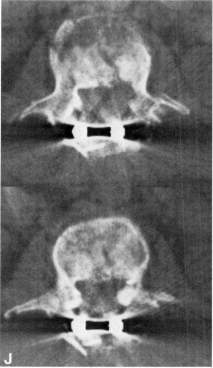

Figure 8-6. *(Continued)* (F) Midsagittal spinal sonogram after posterolateral decompression and insertion of the Harrington distraction rods shows there is now a continuous anterior subarachnoid space (arrows). No bone fragments are now seen in the spinal canal. (G) A transverse intraoperative sonogram shows that after decompression there is now an anterior subarachnoid space (arrows). (H) A lateral roentgenogram shows the Harrington distraction rods in place and maintenance of spinal alignment. Some lumbar lordosis has been bent into these Harrington rods; even more lordosis than this would have been appropriate. (I) An anteroposterior roentgenogram shows the Harrington rods in place. Longer rods should have been used and then cut in order to reduce the distance from the upper hook to the rod–rachet junction. (J) A postoperative CT scan verifies that an adequate neural decompression has been performed. (Reprinted from Eismont FJ, Green BA: Surgical treatment of spinal injuries: Anterior vs. posterior approaches. Adv Orthop Surg 8:24–34, 1984. With permission.)

173

with a vise-grip clamp to maintain the exposure. An assistant at the posterior aspect of the incision can use a Deaver retractor under the edge of the psoas muscle to allow exposure of the lumbar vertebra. An alternative to this retractor system is the Bwokwalter retractor. This is a large ring that is placed over the flank incision. It is clamped to the side of the operating room table. Various styles of retractor blades are available and can be attached to the suspended ring. A Richardson-type retractor may be used to retract the eleventh rib at the cephalad and caudad edges of the incision and a malleable retractor may be placed at the anterior aspect of the lumbar spine and attached to the Bwokwalter ring with a vise-grip clamp. A self-retaining Deaver-type retractor is placed under the psoas muscle and clamped to the Bwokwalter ring, thereby providing excellent exposure.

If the vertebral body is to be excised, the soft tissue is removed from the superior and inferior edge of the intervertebral disc posterolaterally. After this is accomplished, the junction between the vertebral body and the cartilaginous endplate can be seen clearly. A Cobb elevator is inserted into this space and the disc is pried away from the vertebral body. The technique is performed on each endplate. The annulus is cut posteriorly in a coronal direction and a wide rongeur can be used to remove the intervertebral disc. Because the patient has been positioned in a completely decubitus position, a scalpel can be used perpendicular to the floor with care being taken that the spinal canal is not violated. Once its cartilaginous endplate is detached, the disc can be removed readily. After the disc above and below the pathologically involved vertebral body have been removed to the posterior ligament, the anterior two thirds of the vertebral body is removed. In cases of diffuse involvement with metastatic tumor, this can often be accomplished with a scalpel or with large curettes. The posterior one third of the vertebral body is then removed with small curettes or with a high-speed burr. These instruments are used to expose the white cortical surface of the posterior vertebral body in an area where there is minimal neural compression. With loupe magnification and headlight illumination, a hole is made through the posterior cortex and is then enlarged by removing the posterior cortex on the dependent side and the cephalad and caudad cortex of the posterior vertebral wall with a long Kerrison rongeur with a thin footplate. A reverse Kerrison rongeur is used to remove the lateral aspect of the posterior vertebral body on the side from which the decompression is being performed. Care should be taken to decompress laterally until the pedicle is reached and palpated. The nerve roots at that same level should be visible just caudal to the pedicle. In cases of trauma, the posterior longitudinal ligament is removed since occasionally fragments of disc and bone are extruded through this ligament and can cause residual neural compression if the ligament is not removed. In cases of neoplastic disease, the posterior longitudinal ligament is removed if involved by the lesion, whereas in cases of infection, the posterior longitudinal ligament is usually adherent to the dura and removing the disc and adjacent bone allows adequate decompression without removal of the ligament.

Stabilization Procedures Via the Retroperitoneal Approach

In patients with lumbar instability resulting from neoplastic involvement of the anterior vertebral body or vertebral osteomyelitis, the posterior elements are usually intact. Under these circumstances, a tricortical bone graft obtained from the iliac crest and inserted into the defect created may be sufficient to restore the height of the anterior vertebral column and stabilize the spine. This also applies to patients with burst fractures of the lumbar spine without significant injuries to the posterior complex.[3] In these cases, the autogenous iliac bone graft may be obtained through the same incision by simply dissecting through the subcutaneous fat just peripheral to the external abdominal oblique muscle. The inner and outer aspects of the iliac crest are exposed with a combination of subperiosteal dissection and sharp dissection to detach the origins of the abdominal muscles. Osteotomes can then be used to remove a tricortical bone graft. A very thick graft can be obtained from the middle portion of the iliac crest and a thin one can be obtained from the anterior third of the iliac crest. Care must be take not to remove bone closer than 1 inch to the anterior superior iliac spine, otherwise the patient may fracture the iliac crest with contraction of the sartorius muscle while flexing the hip.

Osteotomes or a high-speed burr are used to cut a trough into the inferior endplate of the cephalad vertebral body and the superior endplate of the caudad vertebral body. The bone grafts are inserted and tamped in as far as the opposite side and additional bone grafts are added to the interspace. Even distribution of compressive loads across the interspace is thus attained, and asymmetric collapse of the interspace is prevented.

Methylmethacrylate has been used to achieve immediate spinal stability, and the technique has been described by many authors including Harrington[19] and Clark.[6] Methylmethacrylate is strong in compression, weak in tension, and of intermediate strength in resisting shear forces. From this we conclude that it is most useful for vertebral body replacement since it would be subjected to compression forces and less appropriately used in the posterior spinal column because these elements are often in tension. Methylmethacrylate constructs are strongest immediately after surgery and in most cases weaken with time particularly at the bone–cement interface. We believe that methylmethacrylate is contraindicated in cases of spinal infection and its use in trauma is controversial. We discourage its use in cases of trauma because these usually involve younger patients in whom the temporary support provided by methylmethacrylate is not nearly as desirable as achieving solid bony fusion.[9] Similarly, its use in patients with benign tumors of the spine is discouraged, since methylmethacrylate is unlikely to continue to provide adequate support over a long period of time. Methylmethacrylate is best suited for use in patients with malignant tumors who have a life expectancy of several months to 2 years (Figure 8-7).

Metastatic tumors to the spine usually involve the vertebral bodies with relative sparing of the posterior segments. This involvement may extend over several vertebral segments and is usually associated with a moderate kyphosis. The alternative surgical approaches to these lesions can be either (1) a retroperitoneal approach for access to the middle lumbar spine, or (2) a transthoracic, transdiaphragm, retroperitoneal approach for access to the upper lumbar and lower thoracic spine.

After the involved vertebra is exposed, the intervertebral discs are removed to the anterior aspect of the spinal canal. With the posterior longitudinal ligaments visualized at both the superior and inferior margins of the involved spine, the vertebral body or bodies are removed as previously described.

A Harrington distraction rod system using 1254 hooks inferiorly and 1253 hooks superiorly can be used at this juncture to distract the remaining normal superior and inferior vertebral bodies and correct the kyphosis. Care must be taken not to overdistract the neural elements. This can be determined by realtime ultrasound or by

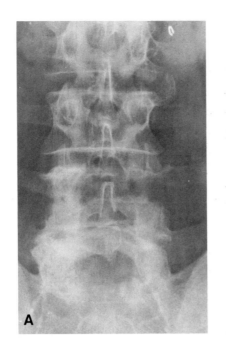

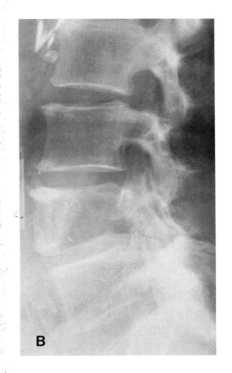

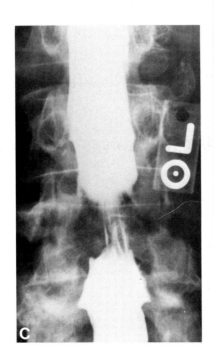

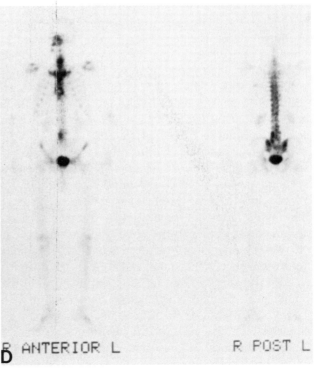

palpating the posterior longitudinal ligament and the dura to make certain that it is not excessively taut.

After the vertebral bodies are removed and the kyphotic deformity is corrected, the area is prepared for the introduction of methylmethacrylate into the defect created by removal of the vertebral bodies. A high-speed burr is used to create a hole through the central portion of the vertebral endplates both superiorly and inferiorly. A 6.5-mm cancellous screw is then selected that is 1 cm longer than the height of the adjacent

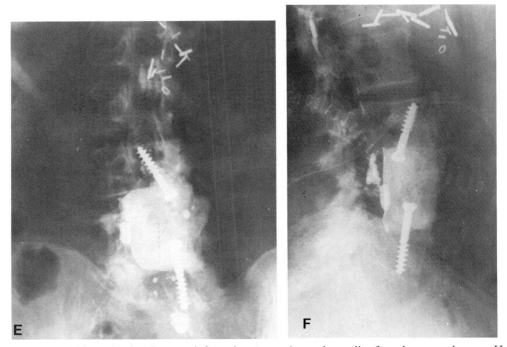

Figure 8-7. This patient underwent left nephrectomy 6 months earlier for a hypernephroma. He has now had severe back and right leg pain that has prohibited him from getting out of bed. Neurologically he has remained normal. (A) An anteroposterior roentgenogram shows absence of the left L4 pedicle. (B) A lateral roentgenogram shows a lucent defect in the posterior one half of the vertebral body at L4. The patient had been irradiated at the L4 level for presumed metastatic hypernephroma without significant relief of his pain. (C) An anteroposterior metri-zamide myelogram revealed a nearly complete blockage at the L4 level. (D) A bone scan reveals the L4 vertebral body to be the only area of abnormal uptake. Because of its solitary nature, the fact that it had been refractory to radiation with no cessation of the patient's pain, and because of his inability to ambulate because of this, it was decided to proceed with an anterior retroperitoneal operation to excise this vertebral body and replace it with methylmethacrylate. (E) An anteroposterior roentgenogram postoperatively reveals cancellous screws into the vertebral bodies of L3 and L5 and a mesh methylmethacrylate construct. Alignment of the spine has remained acceptable. (F) A lateral roentgenogram postoperatively reveals the wire mesh lying anterior to the spinal canal and shows cancellous screws that have been driven into the L3 and L5 vertebral bodies to aid in fixation of the methylmethacrylate. This was not supplemented with any posterior stabilization procedures since the life expectancy of this patient with metastatic hypernephroma was relatively short.

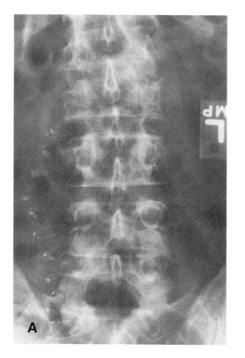

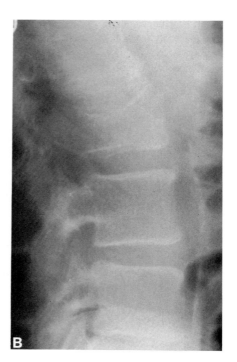

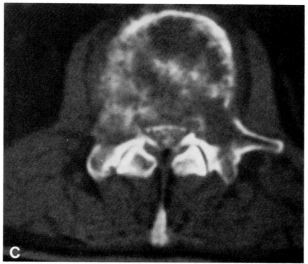

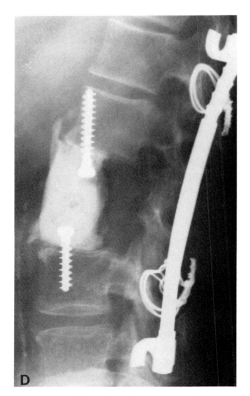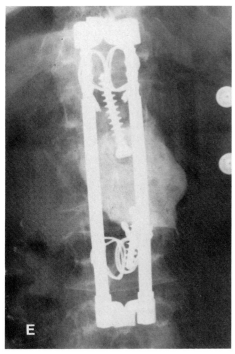

Figure 8-8. This patient had a several-month history of low back and leg pain. With no history of trauma, he had a sudden onset of excruciating pain that would not allow him to assume the erect position. (A) An anteroposterior roentgenogram reveals moderate collapse of the L2 vertebral body. The pedicles of the L2 vertebral body are less distinct than normal bilaterally. (B) A lateral roentgenogram reveals a compression fracture of the L2 vertebral body. (C) A CT scan at the level of the L2 vertebral body reveals severe destruction of the vertebral body consistent with tumor. There has been complete erosion of the transverse process on the right side. The spinal canal has been reduced to a small fraction of normal. A needle biopsy of this vertebral body was consistent with plasmacytoma. Complete medical evaluation including bone marrow aspiration was negative, indicating that this was not a disseminated malignancy. (D) The patient was taken to surgery and a simultaneous anterior vertebrectomy and anterior and posterior stabilization with methylmethacrylate anteriorly and Harrington distraction rods and autogenous bone graft posteriorly was performed. The posterior stabilization was used in this case since his life expectancy was longer than would be expected with most malignant tumors and this treatment would allow him to remain asymptomatic without loosening of the methylmethacrylate with time. The anterior cancellous screws were added to increase the fixation to the adjacent vertebral body and the posterior segmental wiring was added to increase stabilization. Note that lordosis has been bent into these Harrington distraction rods to preserve the normal lumbar lordosis. (E) An anteroposterior roentgenogram postoperatively reveals the methylmethacrylate and Harrington rod constructs. This patient was allowed to ambulate immediately after surgery in a total-contact body jacket. This was continued for 3 months. The patient's pain dramatically decreased with this treatment.

179

normal vertebral body. While an assistant applies pressure to the screw with a 90-degree fine clamp, the screw is threaded into the vertebral body with a Kocher clamp gripping its shank. This screw is advanced to the endplate of the adjacent vertebral body. After cancellous screws are placed into the superior and inferior vertebral bodies, fine wire mesh is cut to the exact height of the vertebral segment to be replaced. The mesh should be wide enough to cover the exposed spinal canal posteriorly as well as one half the thickness of a vertebral body anteriorly on each side. A small amount of methylmethacrylate is placed on the superior and inferior vertebral bodies and on any remaining bone from the vertebral bodies that have been removed. The precut mesh is inserted to form a trough. This mesh should be kept 5 to 10 mm away from the dura. A small amount of methylmethacrylate is smeared over the mesh to seal its holes, and this construct is allowed to cure. A second batch of methylmethacrylate is then used to fill the remaining trough. This cement incorporates the ends of the cancellous screws in the adjacent vertebral bodies as well as anteriorly situated Harrington rods. The methylmethacrylate is continually irrigated as it is curing to dissipate the heat of polymerization. Since the methylmethacrylate used for cranioplasty requires a longer time to set and hence generates less heat, this compound is used in preference to the orthopedic compound.

In patients with slow-growing malignant or quasimalignant tumors consideration may be given to the advisability of performing posterior stabilization with rods and iliac bone grafts at the time of anterior stabilization with methylmethacrylate or at a second stage procedure 7 to 10 days later. This combined approach achieves immediate early stability; the posterior rods and autogenous bone graft become solid coincident with the tendency of the methylmethacrylate to loosen anteriorly (Figure 8-8). The spine must be stabilized posteriorly with either Luque segmental fixation[11] or Harrington compression rods if these are inserted at a second stage. If Harrington distraction rods were to be used, they would tend to distract the bone from the cement. If an anterior and posterior stabilization are done at the same time, then Harrington distraction rods may be inserted first followed by introduction of the cement anteriorly.

Anterior Spine Instrumentation

Several methods recently have been introduced for performing anterior instrumentation of the thoracolumbar and lumbar spine. For example, the Dunn device allows rigid uprights to be fixed between normal superior and inferior vertebral bodies (Figure 8-9). Curved plates in various diameters are available that fit over the central portion of the vertebral body from just anterior to the vertebral foramina on the exposed side to just slightly past the midline on the opposite side of the spine. These plates are fastened to the normal vertebral bodies with self-tapping cancellous screws that are inserted parallel to the front of the spinal canal. When the plate is in proper alignment there is bone cephalad and caudad to the edges of the plate. The screw starter instrument is driven into the vertebral body and a screw of appropriate length is inserted into the vertebral body. The screw should not protrude excessively through the opposite side of the vertebral body. The tip of the screw should just be palpable with the fingertip. A staple is impacted over the plate anteriorly to complete the fixation to the vertebral bodies.

When properly inserted, the planes of the screw and the staple should be situated approximately 70 degrees from each other. Before the plates are attached to the vertebral body, the posterior threaded rod and anterior bolt and locking nuts are selected for proper length and inserted into the plates. Any kyphosis should be corrected with a laminar spreader before application of the plate. Once an anterior tricortical iliac bone graft has been driven into place, the Dunn device can be tightened down to provide compression over this injured segment and enhance bone healing. Small bits of remaining bone graft are then placed anterior to the tricortical iliac graft.

This device is best used in cases of burst fractures of the lumbar spine with marked narrowing of the spinal canal by retropulsed fragments of vertebral body[8] without significant posterior instability or minimal instability secondary to undisplaced laminar fractures. The anterior decompression allows excellent visualization of the pathologic situation, and insertion of adequate bone grafts and the Dunn device provides enough fixation to mobilize these patients in a total-contact body jacket. This approach should not be used to treat patients with primary dislocations because these dislocations are accompanied by severe posterior bony and ligamentous injuries. The anterior approach including vertebrectomy will aggravate the instability and the Dunn device will be unable to compensate for this. This approach is also contraindicated in cases of infection, which should be treated by anterior debridement and bone grafting (Figure 8-10). If instrumentation is required, it is best to use posterior rods (Figure 8-11).

In patients with malignant spinal tumors, the Dunn device does not offer any particular advantage over methylmethacrylate but may be a helpful adjunct in treating extensive benign tumors involving the vertebral bodies or low-grade malignancies involving the spine.

There are several variations of anterior instrumentation systems. Even though these systems appear to be extremely solid after their insertion, they cannot be relied upon to support the spine for prolonged periods of time without adequate bony fusion. Without such fusion, these systems will fail either because the screws and staples break or lose their attachments to bone. The Dwyer and Zielke systems involve fixation of a staple or plate to the vertebral body with a cancellous screw and connection of these staples or plates to each other with either a flexible cable, as in the Dwyer system, or a semiflexible rod, as in the Zielke system. Both of these systems apply compression over several vertebral bodies anteriorly, and although they were not intended for use with radical vertebral body excision, they have subsequently been used in this fashion.[22]

Transthoracic Approach to the Lumbar Spine

The transthoracic approach to the lumbar spine has been described in another chapter, but it is worth emphasizing that by using the transthoracic approach and by detaching the diaphragm and developing the retroperitoneal space, the lumbar spine from L1 to L5 can be exposed.[5]

The positioning of the patient is as described for the retroperitoneal sympathetic approach to the lumbar spine with the patient in a straight lateral decubitus position. The side chosen for the approach is based on the location of the great vessels. The left side is usually used if the level of major interest is at or below the ninth thoracic level. The incision is centered over the tenth rib and extended from the costovertebral angle posteriorly to the costochondral junction anteriorly. The overlying muscles are cut in line with this incision. The periosteum is stripped from the rib, which is cut at the

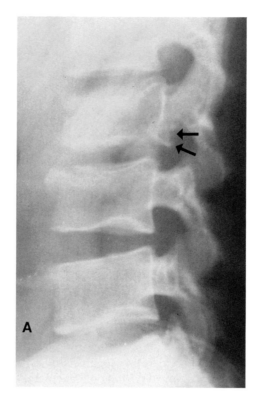

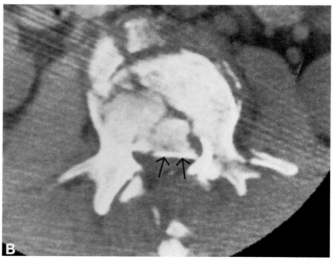

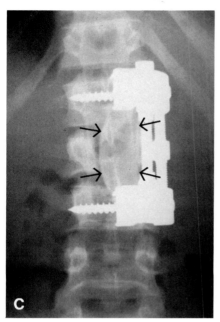
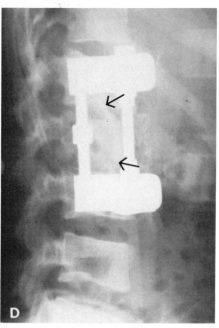

Figure 8-9. This patient fell four stories and sustained fractures of his L2 and L3 vertebral bodies in addition to multiple injuries to his lower extermities. This was associated with an incomplete paraparesis with weakness of both lower extremities. He appeared to have normal bowel and bladder function. (A) The lateral roentgenogram reveals mild compression of the L2 vertebral body with the suggestion of bone retropulsed into the spinal canal at the inferior position of the L2 vertebral body (arrows). There is also a compression of the L3 vertebral body that appears less significant. (B) A CT scan of the level of the L2 vertebral body reveals bone fragments retropulsed from the vertebral body back into the spinal canal (arrows). The spinal canal is narrowed to approximately 40 percent of normal. (C) This fracture was treated with an anterior retroperitoneal vertebrectomy and decompression of the spinal canal. An autogenous iliac bone graft was then inserted between the L1 and L3 vertebral bodies and can be seen on this postoperative anteroposterior roentgenogram (arrows). Stabilization was added by the use of the Dunn device with cancellous screws and staples inserted into the L1 and L3 vertebral bodies. (D) A lateral roentgenogram postoperatively reveals the Dunn device fixed to the L1 and L3 vertebral bodies with threaded rods allowing restoration of normal alignment. The iliac bone graft (arrows) is rigidly held in place by slight compression using this device. This patient had a full recovery of his neurologic function. He was not able to be ambulated until 6 weeks after surgery because of his multiple lower extremity fractures

183

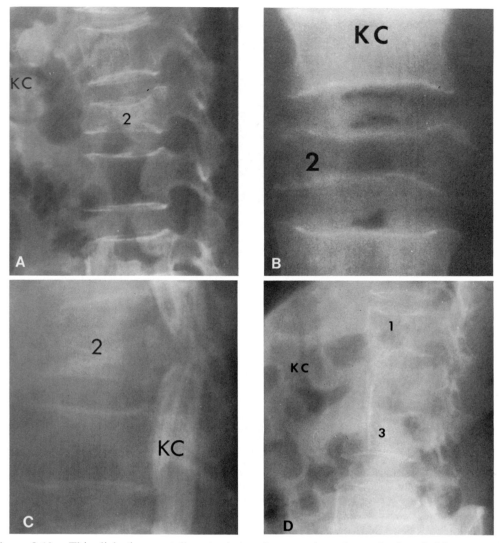

Figure 8-10. This diabetic, mentally retarded patient was brought to the hospital because of intermittent fevers, severe low back pain, leg weakness, and refusal to ambulate. (A) The initial roentgenogram was interpreted as showing only a compression fracture of the L2 vertebra since the vertebral endplates appear to be intact. (B) Anteroposterior tomograms revealed rarefaction of the L2 vertebral endplates and also gas present within the L1 and L2 intervertebral discs and within the L2 vertebral body suggestive of vertebral osteomyelitis and disc space infection. (C) A lateral roentgenogram of the myelography procedure revealed anterior extradural compression at the L2 vertebral body level. Even though this is below the level of the conus medullaris, there has been too much bone destruction to allow treatment with only a posterior laminotomy approach. (D) A follow-up lateral roentgenogram shows incorporation of the iliac graft and preservation of normal spinal alignment. The patient underwent an anterolateral retroperitoneal approach to the spine and a 100-cc abscess was encountered in the psoas muscle and within the L2 vertebral body and adjacent discs. The spine was debrided, the neural elements decompressed, a full-thickness iliac graft inserted from L1 to L3, and the wound left open with Penrose drains down to the spine. After a 6-week course of antibiotics, her infection was resolved and her weakness improved.

costovertebral angle posteriorly and is separated from the cartilage anteriorly. The parietal pleura and periosteum behind the rib are incised and the pleural cavity is entered. The diaphragm is readily visible. With a chest retractor in place the cartilaginous extension from the tenth rib is incised longitudinally for several centimeters and is then cut inferiorly, thereby detaching this piece of cartilage from the remainder of the costal cartilage. Blunt dissection between these two pieces of cartilage exposes the retroperitoneal cavity. The diaphragm is cut approximately 5 mm from its attachment to the chest wall and this is continued posteriorly until the attachment of the diaphragm to the spine is encountered. At this point electrocautery may be used to cut the attachment of the diaphragm to the spine. The surgeon, however, should have his or her fingers on the aorta in order to ascertain its exact location and avoid injuring it. If the lower lumbar spine is to be exposed, the skin incision is curved distally at its anterior margin in a plane halfway between the lateral rectus sheath and the anterior border of the iliac crest. The subcutaneous tissue is incised and the abdominal muscles are incised in line with the skin incision. If the thoracic duct is torn during the procedure, its ends should be oversewn to prevent a persistent chylous drainage into the chest postoperatively.

The Transabdominal Approach to the Lumbar Spine

The transabdominal approach to the lumbar spine is best suited for problems at or below the L4-5 disc level. This approach also provides good access to the sacrum (see Figure 8-1). Performed through a midline incision, this approach allows mobilization of the bifurcation of the aorta, of the iliac arteries, and of the inferior vena cava and the common iliac veins and an excellent exposure of the sacrum and the L5 vertebral body. This exposure should be avoided in cases of infection and malignancy since this will allow contamination of the peritoneal contents.

Combined Anterior and Posterior Spine Reconstruction

Both an anterior and posterior exposure of the lumbar spine may be required for patients with a significant spinal deformity and anterior neural compression (Figure 8-12). This procedure is designed to supplant a series of operations: an initial procedure for anterior release and neural decompression; a second operation for posterior spine instrumentation; and a third operation for anterior bone grafting.

The patient is operated upon in the straight lateral decubitus position and often by two full surgical teams, one of which completes the anterior operation and the other the posterior operation. The table should be raised as high as possible, the patient should be positioned so the back is as close to the edge of the table as possible since the surgical team performing the posterior exposure and instrumentation usually has more difficulty in terms of visualization than does the anterior (abdominal) team. The anterior decompression is completed before the insertion of posterior instrumentation to correct the deformity. This is then followed by placement of the anterior bone grafts. The instrumentation, bone grafting, and closure are performed as previously described. With the advent of adequate anterior spinal instrumentation, this combined approach is currently indicated less often.

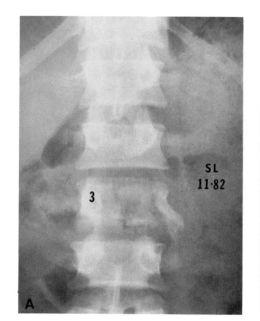

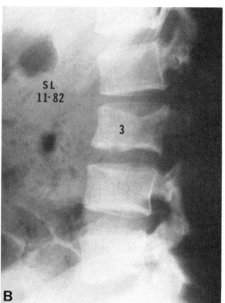

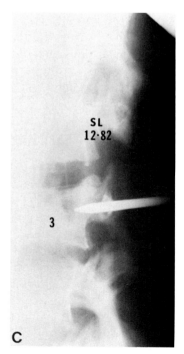

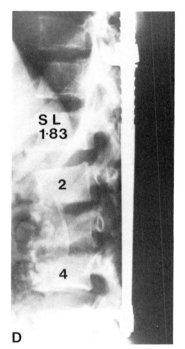
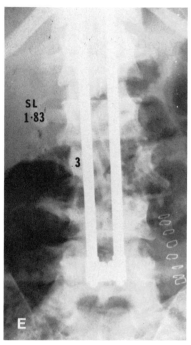

D

E

Figure 8-11. This patient had a grossly contaminated penetrating injury to the L3 vertebra that required radical initial surgical debridement. He subsequently developed a refractory vertebral osteomyelitis. (A) An anteroposterior roentgenogram shows the severe destruction of the L3 vertebral body as a result of the penetrating injury. The extent of surgical posterior bone removal can also be seen. (B) A lateral roentgenogram demonstrates the extent of removal of the posterior elements that was necessary for initial wound debridement. (C) The patient developed a persistent fever and increasing back pain 1 month after injury. Vertebral osteomyelitis was suspected and a Craig needle biopsy of the L3 vertebra was performed; it confirmed the diagnosis. The patient was treated for the bacteria isolated but he remained febrile with a markedly elevated sedimentation rate. (D) Since he was judged to have a refractory vertebral osteomyelitis, he underwent a combined anterior retroperitoneal and a posterior approach for debridement of the spine and simultaneous stabilization. A lateral roentgenogram shows the anterior full-thickness iliac graft and the posterior Harrington distraction rods. Retrospectively, it is apparent that lumbar lordosis should have been bent into these rods rather than using straight rods. (E) An anteroposterior roentgenogram shows the two Harrington distraction rods in place. The patient resolved his spine infection with prolonged antibiotic treatment and his spine stability was adequately restored to allow immediate mobilization in a total-contact body jacket.

187

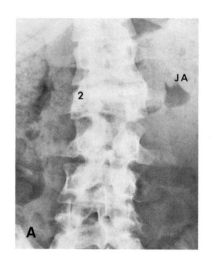

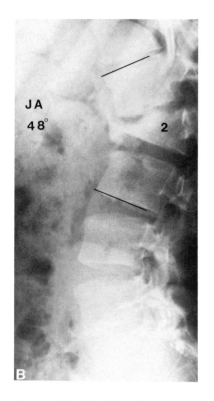

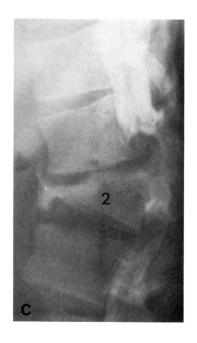

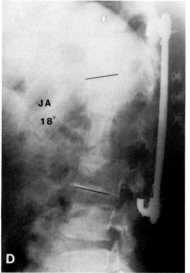

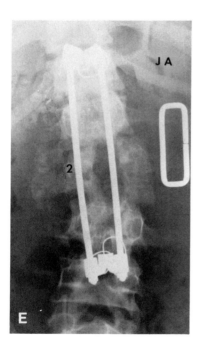

Figure 8-12. This patient sustained an L2 fracture with severe paraparesis and complete loss of bowel and bladder control. He was initially treated with an L2 laminectomy, which did not alter the severe anterior neural compression and an iliac bone graft was placed posteriorly from L1 to L3. No internal fixation device was used. (A) When first seen several months later, there had been no neurologic improvement and the patient had persistent back pain. An anteroposterior roentgenogram shows a minimal scoliosis. (B) A lateral roentgenogram shows a significant 48-degree kyphosis from L1 to L3. (C) A myelogram was performed and a complete blockage was found at the L1-2 interspace. This necessitated injection of dye above and below the L2 level. (D) Anterior L2 vertebral body resection and L1–L3 fusion with iliac autografts was performed and the patient simultaneously underwent a posterior approach to the spine for placement of dual Harrington compression rods and autogenous bone grafts from T12 to L3. At surgery, a pseudoarthrosis was found in the posterior fusion at the L1-2 level; this was curetted and new bone grafts were placed. A lateral roentgenogram shows correction of the patient's kyphosis from 48 degrees to 18 degrees and complete neural decompression is evident. (E) An anteroposterior roentgenogram shows the Harrington compression rods in place. The patient's pain was improved postoperatively and he had slight motor neural improvement and became ambulatory with braces.

REFERENCES

1. Allen BL Jr, Ferguson RL: The Galveston technique of pelvic fixation with L-rod instrumentation of the spine. Spine 9:388, 1984
2. Allen BL Jr, Ferguson RL: The Galveston technique for L-rod instrumentation of the scoliotic spine. Spine 7:276, 1982
3. Bohlman HH, Eismont FJ: Surgical techniques of anterior decompression and fusion for spinal cord injuries. Clin Orthop 154:57, 1981
4. Bryant CE, Sullivan JA: Management of thoracic and lumbar spine fractures with Harrington distraction rods supplemented with segmental wiring. Spine 8:532, 1983
5. Burrington JD, Brown C, Wayne ER, Odom J: Anterior approach to the thoracolumbar spine. Arch Surg 11:456, 1976
6. Clark CR, Keggi KJ, Panjabi MM: Methylmethacrylate stabilization of the cervical spine. J Bone Joint Surg 66A:40, 1984
7. Dickson JH, Harrington PR, Erwin WDL: Results of reduction and stabilization of the severely fractured thoracic and lumbar spine. J Bone Joint Surg 60A:799, 1978
8. Dunn HK: Anterior stabilization of thoracolumbar injuries. Clin Orthop Rel Res 189:116, 1984
9. Eismont FJ, Bohlman HH: Posterior methylmethacrylate fusion in cervical trauma—a review of six cases with emphasis on complications. Spine 6:347, 1981
10. Eismont FJ, Green BA: Surgical tratment of spinal injuries: Anterior versus posterior approaches. Adv Orthop Surg 8:24, 1984
11. Flatley TJ, Anderson MH, Anast GT: Spinal instability due to malignant disease. Treatment by segmental spinal stabilization. J Bone Joint Surg 66A:47, 1984
12. Flesch JR, Leider LL Jr, Erickson DD, Chou SN, Bradford DS: Harrington instrumentation and spine fusion for unstable fractures and fracture dislocations of the thoracic and lumbar spine. J Bone Joint Surg 57A:143, 1977
13. Fountain SS: A single-stage combined surgical approach for vertebral resections. J Bone Joint Surg 61A:1011, 1979
14. Frederickson BE, Yuan HA, Miller H: Burst fractures of the fifth lumbar vertebra. A report of four cases. J Bone Joint Surg 64A:1088, 1982
15. Gertzbein SD, Macmichael D, Tile M: Harrington instrumentation as a method of fixation in fractures of the spine. J Bone Joint Surg 64B:526, 1982
16. Green BA, Callahan RA, Klose KJ, de la Torre J: Acute spinal cord injury: Current concepts. Clin Orthop 154:125, 1981
17. Green BA, Green KL, Klose KJ: Kinetic therapy for spinal cord injury. Spine 8:722, 1983
18. Gumley G, Taylor TK, Ryan MD: Distraction fractures of the lumbar spine. J Bone Joint Surg 64B:520, 1982
19. Harrington KD: The use of methylmethacrylate for vertebral body replacement and anterior stabilization of pathological fracture-dislocations of the spine due to metastatic malignant disease. J Bone Joint Surg 63A:36, 1981
20. Jacobs RR, Asher MA, Snider RK: Thoracolumbar spinal injuries—a comparative study of recumbent and operative treatment in 100 patients. Spine 5:463, 1980
21. Kestler OC: Overgrowth (hypertrophy) of lumbosacral grafts, causing a complete block. Bull Hosp Joint Dis 27:51, 1966
22. Kostuick JP: Anterior spinal cord decompression for lesions of the thoracic and lumbar spine—techniques, new methods of internal fixation, and results. Spine 8:512, 1983
23. Kurland LT: The frequency of intracranial and paraspinal neoplasms in the resident population of Rochester, Minn. J Neurosurg 15:627, 1958
24. MacNab I, Dall D: The blood supply of the lumbar spine and its application to the technique of intertransverse lumbar fusion. J Bone Joint Surg 53B:628, 1971
25. Mesard L, Carmudy A, Manarino E, Ruge D: Survival after spinal cord trauma. Arch Neurol 35:78, 1978
26. Purcell GA, Markolf KL, Dawson EG: Twelfth thoracic-first lumbar vertebral mechanical stability of fractures after Harrington rod instrumentation. J Bone Joint Surg 63A:71, 1981
27. Slabaugh PB, Nickel VL: Complications associated with the Stryker frame. J Bone Joint Surg 60A:1111, 1978
28. Smith TK, Whitaker J, Stauffer EJ: Complication associated with the use of the circular electric turning frame. J Bone Joint Surg 57:711, 1975
29. Southwick WO, Robinson RA: Surgical approaches to the vertebral bodies in the cervical and lumbar regions. J Bone Joint Surg 39A:631, 1957

Henry H. Schmidek
Donald A. Smith
Thomas K. Kristiansen

9

Sacral Fractures: Issues of Neural Injury, Spinal Stability, and Surgical Management

The sacral spine has received relatively little attention in the orthopedic and neurosurgical literature, in part because of the infrequency of developmental, degenerative, or neoplastic conditions of the sacrum requiring surgical intervention. This neglect is unwarranted in trauma, however, because sacral fractures and associated neural deficits are both common and often complex problems. The sacrum and pelvis behave as a single functional unit; an understanding of the principles of sacropelvic stability has obvious relevance in planning the occasional resection of a sacral tumor and in dealing with the common problem of massive pelvic trauma. In this chapter, a classification of sacral fractures is reviewed along with the usual patterns of neurologic involvement. Through an analysis of an institutional series of cases, a specific attempt is made to correlate varying types of vertical sacral fractures with differing types of pelvic injury. The radiographic and physiologic investigation of sacral fractures is reviewed, as are the various options for achieving their reduction, decompression, and stabilization.

ANATOMY OF THE SACRUM

The sacrum is a virtually motionless spinal segment that develops from five fused vertebrae. Each of these vertebrae is formed from three primary ossification centers that give rise to anterior and posterior elements. At about 15 years of age, the fibrocartilaginous disc between the last two sacral vertebrae ossifies. This process continues in a cephalad direction until the sacrum achieves its mature form as a single, solid, roughly triangular shaped bone by age 25, when intersegmental fusion is complete.

The sacrum is locked into the posterior pelvic ring, where it receives and

THE UNSTABLE SPINE
ISBN 0-8089-1757-9

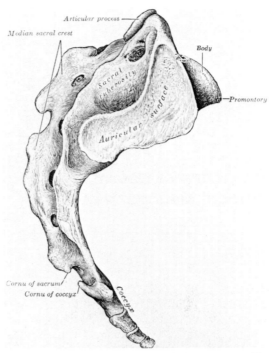

Figure 9-1. The lateral aspect of the sacrum. (Reprinted
from Goss CM (ed): Gray's Anatomy. Philadelphia, Lea &
Febiger, 1966. With permission.)

distributes loads between the pelvis and the mobile portion of the axial skeleton. The
superior surface or "base" of the sacrum is attached to the lumbar spine at the L5-S1
disc and through the anterior and posterior longitudinal ligaments; the posterior
elements are joined by the paired L5-S1 facet joints, their capsular ligaments, the
ligamentum flavum, and the interspinous and supraspinous ligaments. In addition,
iliolumbar ligaments extend from the L5 transverse processes to insert onto the pelvis
in two slips, one blending with the anterior sacroiliac ligament and the other attached
to the anterior aspect of the iliac crest.

Laterally, the large and irregular "auricular surface" of the sacrum is apposed on
each side against the congruent surface of the innominate bones to form the sacroiliac
joints (Figure 9-1). These joints are virtually motionless and derive their extreme
stability from the strong anterior and posterior sacroiliac ligaments and the intrinsic
wedgelike geometry of the sacrum, which causes it to seat into the apex of the
weight-bearing posterior pelvic ring much like the keystone of an arch (Figure 9-2). In
the standing position the pelvis is inclined about 40 degrees to the horizontal. Further
vertical loading will promote rotational stresses through the horizontal axis of the
sacroiliac joint, which are counteracted by the sacrotuberous and sacrospinous
ligaments acting as a tie bar through the lever arm of the sacrum itself (Figure 9-3).

The ventral surface of the sacrum is concave and is creased by four transverse
ridges at the sites of intersegmental fusion. Each of these horizontal ridges terminates
laterally in four paired ventral sacral foramina that transmit the ventral sacral nerves

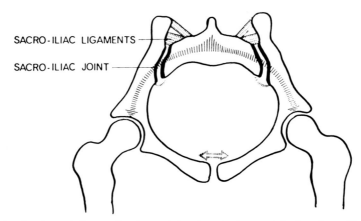

Figure 9-2. Distribution of forces in the pelvic ring during weight-bearing. (Reprinted from Huittinen VM, Slatis P: Fractures of the pelvis. Acta Chir Scand 138:565, 1972. With permission.)

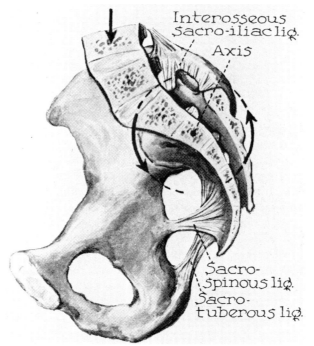

Figure 9-3. Rotational forces acting on the sacrum through the horizontal axis of the sacroiliac joints. (Reprinted from Thorek P: Anatomy in Surgery. Philadelphia, J.B. Lippincott, 1951, pp 552–553. With permission.)

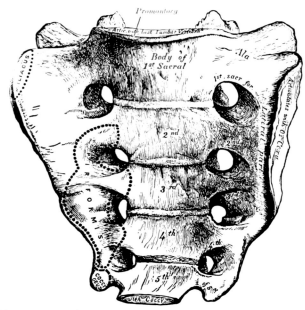

Figure 9-4. The ventral aspect of the sacrum. (Reprinted from Goss CM (ed): Gray's Anatomy. Philadelphia, Lea & Febiger, 1966. With permission.)

and sacral arteries. The S1 foramina, which transmit the S1 nerves, are the largest of these openings. The foramina narrow at successively more caudal levels, yet exceed the diameter of the contained neural elements by roughly two fold (Figure 9-4).

The bone lateral to each of the sacral foramina is formed from the fused rudimentary costal and transverse processes. Superiorly and down to the region of the S2 foramina this forms the "lateral sacral mass," connecting the centrum of the S1 and S2 vertebrae to the sacroiliac joint. On an anteroposterior roentgenogram of the sacrum, the lateral masses or "alae" have the appearance of a "bow tie." Their contained bony trabeculations have a radiate pattern that runs at right angles to the plane of the sacroiliac joint. The lateral surface is the sacral aspect of the sacroiliac joint and extends only to the level of S3 foramina so that forces exerted through this articulation are particularly prone to affect the sacrum at or above the level of S3. Below this level the lateral margins of the sacrum broaden slightly opposite the S4 foramina where the strong sacrotuberous and sacrospinous ligaments insert. Inferiorly, the apex of the sacrum is joined to the coccyx by a fibrocartilaginous disc, which frequently ossifies.

The dorsal surface of the sacrum is convex. Its midline is marked by a vertically oriented middle sacral crest, which is formed from the fused vestigial spinous processes. Inferiorly this crest ends at the S4-5 level in the sacral hiatus where dorsal arch fusion is incomplete. There are shallow troughs or "sacral grooves" on either side of the midline crest that represent the fused laminae of S1 through S4. The lateral edge of each groove is slightly raised to form the "intermediate crest" created from the intersegmental fusion of the rudimentary apophyseal joints. This ridge is also a line of

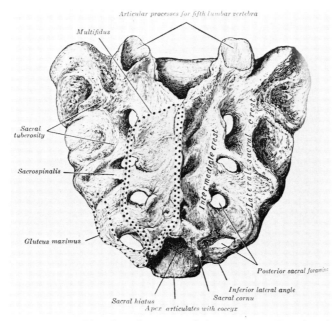

Figure 9-5. The dorsal aspect of the sacrum. (Reprinted from Goss CM (ed): Gray's Anatomy. Philadelphia, Lea & Febiger, 1966. With permission.)

insertion for the dorsal sacroiliac ligaments. Superiorly the intermediate crest is surmounted by the superior articulating process for the L5-S1 facet joint on the basal surface of the sacrum. On each side and just lateral to this process is a small indentation in the superior edge of the lateral sacral mass termed the *sacral notch*. Lateral to each intermediate crest are a series of four paired dorsal sacral foramina through which pass the paired dorsal sacral rami. These are smaller than the corresponding ventral foramina, as are the contained neural elements. There are usually no foramina for the S5 roots that exit ventrally and dorsally between the sacrum and coccyx (Figure 9-5).

The sacral spinal canal has a roughly triangular inlet at S1. The cross-sectional configuration changes to that of an ellipse by the level of the S2 body and retains this shape to the level of the outlet of the canal at the sacral hiatus. Except for the ventral and dorsal foraminal apertures, the sacral canal is completely enclosed by bone. Within the sacral canal are contained neural elements, blood vessels, and fibrofatty tissue.

The dural tube terminates at the level of S2. Its blind end is penetrated by the filum terminale, which continues caudally to insert onto the coccyx. Paired ventral and dorsal roots emerge from the dural tube and unite just distal to the dorsal root ganglion to form spinal nerves. Each spinal nerve in turn divides almost immediately to form ventral and dorsal primary rami. Each of these is composed of afferent and efferent elements and exits from the spinal canal through its respective ventral and dorsal foramina. The ventral rami S1 through S4 join with the lumbosacral trunk derived from the L4 and L5 roots to form the sacral plexus (Figure 9-6). This plexus overlies the sacroiliac joint on the dorsal wall of the pelvis between the pyriformis muscle and its investing fascia and also lies in close relation to the ureters and internal iliac vessels (Figure 9-7). The main

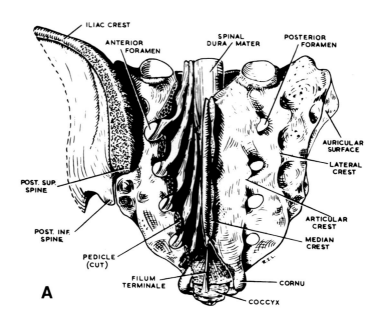

ILIAC CREST

ANTERIOR
FORAMEN

SPINAL
DURA MATER

POSTERIOR
FORAMEN

AURICULAR
SURFACE

LATERAL
CREST

POST. SUP.
SPINE

POST. INF.
SPINE

PEDICLE
(CUT)

FILUM
TERMINALE

ARTICULAR
CREST

MEDIAN
CREST

CORNU

COCCYX

A

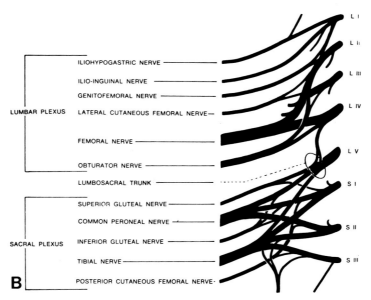

LUMBAR PLEXUS	ILIOHYPOGASTRIC NERVE
	ILIO-INGUINAL NERVE
	GENITOFEMORAL NERVE
	LATERAL CUTANEOUS FEMORAL NERVE
	FEMORAL NERVE
	OBTURATOR NERVE
	LUMBOSACRAL TRUNK
SACRAL PLEXUS	SUPERIOR GLUTEAL NERVE
	COMMON PERONEAL NERVE
	INFERIOR GLUTEAL NERVE
	TIBIAL NERVE
	POSTERIOR CUTANEOUS FEMORAL NERVE

L I
L II
L III
L IV
L V
S I
S II
S III

B

Figure 9-6. (A) Sacral hemilaminectomy showing the neural elements within the spinal canal. (B) The extraforaminal confluence of spinal roots to form the lumbar and sacral plexuses in the retroperitoneum. (Reprinted from Huittinen VM: Lumbosacral nerve injury and fracture of the pelvis: A postmortem radiographic and pathoanatomical study. Acta Chir Scand 429:8, 1972. With permission.)

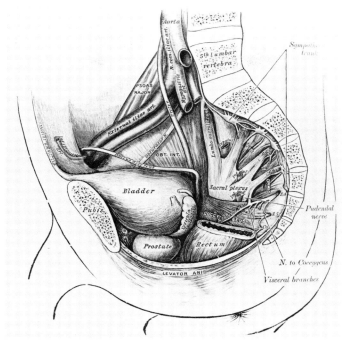

Figure 9-7. Relationship of the sacral plexus to the pelvic viscera. (Reprinted from Goss CM (ed): Gray's Anatomy. Philadelphia, Lea & Febiger, 1966. With permission.)

branches of this plexus are the superior and inferior gluteal nerves, the sciatic nerve, and the pudendal nerve. The fourth and fifth ventral sacral rami join the coccygeal nerve to form the much smaller coccygeal plexus. The corresponding dorsal rami S1 through S5 give sensorimotor innervation to the overlying skin and paraspinal muscles. The sympathetic ganglia lie slightly medial to the ventral sacral foramina. At each level a gray ramus communicans is distributed to the corresponding ventral ramus. The second and third sacral ganglia also contribute sympathetic innervation to the inferior hypogastric plexus via small sacral splanchnic nerves. Pelvic and sacral splanchnic nerves intermingle with descending branches from the superior hypogastric plexus to form the inferior hypogastric plexus, which is contained within the loose areolar tissue posteriorly on either side of the rectum. Together with the pudendal nerves, terminal branches distributed from this site are responsible for the maintenance of urinary and fecal continence and for proper sexual function.

CLASSIFICATION OF SACRAL FRACTURES

Fractures of the sacrum are relatively common injuries that in the past have been frequently overlooked or ignored. They were first mentioned in 1847 by Malgaigne in *Traite des Fractures et des Luxations*.[25] In 1945 Bonnin published a paper on this subject wherein he outlined a classification of sacral fractures.[1] Since Bonnin's article, some meaningful information has appeared, mainly in the form of small series and cases

Table 9-1.
Classification of sacral fractures

Mechanism of Injury	
Direct trauma	
Penetrating	
Low Transverse Fracture (S3 and below)	
Indirect trauma	
High Transverse Fracture (S1 and S2)	
Lumbosacral Fracture Dislocation	
Lateral Mass Fracture	Associated with
Juxta-articular Fracture	Pelvic Ring
Cleaving Fracture	Disruption
Avulsion Fracture	
Combination Fracture	

reports concerning unusual types of sacral injury.[2,3,4,5,7,9–13,19,29,36,38,45,48,49] After reviewing these sources and our own clinical material, a comprehensive classification of sacral fractures relating to mechanism of injury has been devised (Table 9-1). As with all fractures, the potential for variability is infinite, and complex injury forces may defy discrete pattern resolution. All efforts to exhaustively systematize fractures are therefore somewhat contrived yet are necessary to provide a framework for organized thinking and a logical approach.

Sacral Fractures Resulting from Direct Trauma

Direct trauma to the sacrum may result in an open or closed fracture. Gunshot wounds are the most common cause of penetrating injury and are often complicated by extensive visceral damage. The extent of sacral derangement is obviously variable, but in the majority of cases fracture is confined to the posterior pelvic ring. As discussed below, this usually implies a stable structural condition so long as the sacrum and sacroiliac joints above the level of the S1 foramina remain intact.

Hard falls onto the buttocks or a direct blow administered to this area are also occasional causes of sacral fracture. Typically, these injuries result in a low transverse fracture near the kyphus of the sacrum. In these cases a levering action is exerted through the distal segments of the sacrum below its level of fixation by the sacroiliac joint[1,12,38,45] (Figure 9-8). This usually occurs through the foramina of S4, although any of the lower three vertebrae may be involved. The distal fragment is often displaced anteriorly, sometimes to such an extent as to cause rectal perforation.[45] Cerebrospinal fluid leaks may also occur.[38] Since this part of the sacrum is not involved in transmission of weight from the lower extremities to the spine, these are stable fractures.

Sacral Fractures Resulting from Indirect Trauma

Indirect injuries are caused by forces acting on the sacrum either through the pelvis or through the lumbar spine. According to Nicoll, a high transverse fracture is usually the result of a flexion injury sustained by an person locked in a posture of hip flexion

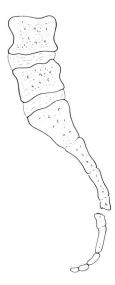

Figure 9-8. Displaced low transverse sacral fracture. (Reprinted from Weaver EN, England GD, Richardson DE: Sacral fracture: Case presentation and review. Neurosurgery 9:725, 1981. With permission.)

with knee extension.[30] A traumatic spondylolisthesis through the level of the S1 or S2 foramina results in forward displacement of the upper spinal segment upon the lower sacrum. Characteristically, this type of injury occurs in younger patients before completion of intersegmental ossification,[2,3,4,17,36,45,49] although exceptions have been reported.[11] A similar mechanism of injury has been proposed for traumatic spondylolisthesis of L5-S1, which often includes fracture of the S1 facets.[4] Historically, transverse fractures have constituted about 5 to 10 percent of all sacral fractures.[1,12,28,44]

A much larger group of sacral fractures can be identified that always occur in conjunction with pelvic fractures. These have been termed *vertical fractures*, both to denote the general orientation of the fracture line and to differentiate them from the group of transverse fractures that often occur as isolated injuries. After a review of the literature and our own case material, we find it useful to distinguish four vertical fracture patterns: (1) lateral mass fracture, (2) juxta-articular fracture, (3) cleaving fracture, and (4) avulsion fracture (Figure 9-9).

Lateral mass fractures typically extend from the area of the sacral notch inferiorly through the first, second, or third ventral foramina on one side to exit just caudal to the sacroiliac joint. The injuring forces typically compress and impact the fracture fragment against the main sacral body. Juxta-articular fractures also involve the lateral sacral mass adjacent to the sacroiliac joint, but the fragments are dissociated from the main sacral body, often giving the appearance of free floating islands of bone in the periarticular region. Cleaving fractures are oriented vertically and extend from the area of the sacral notch to exit inferiorly near the coccyx. They may incorporate one or more neural foramina and tend to be noncomminuted. Avulsion fractures occur along the convex sacral margin at the insertion sites of the sacrotuberous and sacrospinous ligaments. At least one of these sacral fracture patterns has been estimated to occur in 4 to 74 percent of major pelvic trauma.[15,44] Further appreciation of the mechanism of their production and the criteria of their stability will depend upon a more general understanding of the mechanics of pelvic fracture and pelvic stability.

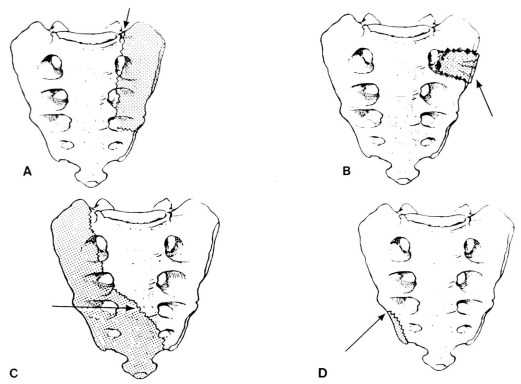

Figure 9-9. (A) Lateral mass fracture. (B) Juxta-articular fracture. (C) Cleaving fracture. (D) Avulsion fracture.

PELVIC FRACTURES AND PELVIC STABILITY

The pelvic ring is a relatively rigid structure whose traumatic disruption results in discontinuity in at least two places.[16] Pelvic ring discontinuity may occur either as a fracture or as a ligamentous disruption. During the past decade, new concepts have emerged in the understanding of pelvic ring injuries that are central to an understanding of vertical sacral fractures. Pelvic fractures are now classified into three radiographically identifiable groups based on mechanism of injury[33] (Figure 9-10). In each of these fracture groups, there is an anterior and a posterior discontinuity in the pelvic ring. The anterior lesion may involve a diastasis of the symphysis pubis, a fracture of the pubic rami, or occasionally a transacetabular fracture. The posterior lesion may include a sacral fracture, a dislocation of the sacroiliac joint, or a fracture of the ilium. In addition to identifying fracture type, a determination of stability must be made. Stability in a clinical sense is defined by the ability of the patient to bear weight without further displacement of the fracture fragments occurring.

Anteroposterior and lateral compression-type injuries may be associated with either a stable or unstable hemipelvis, whereas vertical shear fractures are universally unstable. The best index of instability in these fractures is provided by the disruption and displacement of the sacroiliac joint. This finding has been similarly associated with

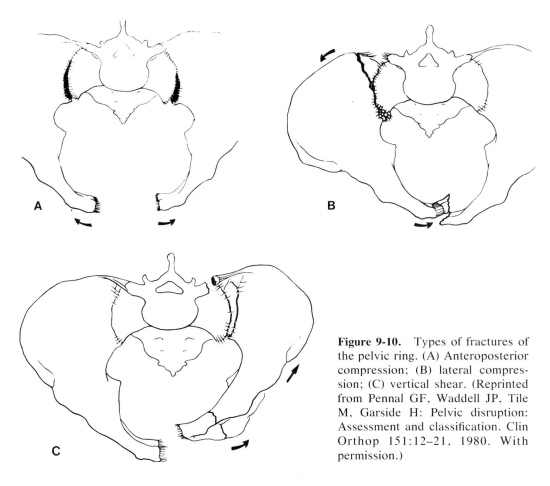

Figure 9-10.   Types of fractures of the pelvic ring. (A) Anteroposterior compression; (B) lateral compression; (C) vertical shear. (Reprinted from Pennal GF, Waddell JP, Tile M, Garside H: Pelvic disruption: Assessment and classification. Clin Orthop 151:12–21, 1980. With permission.)

increased blood loss and has proved extremely important as a resuscitative and prognostic indicator.[33]

Anteroposterior Compression Injuries of the Pelvic Ring

Typically an anteroposterior compression injury consists of a separation of the symphysis pubis associated with disruption of the anterior sacroiliac ligaments as the two halves of the pelvis are pried apart. The strong posterior sacroiliac ligaments remain intact, acting as hinges except in extreme degrees of trauma, when they too may be disrupted. Less frequently, one encounters a juxta-articular fracture through the posterior ilium or a vertically oriented fracture through the sacrum should the bone yield in advance of the ligamentous structure. As long as the sacrum and ilium remain intact, pelvic stability depends on the integrity of the posterior sacroiliac ligaments, which is inferred from the absence of superoposterior displacement of the ilium relative to the sacrum in anteroposterior and lateral roentgenograms. When the posterior component of injury consists of vertical sacral fracture, the pelvis is best considered unstable despite an intact posterior sacroiliac ligament.[20] Rupture of the sacrospinous ligament or avulsion of the sacral margin or ischial spine by this ligament also indicates instability.

Lateral Compression Injuries of the Pelvic Ring

Lateral compression is the most common mechanism of injury to the pelvic ring. Forces directed centripetally from the lateral aspect of the ilium cause an inward rotation of the anterior hemipelvis and injury to the pubic rami and symphysis pubis. Concurrently, a compressive force is produced on the anterior half of the sacroiliac joint while tensile stresses are developed in the posterior sacroiliac ligaments. Posterior ligamentous failure may ensue, or the anterior portion of the lateral mass of the sacrum may be crushed and impacted by compressive forces. In severe cases, both types of injury may result.

Vertical Shear Injuries

A vertical shear fracture of the pelvic ring typically results from an upward force transmitted through one of the lower extremities and occurs in association with severe trauma, such as falls from a height or injury in vehicular accidents. The fracture pattern includes a break through the pubic rami or the symphysis pubis anteriorly and through the sacrum, sacroiliac joint, or ilium posteriorly. The hemipelvis is driven superior and posterior to the main sacral body with complete disruption of the posterior pelvic ring. All vertical shear injuries are therefore unstable. They are attended by a high incidence of associated injuries, which in addition to neural deficit include long bone fractures, urethral and bladder trauma, hepatic and splenic lacerations, and massive retroperitoneal hemorrhage.

SACRAL FRACTURE REVIEW, MEDICAL CENTER HOSPITAL OF VERMONT

This system of pelvic fracture classification is useful both diagnostically and therapeutically.[33,42] Since a majority of injuries do in fact conform to these relatively simple mechanistic conceptions, it would seem probable that specific patterns of sacral fracture might emerge in association with each pelvic fracture type. To explore this possibility and to delineate associated neural injuries, we have reviewed a series of 15 cases of sacral fracture at the Medical Center Hospital of Vermont during the past 5 years (Table 9-2).

The number of cases does not permit broad generalization, yet some preliminary observations can be made relevant to sacropelvic fractures that may warrant further validation in a larger series. Two cases of anteroposterior pelvic compression injury with associated sacral fracture were identified. As the hemipelves are rotated outward, tensile force develops in the anterior sacroiliac as well as the sacrotuberous and sacrospinous ligaments. Failure may occur within the substance of the ligaments or, as is seen in case 3 (Figure 9-11) in the lateral margin of the sacrum, which is avulsed at the point of ligamentous insertion. Once these and the anterior sacroiliac ligament fail, there is little to resist further outward rotation of the hemipelvis. Case 4 (Figure 9-12) demonstrates a long vertical cleaving fracture exiting near the midline distally. A

Table 9-2.
Sacral fractures, Medical Center Hospital of Vermont, 1979–1984

Case Number	Sacral Fracture Type	Pelvic Fracture Type	Sacroiliac Joint Displaced	Stable	Neurologic Deficit
1	Penetrating	—	No	Yes	Yes
2	L5/S1 Fracture-Dislocation	—	No	No	Yes
3	Avulsion	AP Compression	No	No	Yes
4	Cleaving	AP Compression	No	No	No
5	Lateral Mass	Lateral Compression	No	Yes	No
6	Lateral Mass	Lateral Compression	No	Yes	No
7	Lateral Mass	Lateral Compression	No	Yes	No
8	Lateral Mass	Lateral Compression	No	Yes	No
9	Lateral Mass	Lateral Compression	No	Yes	No
10	Lateral Mass	Lateral Compression	No	Yes	Yes
11	Lateral Mass	Lateral Compression	No	Yes	Yes
12	Lateral Mass	Lateral Compression	Yes	No	Yes
13	Lateral Mass	Lateral Compression	Yes	No	Yes
14	Juxta-articular	Lateral Compression	Yes	No	Yes
15	Combination	Verticle Shear	Yes	No	Yes

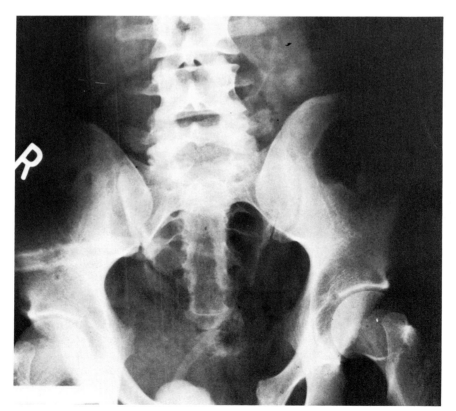

Figure 9-11.   Avulsion fracture of the right lower sacral margin.

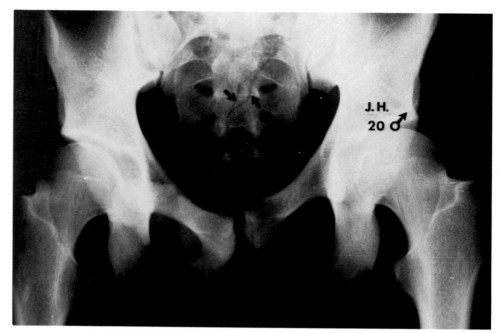

Figure 9-12.   Cleaving fracture of the sacrum.

comparable sacral fracture also in combination with diastasis of the symphysis pubis has been reported by Wiesel et al.[48] This type of fracture is thought to result from tensile forces developed across the anterior sacrum by the anterior sacroiliac ligaments as the pelvis is pried open. If ligamentous structures remain intact, failure of the sacrum is initiated anteriorly by tensile stress and propagates distally to longitudinally cleave the sacrum.

The sacral fractures associated with lateral compression injuries of the pelvis were predominantly of the lateral mass type in our series. Inward rotation of the hemipelvis generates tensile stress on the posterior sacroiliac ligament and compressive stress on the anterior intra-articular portion of the lateral mass. Failure evidently occurs in one of three modes: (1) compression-type fracture of the lateral mass; (2) a combination of lateral mass fracture and rupture of the posterior sacroiliac ligaments; (3) sacroiliac joint dislocation with resultant juxta-articular fractures. Of 10 patients with lateral compression injuries, in 6 the sacrum failed according to the first mode; these were regarded as stable lesions. In 3 the sacrum failed according to the second mode; these were unstable because the bony and ligamentous integrity of the posterior pelvic ring was disrupted. In this type of injury the lateral mass fragments migrate superiorly and posteriorly because of the insertion of the abdominal musculature is maintained. In one case the sacrum failed according to the third mode with gross derangement of the sacroiliac joint and accompanying periarticular fractures not of the lateral mass type. It is presumed that the posterior ligamentous complex fails in tension before a major anterior compression fracture of the lateral mass occurs. The sacroiliac joint dislocates under further stress resulting in avulsion fractures either at attachment sites of the interosseous ligaments or where the two joint surfaces shear over one another.

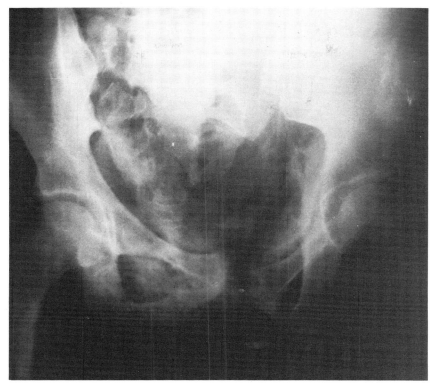

Figure 9-13.   Vertical shear injury of the pelvis with complex sacral fracture.

According to Huittinen, the third pattern of juxta-articular fracture is more common than our experience suggests.[20,21]

The single vertical shear fracture in our series was a severe injury consisting of bilateral sacroiliac joint disruption and a complex fracture of the sacrum (Figure 9-13). The types of sacral fracture resulting from vertical shear injuries defy precise analysis, but it is speculated that the orientation of the resolved injuring force determines the fracture pattern. If the force is directed mainly posteriorly, sacroiliac dislocation with or without juxta-articular fractures is more likely to ensue. As the the resolved force is directed more superiorly, the lateral mass of the sacrum is apt to be engaged by the ilium in the process of dislocation resulting in extensive fractures of the lateral mass. Table 9-3 summarizes the usual patterns of sacral and posterior ring pathology for each of the pelvic fracture types.

Patterns of Neural Injury Occurring in Association with Sacral Fractures

Sacral fractures occur in conjunction with pelvic fractures in 90 percent of cases, and almost one fourth of these cases will be attended by a neurologic deficit.[1,12,44] In the smaller group of isolated transverse sacral fractures, accompanying neural injury is almost invariable. Deficits may take the form of cauda equina injuries, radiculopathies, and plexopathies. Are specific patterns of neural injury associated with specific kinds of sacral and pelvic trauma?

Table 9-3.
Patterns of sacral and posterior pelvic ring injury in the various types
of pelvic fracture

Pelvic Fracture Type	Sacral Fracture Type	Other Posterior Pelvic Ring Injuries	Stable
AP Compression	Cleaving		No
	Avulsion		No
		Anterior Sacroiliac Ligament injury	Yes
Lateral Compression	Lateral Mass		Yes
	Juxta-articular		Yes
		Posterior Sacroiliac Ligament Injury	No
Vertical Shear	Juxta-articular Combination	Anterior and Posterior Sacroiliac Ligament Injury Ileal Fracture	No

Our knowledge of the pathologic anatomy and neurologic sequelae of these injuries is currently fragmentary. Frequently, when series of pelvic fractures are reported, the details of the sacral injury and associated neurologic deficits are insufficiently characterized to permit meaningful analysis. The circumstances of such trauma usually mitigate against anterior operative exposure and direct visualization of the injury site during life is only seldom afforded. Much of our present understanding of the subject derives from a well-studied group of 42 pelvic fractures reported by Huittinen in an autopsy series.[20] Thirty-eight patients of this group had "double vertical fractures" involving both anterior and posterior disruption of the pelvic ring. The exact number of sacral fractures is unspecified. A total of 40 neural lesions were identified among 22 cases of this group (Figure 9-14). Traction injuries that affected primarily the lumbosacral trunk and superior gluteal nerve as each crossed the sacroiliac joint accounted for one half of these lesions. The majority of these injuries were associated with gross hemipelvic dislocation. Nerve root avulsions constituted about 40 percent of lesions and most commonly involved the cauda equina, the superior gluteal nerve, the obturator nerve, and the L5 root. Of the six cases of root avulsion within the cauda equina, five were associated with transverse sacral fracture. Multiple roots were usually affected, and although the site of avulsion occurred intradurally between the dorsal root ganglion and the lumbar enlargement, the distal ends could migrate beyond the neural foramina to lie within the pelvis. Goodell independently corroborated some of these observations during his exploration of a transverse fracture through a sacral laminectomy.[17] Purely compressive injuries accounted for about 10 percent of lesions and were restricted to the ventral rami of sacral nerves S1–S3 as they traversed comminuted fracture sites through the anterior foramina. Operative confirmation of similiar pathologic conditions is available in the reports of Weaver, Fountain, and Fardon, who have also explored patients through a sacral laminectomy.[9,12,45] These authors emphasized the role of hematoma and a ventral gibbus deformity in the case of transverse fractures as additional sources of neural compression within the sacral

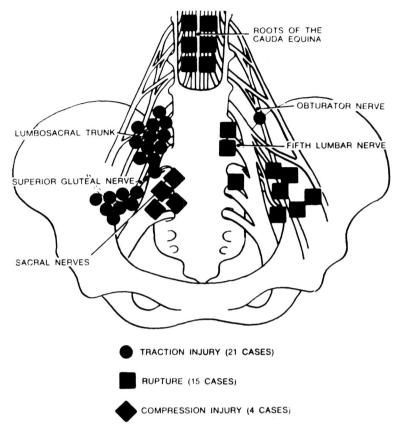

Figure 9-14. Sites of neural injury in 22 patients with pelvic fracture as determined at postmortem. (Reprinted from Huittinen VM, Slatis P: Fractures of the pelvis. Acta Chir Scand 1348:574, 1972. With permission.)

canal. Direct injury to the dorsal rami of the sacral nerves was not described in these studies.

The autopsy findings and isolated clinical observations demonstrate that neural injury accompanying sacral fractures occurs either intradurally or extradurally within the sacral canal, within the neural foramina, extraforaminally in the roots and divisions that contribute to the formation of the sacral plexus, and within the various nerves derived from the lumbar and sacral plexuses. Intraspinal and intraforaminal injury are particularly associated with transverse sacral fractures, while extraforaminal injuries are characteristically associated with fracture or displacement of the sacroiliac joint. The functional deficits resulting from the differing types of sacral injury should therefore be quite predictable, yet this problem has never been analyzed in large clinical series.

Detailed review of the literature and of our own case material reveals siginificant differences in the likelihood and pattern of neural injury, depending upon the orientation of the sacral fracture and the associated injuries to the posterior ring. In Table 9-4 are summarized the neurologic findings and outcomes in 23 cases of transverse sacral

Table 9-4.
Neurologic findings and outcome in a collected series of transverse sacral fractures

Reference	Displaced	Neural Deficit	Decompressed	Follow-up (months)	Condition
Fardon	Yes	S1, B/B*	Yes	9	Improved
Fardon	No	S1	No	3	Improved
Fountain et al.[15]	Yes	S1, B/B	Yes	5	Improved
	Yes	N, B/B	Yes	6	Improved
	Yes	N, B/B	Yes	4	Improved
	Yes	B	Yes	4	Improved
	Yes	N, B/B	Yes	1½	Improved
	Yes	B	No	1	Improved
Purser[40]	Yes	none	No		
Bynes et al.[4]	Yes	BB, S2	Yes	9	Unchanged
	Yes	B minimal	No		Normal
Woodward and Kelly[56]	Yes	L5	No	3	Improved
Weaver et al.[52]	Yes	S1/S2, B/B	Yes		Improved
Heckman and Keats[23]	Yes	B/B	No	14	Normal
Ferris and Hutton[14]	Yes	L5S1, B/B	No	18	Improved
	Yes	L5	No	1½	Abnormal
Bucknill and Blackburne[3]	Yes	L5/S1	No	18	Improved
	Yes	L5/S1	No	3	Normal
	Yes	S1	No	12	Improved
Meyer and Wilkberger[33]	Yes	B	Yes	1½	Normal
	Yes	B	Yes	3	Improved
Goodell[20]	Yes	B/B	Yes	3	Improved
Rowell[44]	Yes	sensation	No	18	Improved
	22/23	22/23	11/23		
	Displaced	With Deficit	Decompressed		

* B = bladder; B/B = bladder and bowel; N = other, unspecified neurologic deficit.

fractures assembled from the literature. Only cases in which sufficient detail was provided to enable the determination of neurologic status are included. Of note is the nearly constant association of transverse sacral fracture with neural injury. Approximately two thirds of these patients had a disturbance of bladder function, implying a bilateral deficit, probably within the spinal canal.

Vertical sacral fractures are less consistently associated with neurologic injury than transverse fractures, although this impression has not been systematically examined. Some suggestive information is available in the orthopedic literature where the frequency of neural injury in unselected series of pelvic fractures is estimated at between 0.75 and 11 percent.[1,24,32] In unstable pelvic fractures, particularly among those accompanied by a sacral fracture, the likelihood of neurologic deficit is said to be significantly increased.[17] Huittinen and Slatis reported a group of 68 patients with unstable "double vertical" fractures of the pelvis, 46 percent of which were complicated by neural injury.[21] Sacral fracture constituted the posterior pelvic ring injury in about 60 percent of this group; a sacroiliac joint disruption was noted in the remainder of cases. Deficits were confined to the L5 through S5 roots, with the predominance of

Table 9-5.

Patterns of neural injury in sacral fracture

Sacral Injury		Neural Deficit
	Direct	
Penetrating		Variable
Low transverse		Often Cauda Equina
		Occasional Radiculopathy
	Indirect	
High transverse		Often Cauda Equina,
		Occasional Radiculopathy,
		Plexopathies
Vertical		Usually Radicular (L5) or
		Plexopathy (L5-S1),
		Particularly with
		Dislocation Sacroiliac Joint

injury concentrated in L5 and S1. These findings in a clinical study are entirely consonant with Huittinen's subsequent observations in the autopsy series discussed above. Deficits were attributed to injury at the sacroiliac joint, but some authors were unable to discern any consistent relationship between the type of fracture visualized radiographically and the presence or severity of neural injury. Huittinen and Slatis repeatedly emphasized the poor prognosis of these lesions, a view shared by Patterson and Norton[32] and Raf,[37] but which contradicts the opinions of Froman and Stein,[14] Lam,[24] and others.

Among the 13 cases of vertical sacral fracture in our series at the Medical Center Hospital of Vermont, seven (54 percent) were attended by a neurologic deficit (see Table 9-2). All injuries occurred in a unilateral L5 or S1 distribution with the exceptions of case 5, a vertical shear fracture with complete loss of bladder and bowel function and perineal sensation, and case 3, a lateral mass fracture with unilateral sensory deficit in an S3 dermatome.

Except in the case of vertical shear fractures, there is no obvious relation between the mechanism of pelvic injury and the likelihood of neural involvement. Vertical shear injury is always associated with dislocation of the sacroiliac joint, a finding that is highly predictive of neural injury. In our small series this was present in four of five such instances. However, deficits may occur even in the absence of such dislocation, as was evidenced by cases 10 and 11 in the MCHV series and as has also been observed by Huittinen and others. Common patterns of neural injury associated with specific types of sacral fracture are given in Table 9-5.

Delayed neurologic deficit occurring after sacral fracture is an important complication that has been recognized by Bonnin and others,[1,2,5,7] and has been attributed to both callus and hematoma formation at the fracture site as well as untreated spinal instability. Case 12 is representative of this complication. A 32-year-old woman was injured in a motor vehicle accident in which she sustained a ruptured spleen, liver laceration, rib and wrist fractures, a myocardial contusion, and what was initially intrepreted as a stable pelvic fracture (Figure 9-15). No neurologic deficit was present either on admission or in the early convalescent period after emergency laparotomy. When the patient sat up in bed three days after her accident, she experienced increased

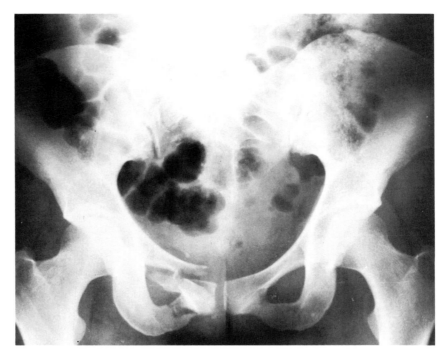

Figure 9-15.   Lateral compression injury with right lateral mass fracture of the sacrum.

pelvic pain and paresthesias along the posterolateral aspect of the left leg. Neurologic examination at this time disclosed sensory and reflex changes referable to the L5 and S1 roots. Repeat roentgenograms of the pelvis disclosed interval migration of the fragments in the anterior fracture site. Because of the ringlike configuration of the pelvis, this necessarily implied motion in the posterior fracture as well. On an emergent basis, a Hoffman-type fixateur was applied to re-establish pelvic reduction. When this was achieved, there was an accompanying restitution of neurologic function (Figure 9-16).

CLINICAL EVALUATION OF PATIENTS WITH POSSIBLE SACRAL FRACTURES

Neurologic Examination and Functional Neuroanatomy

Injury to the superior gluteal nerve is manifest by weakness of hip abduction and internal rotation. Injury to the L5 root may induce sensory alterations in the dorsum of the foot and the lateral aspect of the calf as well as weakness of the muscles of the anterior tibial compartment. Lesions of the lumbosacral trunk produce a summation of these findings. The S1 and S2 roots have myotomal representation primarily in the posterior aspect of the leg, where they are mainly responsible for hip extension, knee flexion, and plantar flexion. The corresponding sensory dermatomes also incorporate the posterior aspect of the leg, the sole and lateral aspect of the foot, and region of the genitalia (S2). The ankle jerk is typically diminished in lesions of the S1 nerve root.

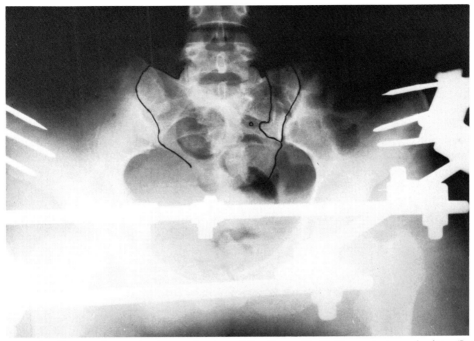

Figure 9-16. Status after reduction and external fixation with Hoffmann's type device. (Image reversed.)

Injury to roots S2 through S5 have been frequently overlooked, perhaps through their failure to precipitate obvious sensorimotor paralysis in the lower limbs. The S2 root participates in innervation of the muscles via the inferior gluteal and sciatic nerves, however, its functional importance for the limb is overshadowed by the predominance of S1 input at these levels. The S2 root plays a major role in the functional integrity of the genitals, bladder, and anorectal area as a main constituent of the pudendal nerve. This nerve, which also receives a contribution from the ventral rami of S3 and S4, innervates the striated musculature that forms the external urethral and external anal sphincters. In addition, the pudendal nerve gives sensory supply to the penis, labia majora, urethra, and anal canal.

Coordinated emptying of the bladder and rectum also requires the functional integrity of the autonomic system. The pelvic splanchnic nerves arise as fine branches in the ventral rami of S2 through S4. They represent the pelvic parasympathetic outflow and are distributed to the bladder and rectum through the inferior hypogastric plexus. Their afferent fibers are mainly responsible for normal awareness of vesical and ampullary filling, while their efferent fibers initiate detrusor and rectal contraction. Local sympathetic input to the inferior hypogastric plexus derives from the small sacral splanchnic nerves arising from the S2 and S3 sympathetic ganglia just medial to their respective ventral foramina. Sympathetic afferents are responsible for pain and thermal sensibilities; the sympathetic efferent limb causes contraction of the internal urethral and anal sphincters and inhibits contraction within the muscular walls of the associated viscus. During ejaculation they initiate contraction in the prostate, seminal vesicles, and ductus deferens to cause the discharge of semen. There is simultaneous activation of the internal vesicle sphincters to block retrograde passage of semen into the urinary bladder.

Neural injury to the sacral roots S2 to S5 is manifest by impairment of urinary and anal continence and sexual function. Clinical studies of patients with spinal dysrhaphism or patients undergoing major resections of sacral neoplasms suggest that functional continence and sexual competence depend upon at least the unilateral preservation of the S2 and S3 nerve roots. Bilateral loss to the S3 level is invariably attended by severe physiologic consequences.[18] With the exception of dermatomal sensory deficits, there are few clues to the discrete localization of injury. Further bedside evaluation includes estimation of anal tone and testing of the bulbocavernosus and anal wink reflexes. These functions depend upon the integrity of the S2 through S5 roots and their central connections in the conus medullaris. Their qualitative diminution does not permit exact localization of the levels affected in injury. Often this phase of the physical examination is neglected, incomplete, or is made impossible by the circumstances of multiple trauma, and the first suspicion of lower sacral injury occurs days later when the patient complains of perineal numbness or is unable to void after an indwelling urinary catheter is removed.

Radiographic Examination of the Sacrum

Bonnin[1] has estimated that sacral fractures should be demonstrable radiographically in approximately 45 percent of cases of pelvic fracture. Conventional anteroposterior roentgenograms of the pelvis do not demonstrate the sacrum optimally because of its curved surface and the lordosis at the lumbosacral junction; furthermore, overlying intestinal gas often obscures or confounds the interpretation of radiologic detail. However, certain findings intimate the presence of sacral fracture and suggest the need for more extensive investigation[1,8,22,23,31]: (1) fracture of a lower lumbar transverse process; (2) patterns of anterior pelvic fracture known to be highly associated with sacral fracture, e.g., four rami fracture; (3) discontinuity or asymmetry in the "sacral notch"; (4) clouding of the trabecular pattern in the lateral sacral mass; (5) irregularity in the "arcuate lines" of the upper three sacral foramina. Arcuate lines are the thin horizontally oriented arches that cap each of the sacral foramina. The foramina are shown to best advantage when the x-ray beam is angled about 50 degrees cephalad into the pelvis to show the sacrum en face (Figure 9-17). Although the patterns of sacral fracture are variable, the majority will traverse ventral foramina, which are then seen indistinctly or asymmetrically. Since breaks are frequently comminuted, they may fail to disclose themselves as single crisp fracture lines. Furthermore, because of the curved surfaces of the sacrum and the obliquity of the fracture, they are sometimes difficult to demonstrate in their entirety radiographically. The lateral view is useful chiefly in evaluating spondylolisthesis or sacral angulation in the case of transverse fractures.[22,23]

Addition radiographic delineation of pathologic sacral anatomy has been sought with oblique views, obstetric views, stereoscopic views, and laminograms. Presently, the CT scan offers superior resolution within the sacral canal and neural foramina[46,47] and will readily demonstrate vertically directed fractures (Figure 9-18). A limitation of this technique is that the intersegmental angulation or displacement that occurs in transverse fractures is not fully appreciated and necessitates conventional lateral roentgenograms or tomograms.

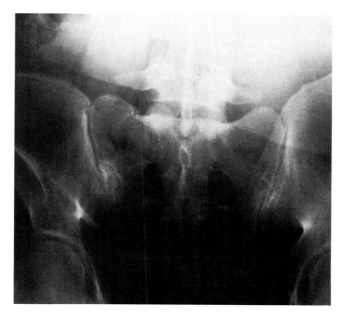

Figure 9-17.   The sacrum shown en face.

When a neurologic injury complicates a sacral fracture, several specialized examinations may be required to define the site of the injury and acquire prognostic information. Sacral myelography plays a lesser role in the investigation of these injuries than in those of the more rostral spine. The termination of the thecal sac at the S2 level together with patterns of neural injury favoring foraminal and extraforaminal injury present strong limitations to its use. The main utility of myelography exists in the evaluation of transverse sacral fractures at the S1 level that through angulation or spondylolisthesis may compress neural elements within the sacral canal. Weaver has demonstrated a mechanical block in this context.[45] Nerve root avulsions within the cauda equina also complicate a high proportion of transverse fractures and can result in traumatic meningoceles at the lumbosacral junction. Myelography may confirm the occurrence and thereby yield valuable prognostic information about the irreversibility of the associated deficit.[17]

Physiologic Investigations

Electromyography provides objective corroboration of the physical examination and is also helpful in localizing the area of injury and in determining prognosis. Degenerative changes (positive sharp waves, fibrillation potentials) confined to the distribution of a single peripheral nerve imply a peripheral injury. Injuries within the lumbar and sacral plexuses formed from the ventral rami of the spinal nerves typically yield more diffuse but patchy changes. Innervation of the paraspinal muscles derives from the early division of the dorsal primary rami. Plexus injuries therefore spare the paraspinal musculature, while in neural damage occurring within the spinal canal they will also participate in the pattern of injury. A normal EMG and nerve conduction study

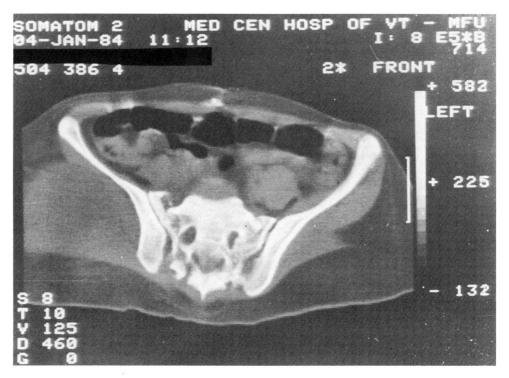

Figure 9-18.   Right lateral mass fracture demonstrated on CT scan.

in conjunction with a physiologic paralysis suggests a neuropractic lesion and ordinarily implies a favorable outlook for functional recovery. The main disadvantage of EMG is its restricted application in the acute phase of injury, since several weeks may be required for electrodiagnostic abnormalities to appear. As conventionally performed, it is useful only in assessing the lumbar and upper sacral roots, since there is no major myotomal representation in the limbs below the S2 level.

Specialized physiologic investigation of the lower sacral roots is accomplished by cystometrography (CMG), which is sometimes performed in concert with sphincter electromyography. Micturition is accomplished by a coordinated sequence of reflex actions that are modulated at suprasegmental and cortical levels. A CMG evaluation of these reflex functions attempts to elicit destrusor contraction through the active instillation of a liquid or gas. Intravesicular pressure is not ordinarily increased much until a volume of about 150 to 200 mL is achieved because of concurrent rises in the sympathetic tone inhibiting muscular contraction within the bladder wall. Once this critical volume is achieved, afferent discharges conducted centrally in the pelvic parasympathetic nerves achieve sufficient intensity to register upon the consciousness. When social circumstances permit, tonic inhibition within the brain stem micturition center is volitionally suppressed and destrusor contraction mediated via the pelvic parasympathetic efferents ensues. This is coupled with reflex inhibition of the pudendal nerve acting on the external sphincter and of the sympathetic outflow working on the internal urethral sphincter and bladder neck. Relaxation of these structures permits opening of the normally acute angulation at the bladder neck by vesicle contraction and permits free egress of urine.

Structural lesions of the sacrum tend to affect both the sympathetic and parasympathetic innervation of the lower urinary tract. On CMG this will be mainfest in destrusor areflexia and uninhibited sphincter relaxation or denervation during simultaneous EMG recording. In a more chronic condition, confirmation of this type of lower motor neuron lesion can be obtained through demonstration of denervation hypersensitivity. In this test, excessive destrusor activity is triggered by the exogenous administration of a parasympathomimetic. The principal usefulness of CMG is in the objectification of the clinical impression. The examination is easily repeated on a serial basis to gauge progress and it can be helpful in distinguishing upper motor neuron and lower motor neuron patterns of dysfunction in occasional cases where a concomitant cerebral or spinal cord injury complicates the sacral lesion. The CMG is also of value in excluding a neurologic component for incontinence when local trauma to the lower urinary tract precludes controlled micturition.

TREATMENT OF SACRAL FRACTURES

There is comparatively little experience in the direct operative decompression of neural injuries resulting from sacral and pelvic fractures. Tabulated in Table 9-4 are treatment results in 23 cases of transverse sacral fracture. Nearly all deficits improve to some degree with time, although only occasionally is the functional restitution complete. Approximately one half of the tabulated cases underwent sacral laminectomy, but the vagaries of case reporting and follow-up preclude a comparison of the results of conservative and operative management in this retrospective review. A direct anterior approach to the sacrum, especially in the acute phase of injury, is frought with hazard, since these injuries are usually accompanied by large presacral hematoma, which is tamponaded within the retroperitoneum. Surgical violation of this space may precipitate massive and sometimes uncontrollable hemorrhage. Neural decompression of acute injuries is best accomplished by obtaining and maintaining reduction of the sacropelvic injury. Patterson reported that 7 of 10 patients with neural deficits secondary to pelvic fracture were substantially improved at a mean follow-up of 18 months, although none were neurologically normal.[32]

Direct internal fixation to stabilize sacral fractures is occasionally possible, but, in general, operative stabilization of the sacrum lags behind the level of sophistication that exists for the remainder of the vertebral column, the appendicular skeleton, and, indeed, the remainder of the pelvis. At least 90 percent of sacral fractures are associated with other disruptions of the pelvic ring,[1,28,44] and in these cases, fixation of the ring may indirectly stabilize the sacrum. The classification of sacropelvic disruption by mechanism of injury as presented above provides the basis for logical evaluation and treatment. Severe pelvic disruption is an acutely life-threatening injury, and as such concerns about resuscitation and general patient management have top priority. In the face of massive hemorrhage, stabilization of the pelvis emergently through external fixation or other means helps to control pain and bleeding and can be a life-saving procedure.

Definitive treatment of sacropelvic fractures rests on a determination of stability as revealed in the patient history, physical examination, and x-ray evaluation. It is clear that the victim of a high-speed vehicular accident is more apt to sustain an unstable sacropelvic disruption than the patient who slips on the bathroom floor. Specific physical signs that suggest instability are asymmetry or prominence about the sacroiliac joint, apparent shortening or malrotation of the lower extremities, tenderness over the sacrum or sacroiliac joint region, or undue motion and pain on compression of the iliac crest. The final determination of stability depends on the roentgenographic analysis of the injury pattern.

An adequately reduced and stable sacropelvic injury is relatively easily managed by initial bedrest with progressive mobilization as patient comfort permits. Unstable fractures are more difficult to treat. If significant displacement is present, reduction must precede stabilization. Generally, reduction can be accomplished by a closed manipulation that reverses the forces producing the injury. The continued maintenance of the reduction often poses an even greater problem, and conventional methods of treatment include rest, skeletal traction, and hip spica casts. As in other types of fracture, it is desirable to achieve early stable fixation. This permits the patient to be mobilized, which leads to improved cardiovascular function, diminished pain, easier nursing care, and shortened hospitalization.[43] Although technical difficulties have impeded the realization of these goals, during the past 20 years great progress has been made in operative stabilization of the pelvis. Application of external fixation to the pelvis has diminished the need for prolonged bedrest.[39] Many different geometric configurations for external fixation frames have been devised that attach to multiple pins placed in the iliac crests anteriorly. However, none of these "anterior frames" can adequately stabilize a major posterior disruption of the pelvic ring to permit weight-bearing.[40]

To overcome this problem, frame designs that attach anteriorly and posteriorly to pins passed through the ilium from front to back have been designed.[27] These frames have been successful in stabilizing major posterior disruptions in both biomechanical and clinical tests. Their major drawback is that the required pin insertion is "technically difficult and requires special instrumentation."[40,42]

If the posterior component of the injury consists of sacroiliac joint dislocation and the lateral mass of the sacrum is for the most part intact, direct internal fixation is possible for the posterior lesion and may be supplemented with a simple anterior external fixation frame. An example is shown in Figure 9-19.

Definitive internal fixation when the substance of the sacrum is comminuted or when there is bilateral sacroiliac joint disruption is extremely difficult, perhaps impossible with the methods presently available. Unfortunately, these injuries are often the result of the greatest violence and pose the greatest threat to life and therefore are in greatest need of stabilization. In such cases, Hansen recommends the application of a bilateral hip spica cast incorporating bilateral distal femoral pins for emergent control of skeletal stability, blood loss, and pain (personal communication).

Extensive experience with sacral fractures that do not involve the remainder of the pelvis is limited and information regarding their treatment is inconclusive. Insofar as penetrating injuries to the sacrum are concerned, the situation is analogous to the pelvis that has undergone sacral resection for tumor, since in either case a portion of the sacrum of variable size and location is functionally absent. Gunterberg's biomechanical studies suggest that removal of the entire sacrum distal to the S1-S2 interspace, including the inferior portion of the sacroiliac joint, weakens the pelvic ring by only 30 percent and that further resection up to the level of S1 including the lower one half of

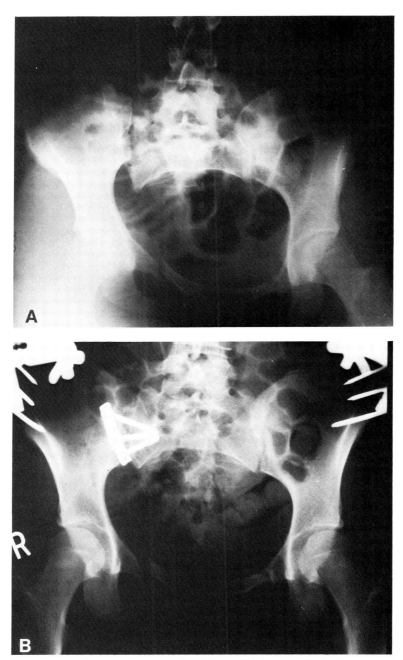

Figure 9-19. (A) Unstable lateral compression injury with juxta-articular fracture of the sacrum. (B) Status after closed reduction and internal fixation.

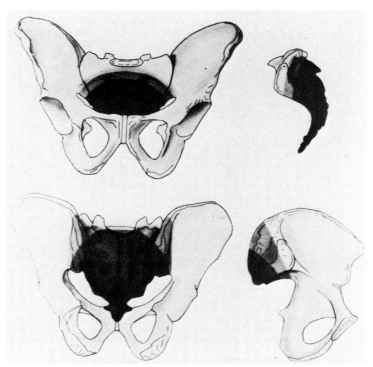

Figure 9-20. Extent of resections in Gunterberg's biomechanical studies of sacral instability. (Reprinted from Gunterberg B: Effects of major resection of the sacrum. Acta Orthop Scand (Suppl 2) 162:5, 1976. With permission.)

the sacroiliac joint weakened it by only 50 percent[18] (Figure 9-20). He concluded that it is safe with regard to the residual strength of the pelvic ring to allow patients to bear their full weight at an early stage after submaximal (trans-S1) resection of the sacrum including adjacent iliac bone. In penetrating wounds the associated nonskeletal injuries often command priority. If instability is present, bedrest with or without femoral pin traction or bilateral hip spica cast incorporating distal femoral pins are treatment options. External fixation with a frame capable of controlling the posterior pelvis, although technically difficult to apply, has the unique advantage of permitting soft tissue access.

In low transverse sacral fractures, the involved portion of the sacrum is not part of the weight-bearing system and is therefore considered a stable fracture. Digital reduction of the angulated distal segment through the rectum is described.[19] Weaver recommends bedrest for 1 to 2 months in treating this injury to promote osseous healing of the fracture site and to avoid pseudoarthrosis.[45] High transverse sacral fractures are rare and experience in their treatment is sparse. Bedrest and traction have been employed with moderate success, although at least one instance of transient neurologic deterioration during closed manipulation has been recorded.[2] Fardon reported a single case treated with operative decompression and Harrington rod instrumentation with good results.[9]

Lumbosacral fracture-dislocation is also quite rare. In this injury the articular facets are typically locked and closed reduction has proved impossible and again may be associated with a worsening of the neurologic picture.[5] Das De reported a series of four such cases treated with open reduction followed by posterior wiring and bone grafting.[4]

REFERENCES

1. Bonnin JG: Sacral fractures and injuries to the cauda equina. J Bone Joint Surg 27B:113, 1945
2. Bucknill TM, Blackburne JS: Fracture-dislocations of the sacrum, report of three cases. J Bone Joint Surg 58B:467, 1976
3. Byrnes DP, Russo GL, Ducker TB, Cowley RA: Sacrum fractures and neurological damage, report of two cases. J Neurosurg 47:459, 1977
4. Das De S: Lumbosacral fracture dislocations. J Bone Joint Surg 63B:58, 1981
5. Dewey P: Fracture dislocations of the lumbosacral spine with cauda equina lesion. J Bone Joint Surg 50B:635, 1968
6. Dunn AW, Morris HD: Fractures and dislocations of the pelvis. J Bone Joint Surg 59A:1639, 1968
7. Fardon DF: Displaced fractures of the lumbosacral spine with delayed cauda equina deficit. Clin Orthop 120:155, 1976
8. Fardon DF: Sacral fractures. J Neurosurg 48:316, 1978 (Letter to the Editor)
9. Fardon DF: Displaced transverse fracture of the sacrum with nerve root injury: Report of a case with successful operative management. J Trauma 19:119, 1979
10. Fardon DF: Intrasacral meningocele complicated by transverse fracture. J Bone Joint Surg 62A:839, 1980
11. Ferris B, Hutton P: Anteriorly displaced transverse fractures of the sacrum at the level of the sacroiliac joint. A report of two cases. J Bone Joint Surg 65A:407, 1983
12. Fountain SS, Hamilton RD, Jameson RM: Transverse fractures of the sacrum. J Bone Joint Surg 59A:486, 1977
13. Frederickson BE, Yuan HA, Miller HE: Treatment of painful long-standing displaced fracture-dislocations of the sacrum. Clin Orthop Rel Res 166:93, 1982
14. Froman C, Stein A: Complicated crush injuries of the pelvis. J Bone Joint Surg 49B:29, 1976
15. Furey WW: Fractures of the pelvis with special reference to associated fractures of the sacrum. AJR 47:89, 1942
16. Gertzbein SD, Chenoweth DR: Occult injuries of the pelvic ring. Clin Orthop 128:302, 1977
17. Goodell CL: Neurological deficits associated with pelvic fractures. J Neurosurg 24:837, 1966
18. Gunterberg B: Effects of major resection of the sacrum. Acta Orthop Scand (Suppl 2) 162:5, 1976
19. Heckman JD, Keats PK: Fracture of the sacrum in a child. J Bone Joint Surg 60A:404, 1978
20. Huittinen VM: Lumbosacral nerve injury in fracture of the pelvis. Acta Chir Scand (Suppl) 429:6, 1972
21. Huittinen VM, Slatis P: Nerve injury in double vertical pelvic fractures. Acta Chir Scand 138:571, 1972
22. Jackson H, Kanon J, Harris H, Harle T: The sacral arcuate lines in upper sacral fractures. Radiology 145:35, 1982
23. Laasonen EM: Missed sacral fractures. Ann Clin Res 9:84, 1977
24. Lam CR: Nerve injury in fractures at the pelvis. Ann Surg 104:945, 1936
25. Malgaigne JF: Treatment of Fractures. (Transl. JH Packard). Philadelphia, J.B. Lippincott, 1859
26. McMurty R, Walton D, Dickinson D, Kellam J, Tile M: Pelvic disruption in the polytraumatized patient: A management protocol. Clin Orthop 151:22, 1980
27. Mears DC, Fu FH: Modern concepts of external skeletal fixation of the pelvis. Clin Orthop 151:65, 1980
28. Mendelman JP: Fractures of the sacrum, their incidence in fracture of the pelvis. AJR 42:100, 1939
29. Meyer TL, Wilkberger B: Displaced sacral fractures. Am J Orthop 4:187, 1962
30. Nicoll EA: Fractures of the dorsolumbar spine. J Bone Joint Surg 31B:376, 1949
31. Northrop CH, Eto RT, Loop SW: Vertical fracture of the sacral ala: Significance of noncontinuity of the anterior superior sacral foraminal line. AJR 124:102. 1975
32. Patterson FP, Norton KS: Neurologic complications of fractures and dislocations of the pelvis. Surg Gynecol Obstet 112:702, 1961
33. Pennal GF, Waddell JP, Tile M, Garside H:

Pelvic disruption: Assessment and classification. Clin Orthop 151:12, 1980

34. Perry JF: Pelvic open fractures. Clin Orthop 151:41, 1980

35. Posner N, White A, Edwards W, Hayes W: A biomechanical analysis of the clinical stability of the lumbar and lumbosacral spine. Spine 7:374, 1982

36. Purser DW: Displaced fracture of the sacrum, report of a case. J Bone Joint Surg 51B:346, 1969

37. Raf L: Double vertical fractures of the pelvis. Acta Chir Scand 131:298, 1966

38. Rowell CE: Fracture of the sacrum with hemisaddle anaesthesia and lumbospinal fluid leak. Med J Australia 1:16, 1965

39. Slatis P, Karaharju EO: External fixation of unstable pelvis fractures: Experiences in 22 patients treated with a trapezoid compression frame. Clin Orthop 151:73, 1980

40. Smith TK, Johnston RM, Browner BC, Bucholz RW: Symposium: External fixation of pelvic fractures. Contemp Orthop 7:81, 1983

41. Solonen KA: The sacroiliac joint in light of anatomical, roentgenological, and clinical studies. Acta Orthop Scand (Suppl 27), 127, 1957

42. Tile M, Pennal GF: Pelvic disruption: Principles of management. Clin Orthop 151:56, 1980

43. Tscherne H, Oestern HJ, Sturm J: Osteosynthesis of major fractures in polytrauma. World J Surg 7:80, 1983

44. Wakeley CPG: Fractures of the pelvis: An analysis of 100 cases. Br J Surg 17:22, 1929

45. Weaver EN, England GD, Richardson DE: Sacral fracture: Case presentation and review. Neurosurgery 9:725, 1981

46. Whelan MA, Gold RP: Computed tomography of the sacrum: Normal anatomy. AJNR 3:547, 1982

47. Whelan MA, Hilaz SK, Gold RP, Luken M, Michelson WJ: Computed tomography of the sacrum, pathology. AJNR 3:555, 1982

48. Wiesel SW, Zeide MS, Terry RL: Longitudinal fractures of the sacrum, case report. J Trauma 19:70, 1979

49. Woodward AA, Kelly PJ: An unusual fracture of the sacrum. Minn Med 57:465, 1974

Carrie L. Walters, Henry H. Schmidek,
Martin H. Krag, Linda Brier

10

The Management of Thoracolumbar Fractures

The goals of maximal neurologic recovery, a stable spine, and freedom from disabling pain have been achieved with varying degrees of success in the treatment of thoracolumbar fractures by a number of different techniques throughout the years. As early as 400 BC Hippocrates taught that a fractured bone must be returned to its anatomic position and stabilized. In the first half of this century the treatment of spinal fractures consisted of manipulation followed by immobilization in plaster as advocated by Watson-Jones, who observed that "perfect recovery is only possible if perfect reduction is insisted upon."[50] Guttman in the 1940s introduced postural reduction without forceful manipulation, while Albee advocated open reduction and fusion of spinal fracture-dislocations.[20,40] During the 1950s the experience with operative treatment increased. Holdsworth, Pennybacker, and others observed that progressive spinal angulation at the fracture site, resulting in neurologic dysfunction and chronic debilitating pain, could be reduced by operative intervention.[26,40] Hardy, Guttman and others continued to emphasize the benefits of nonsurgical treatment into the 1970s.[21,40]

The usefulness of surgical intervention, however, has continued to improve in recent years for a variety of reasons. One of the most important has been the ongoing development of spinal stabilizing hardware. The first really successful implant was the Harrington rod system, originally developed for scoliosis correction[24] and later adopted[8,12,16,25,50] and modified[5,11,14,15,18,51] for fracture stabilization. More recently developed devices[13,22,32,33,48] have been used anteriorly. The most recent implants[13,34,45] actually produce rigid fixation (and not just distraction or compression), and also attach directly at the fracture site, thus substantially reducing the length of spine involved in the fusion.

A second important factor for increased efficacy of surgical intervention has been the improved selectivity made possible by better roentgenographic visualization, such as conventional tomography and, more recently, computer-assisted tomography (CT scans). With these and other developments, evidence is accumulating that surgical intervention, when properly applied, can dependably produce a number of benefits, including reduced spinal pain, improved spinal stability, shortened hospitalization time, and fewer complications related to spinal cord injuries. Although the evidence is less clear cut concerning the benefits of surgery for neurologic improvement in the immediate postinjury period, there is an increasing amount of data suggesting that patients with spines that have not been adequately decompressed do have an increased risk of developing increasing neurologic deficits and pain months to years after the injury.[2,16,28,37,39]

Four years ago a report originated from our Spine Injury Service describing an approach to the treatment of thoracolumbar fractures and the results that had been achieved.[46] The present report describes our current thinking regarding the management of these problems and documents the improved outcome resulting from a number of changes, particularly with regard to stabilization procedures and timing of ambulation.

MATERIALS AND METHODS

The present series comprises 67 surgically treated patients with thoracolumbar fractures treated surgically at the Medical Center Hospital of Vermont from January 1977 to September 1983. The 48 patients treated from 1977 to 1981 constitute group A and have in part been reported upon earlier.[47] The 19 patients treated from 1981 to 1983 are new cases and constitute group B. Thirteen (19 percent) patients had injuries between T1 and T10; 43 (64 percent) had thoracolumbar junction injuries (T11–L2); 5 (7 percent) had lumbar injuries (L3–L5); and 6 (9 percent) had fractures of at least two spinal levels. The L1 vertebra was the most frequently injured among both the single and multilevel injuries, being involved in five of the six multilevel fractures (Figure 10-1). Data on these cases were obtained from hospital charts, outpatient records, and the review of all available roentgenograms and spinal CT scans. Fractures treated by nonoperative means were excluded from this study. There were 43 men and 24 women, ranging in age from 15 to 72 years with a mean age of 27 years (Table 10-1). The injuries were caused by motor vehicle accidents in 24 (36 percent) patients; falls from a height in 21 (31 percent) patients; motorcycle accidents in 6 (8 percent) patients; skiing accidents in 6 (8 percent) patients; motorized hang glider accidents in 2 (3 percent) patients; and miscellaneous causes in 8 (12 percent) patients (Table 10-2). Twenty-five patients were initially treated at the Medical Center Hospital of Vermont: 6 within 4 hours, 1 within 8 hours, and the remaining 18 within 24 hours of the time of injury. Forty-two patients received their initial treatment elsewhere and were then transferred to the Medical Center Hospital: 22 of these patients arrived within 24 hours of injury, 6 within 48 hours, and 14 between 3 days and 5 1/2 months.

Based on the appearance on plain x-ray films and CT scans, the fractures were catagorized as follows:

1. Flexion injury. Disruption of the posterior ligaments without associated bony injury (Figure 10-2).
2. Axial compression injury. Comminuted fracture of the vertebral body with bone retropulsed into the spinal canal. Posterior ligamentous complex intact (Figure 10-3).

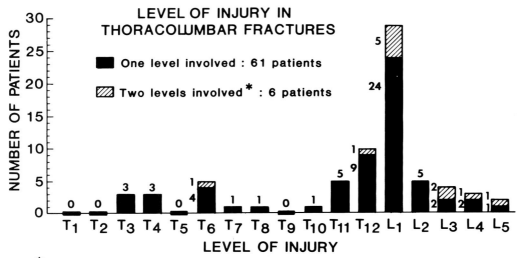

*One patient had a C_5 fracture in addition to a thoracolumbar fracture.

Figure 10-1. The level of injury in thoracolumbar fractures.

3. Flexion. Axial compression injury.
    Type A. Anterior wedge fracture of the vertebral body less than 50 percent of its height, usually with intact posterior spinous elements and ligamentous structures (Figure 10-4).
    Type B. Anterior wedge fracture of the vertebral body exceeding 50 percent of its height, usually with posterior ligamentous disruption with or without posterior bony element fractures (Figure 10-5).
    Type C. Burst fracture-dislocation with vertebral body fragments retropulsed into the spinal canal, disruption of the posterior ligamentous complex and, frequently, with fracture of the posterior bony elements (Figure 10-6).
4. Flexion-rotation injury. Rotational fracture-dislocation with the cephalad vertebral body rotated upon the caudad vertebral body, carrying with it a "slice fragment" of the upper portion of the lower vertebra. The rotational force results in a unilateral facet fracture of the caudal vertebra, while the flexion force often results in a concomitant wedge or burst fracture (Figure 10-7).
5. Hyperextension injury. Anterior ligamentous disruption with posterior displacement of the cephalad vertebral body in relation to the caudal one (Figure 10-8).

Table 10-1.
Thoracolumbar fractures—1977–1983

Total Number of Patients: 67
Thoracolumbar Junction Fractures (T11–L2): 48
Mean Age: 27
Age Range: 15–72
Males: 43
Females: 24

Table 10-2.
Mechanism of injury—Thoracolumbar fractures

Motor Vehicle:	24
Fall from Height:	21
Motorcycle:	6
Skiing:	6
Motorized Hang Glider:	2
Other:	8

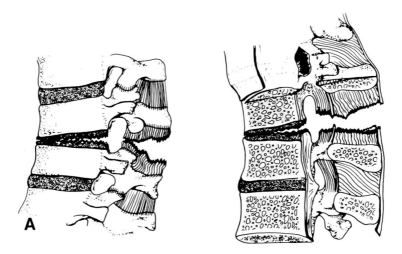

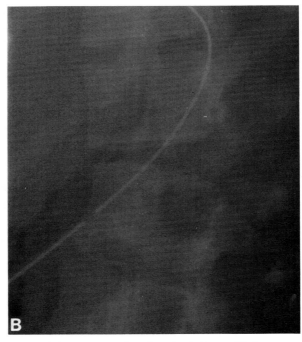

Figure 10-2. (A) A flexion injury in lateral and sagittal views. (B) Lateral x-ray film of a flexion injury.

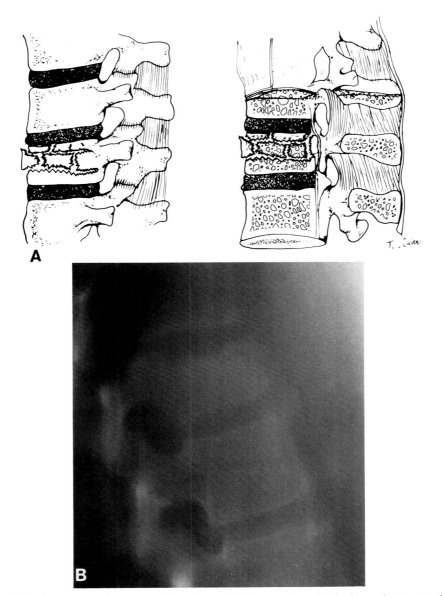

Figure 10-3. (A) An axial compression injury in lateral and sagittal views demonstrating an intact posterior ligmentous complex. (B) Lateral tomogram of an axial compression injury.

6. Flexion-distraction injury (seat belt injury, Chance fracture). A transverse disruption of the vertebral body and neural arch through the pedicles with intact posterior ligamentous structures (Figure 10-9).

This classification system is largely based on that of Holdsworth[26] and Bohlman et al.[3] In addition, other systems have been proposed more recently such as by McAfee et al.[38] and Denis.[10]

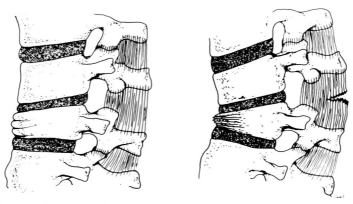

Figure 10-4. An anterior wedge fracture. (Left) less than 50 percent; (right) greater than 50 percent.

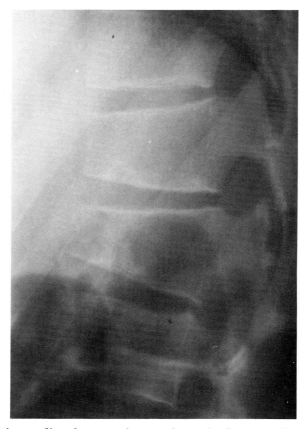

Figure 10-5. Lateral x-ray film of consecutive anterior wedge fractures. Uppermost fracture less than 50 percent; lower fracture greater than 50 percent.

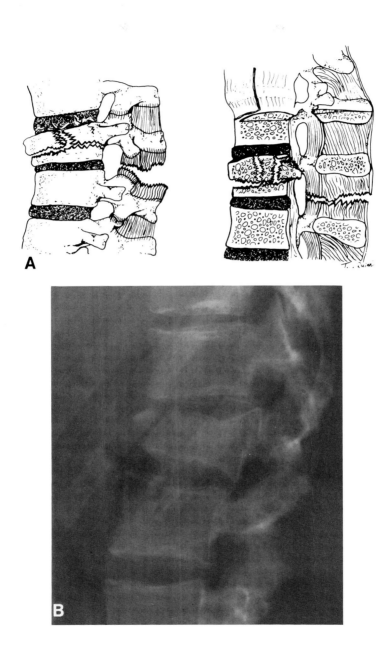

227

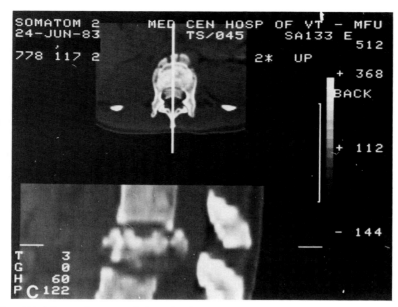

Figure 10-6. (A) A burst fracture-dislocation in lateral and sagittal view. (B) Lateral -ray film of a burst fracture-dislocation. The retrouplsed body fragment is hidden behind the pedicle. (C) A CT scan of a burst fracture-dislocation with sagittal reconstruction demonstrating the retropulsed fragment at the level of the pedicle.

Based on available evidence,[26,39,43,53] we consider the following injury types to be unstable and thus appropriate for strong consideration for surgical intervention: wedge fractures with a 50 percent or greater reduction in vertebral body height; burst fractures involving the pedicles, lamina, or facets, or disruption of the posterior longitudinal ligament; flexion-rotational injuries; hyperextension injuries and flexion-distraction injuries[26,39,43,53] (Table 10-3).

The 67 cases reported upon here consist of one flexion injury, 10 axial compression fractures; 44 flexion-axial compression fractures (3 type A, 15 type B, and 26 type C), 8 flexion-rotation injuries, 1 hyperextension injury; and 2 flexion-distraction injuries (Table 10-4). One case involving multiple thoracic fractures did not fit any one of these categories. Thirty-five of the 67 patients had the following nonspinal injuries: 8 head injuries, 8 limb fractures, 6 rib fractures, often with pulmonary contusions; 1 pelvic fracture, 1 aortic aneurysm, and 11 with more than one other system involved (Table 10-5).

Neural status was graded upon admission and subsequently using the Frankel scale.[17] Category A is no neurologic function below the level of injury, category B is preservation of sensory function below the injury only, category C is motor function below the level of injury that is inadequate for ambulation; category D is motor function below the level of injury allowing ambulation with or without braces, and category E is normal neural status. When examined initially at the Medical Center Hospital, 16 patients were in group A, 2 were in group B, 12 were in group C, 13 were in group D, and 23 were in group E (Table 10-4). Two patients in group E deteriorated neurologically shortly after admission to group B and C, respectively. One patient could not be

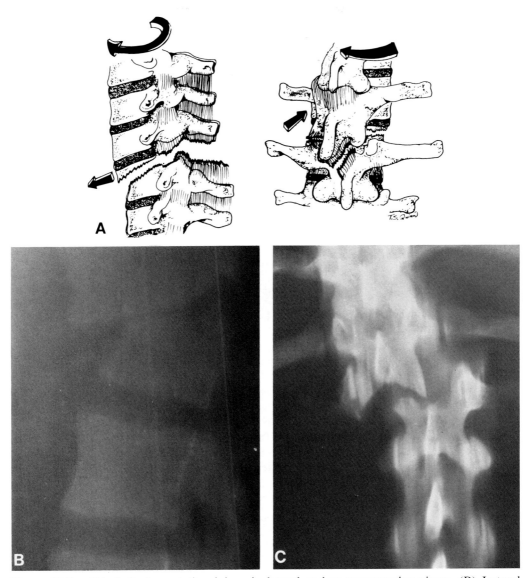

Figure 10-7. (A) A flexion-rotation injury in lateral and posteroanterior views. (B) Lateral tomograms of a flexion-rotation injury. (C) Anteroposterior tomograms of a flexion-rotation injury at T12-L1 demonstrating the fracture and dislocation of the left superior facet of L1.

categorized initially because of a head injury that produced a decreased level of consciousness and hemiparesis.

The current radiographic investigation of patients with thoracolumbar fractures includes anteroposterior and lateral spine roentgenograms to identify the level(s) of injury and computerized tomography with sagittal reconstruction of the injured area. All patients were evaluated with plain roentgenography, 41 patients with CT scans, and

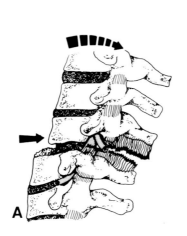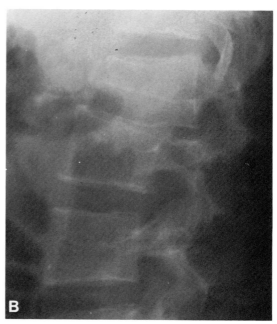

Figure 10-8. (A) A hyperextension injury. (B) Lateral x-ray film of a hyperextension injury.

22 with myelography. Several patients early in the series were investigated with polytomography. More recently we have been using metrizamide-enhanced CT scanning to identify the level of the conus (Figure 10-10) and the relationship of the neural elements to the bony fragments (Figure 10-11).

Since 1982, patients initially have been immobilized on the rotokinetic bed (Roto-Rest Mark I, Kinetic Concepts, San Antonio, TX 73219), which continuously rotates from side to side. Because the patient need not be turned prone, this device is particularly useful when there are concomitant injuries requiring chest tubes, external fixators for limb fractures, and close observation of the abdomen. Patients remain on this bed until surgery, after which they are transferred to a regular bed.

Patients are usually operated upon within 2 weeks of injury depending on their general condition. Fifty of the 67 patients were operated upon within 2 weeks of injury and all but 8 cases within 3 weeks. Only those patients with increasing neurologic deficit underwent emergent surgical decompression and stabilization. Two such patients were encountered in this series. Last, one patient with a thoracic fracture sustained 7 years previously and managed by a posterior bony fusion without decompression required subsequent anterolateral decompression when he experienced increasing pain and a progressive neurologic deficit despite an adequate fusion.

Patients with neural injury received 4 mg of dexamethasone every 6 hours for the first three days after injury. Physical therapy is started within the first three days of hospitalization. Prophylactic anticoagulation is not used.

All patients in this series had unstable fractures as defined above and underwent internal stabilization. Thirty-one patients without bone encroachment on the spinal cord or nerve roots underwent open reduction, internal fixation (usually with Harrington distraction rods), and bone grafting. Thirty-six patients with spinal canal

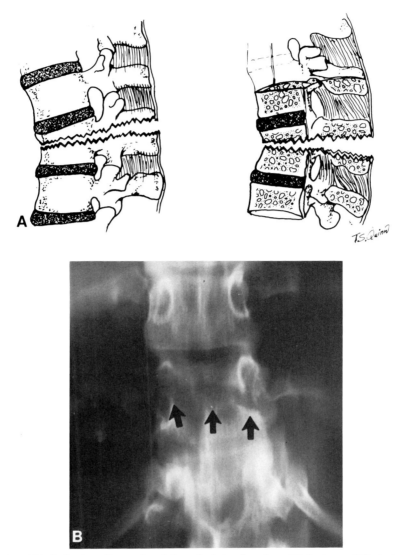

Figure 10-9. (A) A flexion-distraction injury in lateral and sagittal views. (B) Anteroposterior tomograms of a flexion-distraction injury with fracture line (arrows) through the body and both pedicles.

encroachment were managed by a one-stage operation including neural decompression, internal fixation, and bone grafting.

The 48 patients in group A were managed with Harrington rods, using hooks placed under the inferior articular process of the second vertebra above the fracture and into the lamina of the second vertebra below the fracture. A bone graft was placed over the five involved vertebrae. In group B, the approach was modified using the "rod-long fuse-short" technique proposed by Purcell et al.[44] and popularized by Jacobs et al.[29,31] This involves placing hooks farther apart (third level above to third level below the

Table 10-3.
Stability of thoracolumbar fractures

Type of Fracture	Forces Acting on the Spine	Vertebral Body Fracture	Intra-canicular Bone	Ligamentous Disruption	Stability
Pure flexion injury	Flexion	0	0	+	Unstable
Pure burst fracture	Axial loading	+	+	0	?
Anterior wedge fracture	Combination flexion and axial loading	+	0	0	Stable
Anterior wedge fracture (greater than 50 percent)	Combination flexion and axial loading	+	0	+	Unstable
Burst fracture-dislocation	Combination flexion and axial loading	+	+	+	Unstable
Slice fracture or flexion-rotation fracture	Flexion/rotation	+	0	+	Unstable
Hyperextension injury	Hyperextension	0	0	+	Unstable
Chance fracture—seat belt injury	Flexion/distraction	+	0	0	Unstable

fracture) for improved strength[44] and placing a bone graft over only three vertebrae (the injured vertebra, one above, and one below), thereby minimizing the loss of spinal mobility and disruption of normal vertebral levels. A new spinal implant is currently under development[34] that may be implanted through a posterior approach and that has the advantages of spanning only two or three vertebrae and of providing truly rigid multidirectional fixation.

Neural decompression was done before internal fixation and distraction to prevent the neural elements from being stretched over the protruded bone fragments or lacerated by bony spicules. There is little evidence that instrumentation alone produced substantial reduction of bone fragments from the spinal canal (Table 10-6). The selection of the operative approach for the decompression was determined by the location of the compressing bone fragments.

In the case of anterior spinal encroachment, decompression may be accomplished by using any of three different incisions: anterolateral (e.g., thoracotomy), posterior midline, or posterolateral. The anterolateral skin incision for the anterior or transpleural approach to the vertebrae has the advantage of providing access to the full width of the vertebral body without having to retract the dura. Its disadvantage is the potential morbidity arising from manipulation of the great vessels and lung in a patient already at risk of developing pulmonary complications. Furthermore, there are no secure well-tested fixation systems available for implantation through this approach, although various devices are being evaluated.[13,22] The posterior midline incision provides safe and easy access to the laminae, facet joints, and nerve roots, but in order to decompress the full width of the anterior spinal canal, either a laminectomy must be performed and the dura retracted medially on each side; the lateral portion of the laminae, the medial portion of the facet bilaterally and both pedicles must be excised to decompress half of the anterior canal from each side (posterolateral approach); or a single pedicle must be excised after the erector spinae muscles have been transected to allow a sufficiently

Table 10-4.
Thoracolumbar (T1–L5) fracture type and initial clinical grade

Type of Fracture	Total Number by Type	Clinical Grade (Frankel Scale)				
		A	B	C	D	E
		Nonambulatory			Ambulatory	
Flexion	1	0	0	0	1	0
Axial Loading Burst Fracture	10	0	0	2	4	4
Flexion plus Axial Loading	44					
Type A	3	2	0	0	0	1
Type B	15	3	0	2	1	9†
Type C	26*	7	1	5	6	6†
Flexion-Rotation	8	4	1	3	0	0
Hyperextension	1	0	0	0	0	1
Flexion-Distraction	2	0	0	0	1	1
Total	(66)	16	2	12	13	23‡

* One patient with an associated head injury could not be adequately classified with regard to clinical grade.
† One patient deteriorated from grade E shortly after admission.
‡ One patient (Frankel grade E) with multiple thoracic fractures could not be adequately categorized with regard to fracture type.

transverse view for safe decompression across the anterior spinal canal (anterolateral approach).[47]

To overcome these drawbacks, a variety of off-midline skin incisions have been proposed such as those of Capener,[7] Alexander,[1] and more recently, Larson.[36] Since 1982, we have used a posterolateral, muscle-splitting incision for anterior spinal canal decompression, In performing this operation, the patient is placed in a three-quarter lateral position with the side of maximal bone encroachment uppermost. The correct surgical level is identified on x-ray studies. A 10-cm longitudinal incision is made along the lateral margin of the erector spinae muscles (approximately 6 to 8 cm from the midline) and is carried down to the lumbar dorsal fascia, the anterior leaf of which separates the erector spinae and quadratus lumborum muscles. Staying within this fascial plane and dissecting anteromedially, the vertebral transverse process is identified and removed (Figure 10-12). When the fracture occurs in the lower thoracic or first

Table 10-5.
Associated injuries in thoracolumbar fractures

Injury	Number of Patients
Head	8
Thorax—bone	4
Thorax—bone plus Pulmonary	2
Pelvis	1
Upper extremity	3
Lower extremity	5
Aortic aneurysm	1
More than one other system involved	11
No associated injuries	32

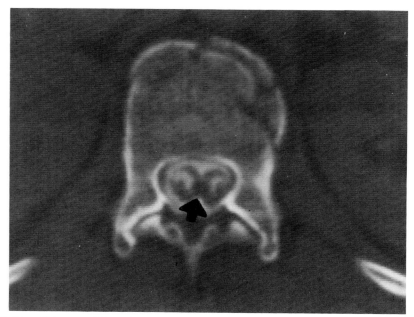

Figure 10-10. CT scan of L1 with intrathecal metrizamide demonstrating the conus (arrow).

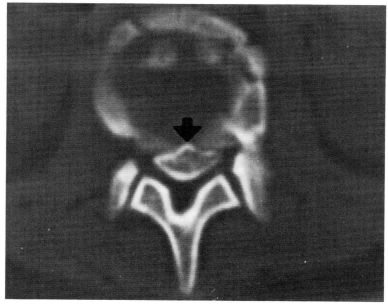

Figure 10-11. CT scan with intrathecal metrizamide showing herniation (arrow) of the dural sac and its contents into the fractured vertebral body.

Table 10-6.
Residual Intracanalicular bone in burst fractures (T1–L5) treated with
Harrington Rods

| Patient | Level | Percentage of Bony Occlusion | | % Δ |
		Preoperatively	Postoperatively	
B-7	T12	30	30	0
A-28	T12	50	30	20
B-14	L1	60	60	0
C-20	L1	70	70	0
A-13	L2	60	33	27
B-15*	L4	90	50	40

* Weiss Springs

lumbar vertebrae 6 to 8 cm of the adjacent rib and occasionally the level above is resected, exposing but leaving intact the neurovascular bundle. The pedicle of the damaged vertebra is then removed with a high-speed air drill.

Magnification either with surgical loupes or the operating microscope is desirable for the remainder of the decompression. The nerve root exiting from the neural foramen at the level of the fracture is frequently trapped between the pedicle and the retropulsed bony fragment. Care must be taken not to damage it further as the dissection continues. In the majority of burst fractures, the retropulsed fragment, located between the pedicles, does not extend below the caudal margin of the pedicle (Figure 10-13A,B,C). Thus, bone removal usually does not need to extend caudally beyond the pedicular level, minimizing the amount of intact bone removed (Figure 10-14). The spinal dura is identified at the junction of the nerve root sleeve and the dural sac.

The decompression is begun by removing bone just anterior to the retropulsed fragment, across the width of the spinal canal, thereby undermining the retropulsed fragment. This allows the residual rim of bone compressing the anterior dura to be depressed anteriorly into the cavity. From this position, the fragment can be removed

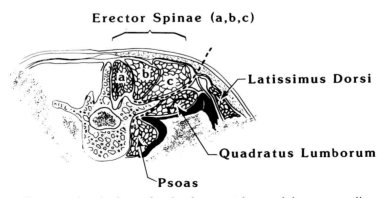

Figure 10-12. Cross-sectional view of a lumbar vertebra and its surrounding musculature showing the plane of dissection (dotted line) between the erector spinae muscles and the quadratus lumborum.

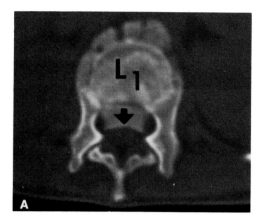

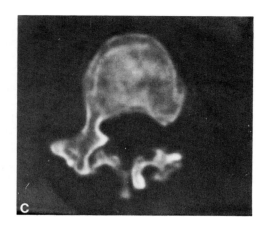

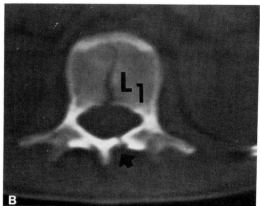

Figure 10-13. (A) CT scan of a L1 burst fracture demonstrating the stellate nature of the body fracture and the retropulsed fragment of bone at the pedicular level. (B) CT scan of the same vertebra as shown in (A) but at the caudal level of the pedicle showing only a vertical fracture in the body, no bony fragment in the canal, and a fractured lamina (arrow). (C) Postoperative CT scan of the L1 burst fracture shown in (A) demonstrating the decompressed canal and the degree of bone removal necessary (pedicle and transverse process) to achieve it.

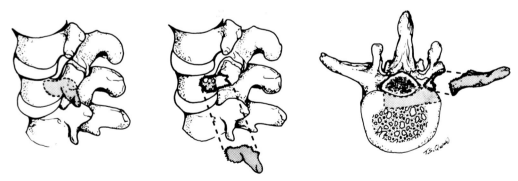

Figure 10-14. Lateral and cross-sectional views of lumbar vertebrae demonstrating the degree of bone removal necessary to decompress an axial compression or burst fracture-dislocation injury.

safely, thereby restoring the cross-sectional configuration of the spinal canal (Figure 10-13D). The intervertebral disc above the fractured vertebra is usually so significantly damaged that it is routinely excised, even though free disc fragments are usually not present. The inferior disc is usually not significantly disrupted and therefore is not surgically disturbed. Tears in the ventral dura caused by bone fragments are frequently present; however, avulsions of nerve roots have not been seen with frequency. No attempt is made to repair the ventral dura, and the leak is managed with a Gelfoam pack. No patient has developed a CSF leak postoperatively.

When the encroachment into the spinal canal is not anterior in nature, there is a combination of posterior and anterior compression and a different surgical approach is used. Fractures of the superior articular process may encroach into the neural foramen, pedicle fractures may cause lateral canal encroachment, or displaced lamina fractures may produce posterior canal encroachment. In these cases, a posterior midline skin incision gives direct and safe access for decompression via a standard laminectomy or posterolateral bony decompression as outlined above.

After the bone fragment has been removed, Harrington instrumentation is performed. Through a separate midline longitudinal incision, electrocautery is used to develop the dissection down to the surface of the supraspinous ligament. If the interspinal ligament has not been torn, longitudinal dissection is then continued 5 to 8 mm off the midline on each side down through the thoracolumbar fascia in order to avoid disturbing the supraspinous and interspinous ligaments. Next, subperiosteal dissection is completed, which allows the erector spinae muscles to be retracted. Further dissection is carried out to the lateral tip of the transverse processes only on the fractured vertebra and the one immediately above and below the injured level.

Using the technique of Jacobs,[31] dissection is carried out in a cephalad direction sufficiently far to allow placement of the superior hooks under the inferior articular processes of the third vertebra above the fractured level, care being taken to minimize damage to the facet capsule. Similarly, dissection is carried in a caudal direction to allow placement of the lower hooks on the superior edge of the lamina of the third vertebra below the fractured level. The facet joint capsules of the superior and inferior articular processes of the fractured vertebra are excised as well as the articular cartilage on both sides of these four facet joints. Decortication is performed at three levels (the fractured vertebra, one above, and one below) out to the tips of the transverse processes. This is done with a steel burr and air drill rather than an osteotome and mallet to reduce the likelihood of neural damage from further bone fragment motion. Decortication is done before rod placement since the lamina is still fully exposed.

After hook placement, the rods are selected such that the ratchet–rod junction is as close to the upper hook as possible, thereby minimizing the stress at this critical location on the rod.[6,14] Rods may either be contoured as needed or Edwards' sleeves may be used. If the rods are contoured, square-ended Moe rods are used to prevent axial rotation of the contoured rod. Bone grafts are then obtained from the iliac crest through a separate incision and placed posterior to the transverse process, facet joints, and laminae so as to incorporate only the fractured level plus one vertebra above and below this level.

Of the 67 patients in this series, 5 underwent a posterior decompression, internal fixation, and transverse process bone grafting; 4 underwent posterolateral decompression, internal fixation, and bone grafting; 22 underwent anterolateral decompression, internal fixation, and bone grafting; 4 underwent transthoracic decompression, internal

Table 10-7.
Surgical procedures in 66 patients with thoracolumbar (T1–L5)
fractures

Surgical Procedure	Neurologic Improvement			
	Two Levels	One Level	Same	Total
Anterolateral Decompression plus I.F. plus Bone	2	4	16*	22
Harrington Rods plus Bone	1	5	16	22
Laminectomy plus I.F. plus Bone	2†	2	1	5
Posterolateral Decompression plus I.F. plus Bone	0	1	3	4
Transthoracic Decompression plus I.F. plus Bone	2†‡	1	1	4
Weiss Springs plus Bone	0	1	8	9
Total	7	14	45*	66

* One patient with hemiparesis preoperatively.
† One patient deteriorated before surgery and then returned to original neurologic status.
‡ One patient improved three levels.
I.F. = Internal Fixation
Bone = Bone Fusion

fixation, and anterior interbody bone grafting; and 31 cases were treated by distraction Harrington rod instrumentation or Weiss springs and bone grafting without a formal neural decompression (Table 10-7). Patients with complete paraplegia (Frankel A) are not routinely subjected to decompressive procedures. One patient with a 70-percent compromise of the spinal canal and a normal neurologic examination elected to undergo stabilization without decompression.

Between 1978 and 1983 somatosensory evoked responses (SSERs) were routinely used preoperatively and intraoperatively in patient with residual neural function. In this series, 21 patients demonstrated no deterioration in the SSERs during the surgical manipulations; however, two of these patients awoke transiently weaker with proprioception preserved. These two patients had undergone anterolateral decompression and the continued presence of normal intraoperative SSERs prompted a more vigorous removal of the retropulsed bony fragments than would otherwise have been attempted. The intraoperative use of SSERs is currently reserved for those patients with evidence of some neural function below the level of the injury in whom realignment is performed without prior decompression.

Repeat CT scans were routinely done postoperatively to document the extent of decompression. The presence of Harrington rods has been shown to still allow adequate visualization postoperatively.[52]

The postoperative management of group A patients consisted of bedrest on a Stryker frame for 6 weeks and then mobilization in a molded spinal orthosis, which was worn for 1 year. In these patients, the Harrington instrumentation was not routinely removed since the bony fusion extended the full length of the rods.

The group B patients were immediately placed onto regular beds postoperatively, fitted with a custom molded bivalved spinal orthosis within 3 to 7 days (molded preoperatively when possible) and mobilized as soon as the orthosis was tolerated. The Harrington rods were removed at 5 or 6 months and the orthosis was continued until 8 or 9 months postoperatively. After removal of the rods, while the patient was still in the orthosis, an exercise program was begun. After the orthosis was removed, spinal mobility exercises were started.

Subsequent to the acute care phase, 35 patients with partial or complete neural deficits continued their care at our rehabilitation facility, 30 patients were discharged home, 1 died of his head injuries, and 1 patient was transferred to the maternity ward.

RESULTS

Twenty-one patients were neurologically intact on admission (grade E) and remained unchanged after surgery; of the 29 with partial deficits at the time of surgery (Frankel grades B,C,D) 12 improved one grade, 3 improved by two grades, 1 improved by three grades, and 13 remained unchanged (Table 10-8). Among the 16 patients with complete lesions (grade A), 3 improved to grade C and 13 remained unchanged. Two grade E patients deteriorated preoperatively to grades B and C, respectively. Both of these patients underwent emergent surgical decompression and stabilization. Postoperatively both patients returned to grade E.

Fractures resulting from either axial loading forces or a combination of axial loading and flexion forces constituted the majority (54) of our cases. Pure flexion, hyperextension, and Chance fractures were rare (see Table 10-4).

The group A patients had an average acute hospital stay of 57 days, while in group B this was reduced to 34 days. The average time from injury to surgery remained essentially the same, 14 and 13 days, respectively. Patients currently (group B) average 33 days in the rehabilitation unit as opposed to the previous (group A) average of 45 days. Total hospitalization has gone from an average of 80 days to 52 days (Table 10-9). Twenty-four complications occurred in 18 patients (35 percent) from group A compared with only five complications in 4 patients (21 percent) in group B (Table 10-10). No complications have occurred because of the earlier mobilization of group B patients. In addition, there has been a reduced incidence of thrombophlebitis (10 percent in group A, 0 percent in group B) although this may be partially explained by a reduced incidence of paraplegic patients (29 percent in group A, 11 percent in group B, as shown in Table 10-11).

Table 10-8.
Neurologic outcome in 66 patients with thoracolumbar (T1–L5) fractures

| | | Postoperative Frankel Grade | | | | |
Preoperative Frankel Grade	Number of Patients	A	B	C	D	E
A	16	13	0	3	0	0
B	3*	0	0	1	1	1
C	13*	0	0	2	9	2
D	13	0	0	0	11	2
E	21	0	0	0	0	21
TOTAL:	66†	13	0	6	21	26

* One patient, initially a grade E, deteriorated before surgery.
† One patient initially hemiparetic and not included.

Table 10-9.

Time course for patients with thoracolumbar fractures (T1–L5)

	Group A*	Group B*	Combined
Time to Surgery	14 days	13 days	14 days
	(N = 45)†	(N = 18)†	(N = 63)
Acute Hospitalization	57 days	34 days	51 days
	(N = 44)‡	(N = 17)§	(N = 61)
Rehabilitative Hospitalization	45 days	33 days	42 days
	(N = 22)	(N = 9)	(N = 31)
Total Hospitalization	79.5 days	51.5 days	72 days
	(N = 44)	(N = 17)§	(N = 61)
Follow-Up	24 months	9 months	20 months
	(N = 44)	(N = 18)	(N = 62)
Range	(0–66 months)	(1–29 months)	(0–66 months)

* Group A: 1977–1981; group B: 1981–present.
† Patients transferred from other hospitals longer than 2 months after their injury were not included.
‡ One patient was transferred to the maternity ward.
§ One patient was in the hospital at the time the series closed.

Table 10-10.

Treatment-related complications in patients with thoracolumbar fractures (T1–L5)*

Complication	Number of Patients
Group A: 48 patients with 0–66 months follow-up	
Harrington rod hook displacement (5 days to 8 months)	4
Harrington rod fracture (1 to 3½ years)	2
Weiss spring fracture (1½ years)	1
Brachial plexus palsy	1
Upper arm paresthesias	1
Progressive kyphosis (1½ months to 12 months)	3
Thrombophlebitis	5
Neurologic worsening secondary to arachnoiditis	1
Pseudarthrosis	1
Fat emboli	1
Superficial wound dehiscence	1
Pneumothorax intraoperatively	1
Marker pin left in place	1
Septicemia/death	1
Total treatment-related complications in 18 patients	24
Group B: 19 patients with 1–29 months follow-up	
Harrington rod hook displacement (6 weeks postoperatively)	1
Brachial plexus palsy (clearing within 10 days)	2
Peroneal nerve palsy (secondary to lower extremity cast)	1
Neurologic worsening secondary to residual bone	1
Total treatment-related complications in 4 patients	5

* Group A: 1977–1981; group B: 1981–present.

Table 10-11.
Initial neurologic grade compared with ambulation time

Frankel Grade	Group A Late Ambulation	Group B Early Ambulation
A	14	2
B	2	
C	7	5
D	7	7
E	18	5
Total	48	19

DISCUSSION

The treatment of thoracolumbar fractures has continued to evolve as we have come to appreciate the unique characteristics of various fracture types and have tailored the surgical approaches specifically to them. The CT scan has provided a major advance by allowing a clear delineation of the full extent of vertebral body damage as well as canal encroachment as in burst fractures and burst fracture-dislocations. In addition, certain fractures of the lamina, pedicles, and facets that often were not appreciated on plain roentgenograms of the spine are much more apparent. Sagittal reconstruction of CT scans has also been helpful by demonstrating the cephalocaudal extent of the bony encroachment into the spinal canal. Metrizamide-enhanced CT scanning provides supplemental information by demonstrating the relationship of the bone elements of the spine to the dura, the location of the conus, and soft tissue encroachment upon neural structures. The latter is particularly important if the bone derangement does not provide an adequate explanation for the neural deficit. Conventional anteroposterior and lateral spinal roentgenograms remain useful for surveying the spine for injuries and for determining the degree of angulation and translation at the fracture site. Re-examination is helpful postoperatively since the majority of the potential complications involve problems with instrumentation, bony alignment, and bony fusion.

The improved visualization of these injuries through improved radiographic technique is exemplified by the increasing frequency of the diagnosis of burst fractures. In 1969, the series reported by Frankel et al. contained only 6 of 394 patients with burst fractures.[17] In 1977, Flesch et al. reported only 2 of 40 patients with this type of fracture.[16] In contrast, 36 of the 67 cases in this series were burst fractures (type 2 or 3C). This increase is probably attributable to increased recognition of these fractures, since the mechanisms of injury (often a fall from a height) and the spinal level involved (usually T12-L1) are relatively constant in the three series. This becomes important when considering the optimal operative approach, since burst fractures are frequently not adequately decompressed with realignment and stabilization alone, whereas the other types of fractures are.[3] Another observation related to improved fracture delineation and more accurate assignment of the injury to a classification system is that there now appears to be some correlation between fracture type and the patient's initial neural state. This finding is in contradistinction to Frankel's series in which it was not possible for such a correlation to be made. In our series, no patient with a flexion-rotation injury was initially ambulatory; while over half of the patients with axial loading and flexion-axial loading injuries were ambulatory. There were too few patients in the other categories to allow comment.

Neural recovery occurred in 31 percent (21 of 67, although 21 were initially grade E and could not improve) of our patients, which is comparable with the results obtained in both operative and nonoperative series suggesting that recovery is determined by the extent of neural damage at the time of injury.[17,27,28,37] Although operative intervention does not increase neurologic recovery, the evidence suggest that realignment and internal fixation decreases spinal deformity and subsequent pain while decompression prevents later deterioration in neurologic function.[2,16,28,37] Bohlman[2] reported the cases of 10 patients, two of whom had had a previous decompressive laminectomy with posterior fusion and who developed increasing pain (8 patients) and progressive new paralysis (6 patients) 9 months to 10 years after thoracolumbar fracture. All 10 required surgical decompression: by a transthoracic approach in one, by an anterolateral (transpedicular) approach with fusion in the other nine. Seven of the eight patients were relieved of pain; four of the six recovered neurologic function while two remained unchanged. No patient lost motor function as a result of the surgery. McAfee et al.[39] reported neurologic deterioration in two nonoperatively treated patients with burst fractures that produced a reduction in vertebral height greater than 50 percent. The patients were originally intact neurologically but then developed progressive vertebral body collapse, kyphosis, and evidence of neural compression (parasthesias, radicular symptoms, and focal deficits). One of these patients improved after spinal decompression. No follow-up information was provided on the other patient. Nash et al.[42] reported two cases of burst fracture in which the patients also developed progressive kyphosis during conservative treatment. One patient developed a Brown-Sequard syndrome, the second developed a progressive kyphotic deformity with spinal angulation increasing from 19 to 30 degrees during treatment in an extension body jacket. Symptomatic premature degenerative spinal stenosis may occur 10 to 15 years after thoracolumbar fractures in the absence of either progressive kyphosis or further protrusion of bony fragments into the spinal canal, especially if the lateral recesses are narrowed by fracture fragments.[39] We have seen four patients with increasing symptoms 9 months to 8 years after their original injury as a result of either inadequate primary surgical decompression, increasing kyphosis, or spinal adhesive arachnoiditis.

The surgical goals in the treatment of thoracolumbar fracture—decompression of neural structures and stabilization of the vertebral column are directed toward preventing the delayed onset of complications of spinal deformity, pain, and neurologic deficit. In addition, early operative intervention allows for a shorter hospital stay, immediate ambulation, and lessened pulmonary, vascular, urologic, and psychologic complications.

Decompression can be accomplished either by realignment if there are no separate bone fragments in the spinal canal, by bone removal in the case of burst fractures, or by a combination of realignment and bone removal as is required for burst fracture-dislocations. When realignment alone is performed, neural compression may be independently produced by disc protrusion or hematoma formation. If the mechanical maneuvering necessary for realignment is especially difficult or an unusual amount of bleeding is encountered, an intraoperative myelogram with 5 to 10 mL of contrast material is useful to define the anatomy of the canal.

While reduction of angular deformities can often be accomplished by closed methods, translational deformities are less often reduced by nonoperative methods.

The advantage of open reduction and internal fixation with the Harrington system is that (1) anatomically realigned bone heals more effectively that bone fixed in an nonanatomic position,[16] and (2) sufficient stability is produced immediately to allow early mobilization. The use of short bone grafts, limited to segments involved by the fracture, allows maximal spinal mobility after removal of the Harrington rod.

While a detailed discussion of spinal stability is beyond the scope of this text,[35] a few points of particular importance to the operative management of these fracture should be made. As experience with long-term follow-up of thoracolumbar fractures increases, the definition of instability has been modified to include "chronic" as well as "acute" instability. In the acutely unstable spine, neurologic function is threatened by displacment during the early phase, while in the chronically unstable spine, progressive spinal deformity leading to pain and neurologic deficit can develop months to years after the injury. White and Panjabi[51] have defined clinical instability as the "loss of the ability of the spine, under physiologic loads, to maintain relationships between vertebrae in such a way that there is neither initial damage nor subsequent irritation to the spinal cord or nerve roots, and, in addition, there is no development of incapacitating deformity or pain due to structural changes." This is clinically significant in that fractures that were previously considered stable such as the burst fractures and wedge compression fractures, are now thought to be potentially unstable.[39] Holdsworth originally described burst fractures as vertebral body fractures with bony fragments retroplused into the spinal canal resulting from a pure compression force with an intact posterior ligamentous complex (i.e., intraspinal ligaments, capsular ligaments, ligamentum flavum) as well as an intact posterior bony complex. He considered these fractures stable.[26] While conventional x-ray films and physical examination can help to determine acute ligamentous rupture, experiences with CT scanning has demonstrated that posterior element fractures are frequently missed on plain x-ray films. Brandt-Zawadski et al.[4] have found that 57 percent of burst fractures have associated posterior element fractures. In our series, 367 patients with burst fractures had CT scans that adequately demonstrated the posterior elements. Twenty-six of 70 percent had posterior or neural arch fractures rendering the burst fracture unstable.[54]

McAfee et al.[39] have called attention to the more chronic situation in which the burst fracture heals with a loss of vertebral body height allowing the intact spinal ligaments to become lax, which in turn leads to a kyphotic deformity and potential injury to the cauda equina as the nerve roots are stretched over the anterior bone fragments. For these reasons, we now consider all burst fractures either unstable or potentially unstable. Wedge compression fractures are considered unstable if there is greater than 50 percent loss of vertebral body height or any evidence of posterior ligamentous complex rupture on plain x-ray films or physical examination (see Table 10-3).

While the functional definition of instability of White and Panjabi accentuates the importance of neurologic function in the criteria for acute and chronic stability, a more anatomic definition is helpful to aid in decision making in the acute phase of the injury. The guidelines that we now follow to determine which patients should be stabilized and whether or not decompression is warranted closely resemble those set forth by Whitesides and Shah[54] and Dickson et al.[12] The spine is considered acutely unstable if two of the following conditions exist: (1) loss of integrity of the vertebral body, (2) loss of integrity of the posterior ligamentous or bony structures, and (3) loss of alignment of the spine in terms of either angulation or translocation. Since roentgenograms do not necessarily reflect the maximal displacement that occurred at the time of injury if the neurologic deficit is greater than expected from the radiographic studies, the patient is treated as having a more unstable spine than a patient with similar x-ray films without a neurologic deficit.

The rational treatment of thoracolumbar fractures is dependent on accurate categorization of the injury using a classification that reflects the varying degrees of both bony and ligamentous injury. The latter is particularly important since ligamentous injury cannot be guaranteed to heal with prolonged immobilization alone. Using the classification described above, a flexion injury is treated by closed or open reduction, Harrington compression rods, and a two-segment bone graft. A burst fracture with or without dislocation is treated by anterior spinal canal decompression through a posterolateral skin incision and an anterolateral approach to the canal, Harrington distraction rods with a three-segment bone graft. Wedge compression fractures of less than 50 percent do not require surgery. Wedge compression fractures of greater than 50 percent are treated with Harrington distraction rods and bone fusion. Flexion-rotation fractures are treated by open or closed reduction, internal fixation, and bone fusion. This is the most unstable of the thoracolumbar fractures and postural alignment can often be accomplished by placing the patient in the supine position. Although these fractures through the vertebral body and articular processes can be anticipated to heal well resulting in spinal stability, the dangerously unstable nature of this fracture puts the patient at high risk for redislocation and further neural damage. Internal fixation and bone grafting is therefore the treatment of choice in most of these cases. Occasionally when the rotatory force fractures the articular process, bone will be displaced into the spinal canal. Decompression is usually best accomplished through a posterior approach. Hyperextension injuries are treated by either open or closed reduction, Harrington instrumentation, and bone grafts. Flexion-distraction fractures may potentially heal without operative intervention, however, we recommend internal fixation and bone grafting to facilitate the patient's early mobilization and rehabilitation.

Although the advantages of realignment, internal fixation, and fusion in dislocations and decompression, internal fixation, and fusion in burst fractures in patients with partial neurologic deficits is reasonably well established, the optimal treatment of a paraplegic patient with a burst fracture and a neurologically intact patient with a burst fracture and significant spinal encroachment remains a problem that we have not fully resolved to our satisfaction. In this series, we had six patients in the former category and nine patients in the latter category. Among the six paraplegics, two were treated by open reduction, internal fixation with Harrington rods, and bone grafts, and four had decompressive procedures performed in addition to the insertion of Harrington rods and bone grafts. One patient who was not decompressed subsequently developed severe burning bilateral pain in the legs; the other is pain free. One of the four patients who underwent decompression has back pain radiating around his abdomen; the other three are pain free. One patient in the decompression group improved to a grade C postoperatively. The management of the nine neurologically normal patients included Harrington rod stabilization and bone grafts in four, one of whom has severe back pain and three of whom are asymptomatic. Of the five patients treated by decompression, Harrington rods, and bone grafts, none have developed a pain problem. There has been no neurologic worsening as a result of the operative procedures.

Continuous intraoperative monitoring of somatosensory evoked responses during decompressive procedures for thoracolumbar fractures in our experience has been of questionable value in alerting the surgeon to compromise of neural function attending the surgical maneuvers. Although SSERs are thought to be transmitted primarily in the dorsal columns,[9] it was thought that particularly in the area of the conus it would be unlikely that significant motor damage could occur without detectable change in the SSERs. However, to date two patients in our series, both with L1 burst fractures subjected to decompression and stabilization have exhibited objective signs of transiently increased motor deficit postoperatively despite an absence of any evidence of alteration of their intraoperative SSERs. Both of these patients had normal proprioceptive function preoperatively and postoperatively. Presently we use SSERs mainly in cases requiring only spinal realignment.

In patients who are neurologically stable and without associated injuries, surgery is performed as an elective procedure after a few days delay to reduce intraoperative blood loss and to ensure optimal operative conditions. In patients with dislocations, realignment is considerably easier if it is accomplished within the first week. Our experience has been that most patients over the first several days actually improved slightly, especially with regard to sensory function. This improvement, however, is not enough to change their Frankel grade. In these patients, surgery is delayed until the improvement plateaus. Patients with major life-threatening trauma to other organ systems are operated upon when their general condition allows. In our series, this has been the primary cause of delay in surgical intervention. In patients who are neurologically deteriorating, emergency surgery is performed after adequate radiologic investigation to determine the cause of deterioration. Epidural hematomas, further dislocation of the spinal vertebrae, further migration of the bone fragment into the canal, infarction of neural tissue secondary to hypotension, and increasing edema have all been implicated in worsening neurologic deficits after thoracolumbar fractures.

There were no life-threatening complications directly attributable to the surgical procedure in the last 67 patients (see Table 10-4). One patient died as a result of a severe head injury. The complications that have necessitated reoperation include dislodged or broken Harrington rods in six patients and inadequate decompression in one patient. The majority of the problems with Harrington rods occurred 6 months or more after placement. Currently, Harrington rods are removed at 5 to 6 months and to date this has prevented these types of complications. The incidence of thrombophlebitis in the lower extremities has been reduced by earlier mobilization, physical therapy from the time of admission, and possibly the use of the rotokinetic bed.[19] We have not used low-dose heparin. Three patients who were positioned in the three-quarter lateral position developed brachial plexus injuries intraoperatively in the dependent arm. This is avoidable with meticulous attention to positioning and padding. We currently are also using SSER monitoring of the arms to help avoid this problem. Psychologic problems, specifically depression, have been reduced by earlier mobilization and transfer to the rehabilitation unit where the patient can take a more active role in his or her recovery process. Psychologic evaluation is done upon admission and the patient and his or her family are followed by either a psychiatrist or psychologist throughout the acute and rehabilitiative hospitalization. Long term counseling is available if necessary. There have been no wound infections. Urinary tract infections remain a problem. Almost every patient unable to void on his or her own had a urinary tract infection at some time during the acute or rehabilitative hospitalization. Intermittent self-catheterization is used. The patients are not routinely started on prophylactic antibiotics. With earlier ambulation we have decreased acute hospitalization from 57 to 34 days and total hospitalization from 80 to 52 days.

New technology continues to improve the care of patients with thoracolumbar fractures. In the area of treatment, newer fixation systems implantable through either an anterior[13,22] or posterior[34] approach should provide improved stability using fewer vertebrae than presently. In the area of diagnosis, a number of developments are occurring. Recently, intraoperative ultrasound has been advocated for visualization of bone fragments and hematomas, but this currently requires laminectomy. Smaller probes may allow more universal application of this technique in the future. Nuclear magnetic resonance imaging promises to allow detailed definition of the ligamentous and neural injuries in these fractures much as CT scanning has helped to define the bony injuries.[23,41] With better definition of the entire pathologic process, it is hoped that operative intervention can be more accurately tailored to the individual situation and thus further improve treatment.

REFERENCES

1. Alexander G: Neurological complications of spinal tuberculosis. Proc R Soc Med 39:730, 1946
2. Bohlman HH: Late progressive paralysis and pain following fractures of the thoracolumbar spine. J Bone Joint Surg 58A:728, 1976
3. Bohlman HH, Ducker TB, Lucas JT: Spine and spinal cord injuries. In Rothman R, Simeone F: The Spine. Philadelphia, W.B. Saunders, 1982, pp 661–757
4. Brant-Zawadzki M, Jeffrey B Jr, Minogi H, Pitto L: High resolution CT of thoracolumbar fractures. AJNR 3:69, 1982
5. Bryant CE, Sullivan JA: Management of thoracic and lumbar spine fractures with Harrington distraction rods supplemented with segmental wiring. Spine 8:532, 1983
6. Burnski JB, Hill DC: Stresses in a Harrington distraction rod: Their origination and relationship to fatigue fractures. In Vivo, Proceedings of the Orthopedic Research Society, 29th Annual Meeting, 1983
7. Capener N: The evaluation of lateral rhachotomy. J Bone Joint Surg 36B:173, 1954
8. Convery FR, Minteer MA, Smith RW, Emerson SM: Fracture dislocations of the dorsal-lumbar spine: Acute operative stabilization by Harrington instrumentation. Spine 3:160, 1978
9. Cusick JF, Myklebust JB, Larson SJ, Sances A: Spinal cord evaluation by cortical evoked responses. Arch Neurol 36:140, 1979
10. Dennis F: The three column spine and its significance in the classification of acute thoracolumbar spinal injuries. Spine 8:817, 1983
11. Dennis F, Ruiz H, Searls K: Comparison between square-ended distraction rods and round-ended distraction rods in the treatment of thoracolumbar spinal injuries. A statistical analysis. Clin Orthop 189:162, 1984
12. Dickson JH, Harrington PR, Erwin WD: Results of reduction and stabilization of the severely fractured thoracic and lumbar spine. J Bone Joint Surg 60A:799, 1978
13. Dunn HK: Anterior stabilization of thoracolumbar injuries. Clin Orthop 189:116, 1984
14. Edwards CC, Griffith P, Levine AM, DeSilva JB: Early clinical results using the spinal rod sleeve method for treating thoracic and lumbar injuries. Orthop Trans 6:345, 1982
15. Edwards CC, York JJ, Levine AM: Determinants of hook dislodgement: Rigidity of fixation, rod clearance, and hook design. International Study of Lumbar Spine, Annual Meeting, Montreal, 1984
16. Flesch JR, Leider LL, Erickson DL, Chou SN, Bradford DS: Harrington instrumentation and spine fusion for unstable fractures and fracture-dislocations of the thoracic and lumbar spine. J Bone Joint Surg 59A:143, 1977
17. Frankel HL, Hancock DO, Hyslop G, Melzak J, Michaelis LS, Ungar GH, Vernon JDS, Walsh JJ: The value of postural reduction in the initial management of closed injuries of the spine with paraplegia and tetraplegia. Paraplegia 7:179, 1969
18. Gaines RW, Breedlove RF, Munson G: Stabilization of thoracic and thoracolumbar fracture-dislocations with Harrington rods and sublaminar wires. Clin Orthop 189:195, 1984
19. Green B, Green K, Klose KJ: Kinetic nursing

for acute spinal cord injury patients. Paraplegia 18:181, 1980

20. Guttman L: Initial treatment of traumatic paraplegia. Proc R Soc Med 47:1103, 1954

21. Guttman L: Spinal deformity in traumatic paraplegics and tetraplegics following spinal procedures. Paraplegia 7:38, 1969

22. Hall JE: Dwyer instrumentation in anterior fusion of the spine: Current concepts review. J Bone Joint Surg 63A:1188, 1981

23. Han JS, Kaufman B, Yousef S, Benson J, Bonstible C, Alfidi R, Hooga J, Yeung H, Husa R: NMR imaging of the spine. AJNR 4:1151, 1984

24. Harrington PR: Treatment of scoliosis: Correction and internal fixation by spine instrumentation. J Bone Joint Surg 44A:591, 1962

25. Harrington PR: Instrumentation in spine stability other than scoliosis. S Afr J Surg 5:7, 1967

26. Holdsworth FW: Fractures, dislocations, and fracture-dislocations of the spine. J Bone Joint Surg 45B:6, 1963

27. Holdsworth FW, Hardy A: Early treatment of paraplegia from fractures of the thoracolumbar spine. J Bone Joint Surg 35B:540, 1953

28. Jacobs RR, Asher MA, Snider RK: Dorsolumbar spine fractures: Recumbent vs. operative treatment. Paraplegia 18:358, 1980

29. Jacobs RR, Asher MA, Snider RK: Thoracolumbar spinal injuries: A comprehensive study of recumbent and operative treatment in 100 patients. Spine 5:463, 1980

30. Jacobs RR, Gertzbein SD, Nordwall A, Mathys R Jr: A locking hook spinal rod: Current status of development. Scoliosis Research Society 17th Annual Meeting, Denver, 1982

31. Jacobs RR, Nordwall A, Nachemson A: Reduction, stability and strength provided by internal fixation systems for thoracolumbar spinal injuries. Clin Orthop 171:300, 1982

32. Kostuick JP: Anterior spinal cord decompression for lesions of the thoracic and lumbar spine, new methods of internal fixation and results. Spine 8:512, 1983

33. Kostuick JP: Anterior fixation for fractures of the thoracic and lumbar spine with or without neurologic involvement. Clin Orthop 189:103, 1984

34. Krag MH, Beynnon B, Weaver D, Pope MH, Frymoyer JW: An internal fixator for a posterior thoracic lumbar or lumbosacral spinal stabilization: Initial mechanical testing and implantation. American Spine Injury Annual Meeting, Atlanta, 1985

35. Krag MH, Pope MH, Wilder DG: Mechanisms of spine trauma and features of spinal fixation methods. I. ''Mechanism of Injury,'' Proceed-ings of NATO Advanced Institute on Spinal Cord Rehabilitation Engineering. Stroke, Mandeville, England, May, 1981. Springfield, IL, Charles C Thomas, 1985

36. Larson SJ: Lateral extrapleural and extraperitoneal approaches to the thoracic and lumbar spine. In Ruge D, Wiltse L: Spinal Disorders. Philadelphia, Lea & Febiger, 1977, pp 137–141

37. Lewis J, McKibbin B: The treatment of unstable fracture-dislocations of the thoracolumbar spine accompanied by paraplegia. J Bone Joint Surg 56B:603, 1974

38. McAfee PC, Yuan HA, Frederickson B, Lubicky J: The value of computed tomography in thoracolumbar fractures. J Bone Joint Surg 65A:461, 1983

39. McAfee PC, Yuan HA, Lasda NA: The unstable burst fracture. Spine 7:365, 1982

40. Miller CA: Thoracolumbar fractures. Contemp Neurosurg 2:1, 1980

41. Mills ND, Brandt-Zawadski M, Yeates A, Crooks LE, Kaufman L: Magnetic resonance imaging of the spinal cord and canal: Potentials and limitations. AJNR 5:9, 1984

42. Nash CL, Schatizinger LH, Brown RH, Brodkey J: The unstable stable thoracic compression fracture. Spine 2:261, 1977

43. Posner I, White AA, Edwards WT, Hayes WC: A biomechanical analysis of the clinical stability of the lumbar and lumbosacral spine. Spine 7:374, 1982

44. Purcell GA, Markof KL, Dawson EA: Twelfth thoracic-first lumbar vertebral mechanical stability of fractures after Harrington rod instrumentation. J Bone Joint Surg 63A:71, 1981

45. Rezaian SM, Dombrowski ET, Ghista TDN, Tavoscoly M, Modaghegh S: Spinal fixator for sugical treatment of spinal injury. Orthop Rev 12:31, 1983

46. Schlicke L, Schulak J: The simultaneous use of Harrington compression and distraction rods in a thoracolumbar fracture-dislocation. J Trauma 20:177, 1980

47. Schmidek HH, Gomes FB, Seligson D, McSherry JW: Management of acute unstable thoracolumbar (T11–L1) fractures with and without neurologic deficit. Neurosurgery 7:30, 1980

48. Schmidek HH, Seligson D, Coffin LH, Gomes FB: The anterior anterolateral approach to the thoracic and thoracolumbar spine. In Schmidek HH, Sweet W: Operative Neurosurgical Techniques, vol II. New York, Grune & Stratton, 1982

49. Trias A, Bourassa P, Massoud M: Dynamic

loads experienced in correction of idiopathic scoliosis using two types of Harrington rods. Spine 4:228, 1979

50. Watson JR: Fractures and Other Bone and Joint Injuries. Baltimore, Williams & Wilkins, 1940, p 211

51. White AA, Panjabi MM: Clinical Biomechanics of the Spine. Philadelphia, J.B. Lippincott, 1978

52. White R, Newberg A, Seligson D: Computer-ized tomographic assessment of the trauma-tized dorso-lumbar spine before and after Har-rington instrumentation. Clin Orthop 146:150, 1980

53. Whitesides TE: Traumatic kyphosis of the thoracolumbar spine. Clin Orthop 128:78, 1977

54. Whitesides TE, Shah SGA: On the manage-ment of unstable fractures of the thoracolumbar spine. Spine 1:99, 1976

Narayan Sundaresan, Joseph H. Galicich,
Joseph M. Lane, H. Scher

11

Stabilization of the Spine Involved by Cancer

Any neoplasm can metastasize to the spine, but the most common primary sites for spinal metastases are the breasts, lungs, prostate, and the hematopoietic system.[1,3,8,30,34] These sites account for over 50 percent of the metastatic tumors producing cord compression. Metastatic malignancies outnumber primary axial tumors of the spine by a 9:1 ratio. The frequency of the occurrence of spinal metastases in cancer patients is difficult to assess, although autopsy studies suggest an incidence of 5 percent in all cancers and 30 to 80 percent for the common solid tumors. Within the skeletal system, metastases are more frequent in the axial skeleton compared with the appendicular skeleton. Spread of tumor to bone is almost exclusively hematogenous, although occasionally paravertebral malignancies invade the spine directly or a tumor spreads into the spine from involved lymph nodes through the intervertebral foramina or along the perineurium of intercostal nerves.

Several factors contribute to the high incidence of vertebral metastases. Batson[1] demonstrated a valveless network of vertebral veins that communicated directly with the intercostal and lumbar veins. Through injection studies, he demonstrated that the prostatic and breast venous systems directly drain into this plexus. The vertebrae are thus exposed to a large number of microemboli, which may favor metastatic deposition in the spine. In addition, unlike bones of the peripheral skeleton, which contain relatively avascular (yellow) marrow, vertebrae contain active red marrow throughout life. Some solid tumors such as breast and prostate cancers have a selective propensity to metastasize to the axial skeleton; this is termed *osteotropism*.[2]

As in the long bones, metastases to the vertebral column are frequently complicated not only by pathologic fractures but also by the pain and morbidity of metabolic derangements such as hypercalcemia. Diffuse infiltration of the marrow also reduces the patient's ability to tolerate radiation therapy; the use of high-dose steroids in such a setting may precipitate a fatal superinfection. Although skeletal metastases are characterized as osteolytic, osteoblastic, or mixed based on radiologic appearance, the basic mechanism is increased bone absorption, which is thought to be mediated by an osteoclast-activating factor released by the neoplastic cells.[2,26]

The clinical diagnosis of spinal cord compression in patients with a known cancer is often straightforward. Ninety percent of patients have progressively severe back pain, often with a radicular component. The progression is usually subacute, and the time from onset to the development of neurologic deficits ranges from 6 to 10 weeks. If not diagnosed at this stage, the condition evolves progressively to a paraplegia or quadriplegia depending on the level of spinal involvement. Approximately 70 percent of spinal metastases involve the thoracic region, and the remaining lesions are distributed equally between the lumbar, cervical, and sacral segments. Occasionally the patient's initial pain is a referred pain, which leads to delay in diagnosis. This is particularly common in patients with thoracolumbar metastases, where a pathologic compression fracture frequently causes pain that radiates to the superior iliac crests or to the groin. Superior sulcus tumors of the lungs similarly produce pain in the shoulder secondary to apical pleural involvement.

Plain roentgenographic evaluation of the spine is the initial diagnostic test that should be performed; localized destruction of a pedicle or a pathologic compression fracture may suggest the presence of metastatic disease. The base of the skull, the sacrum, and the cervicothoracic region are poorly visualized by conventional radiography; therefore, computed tomography is usually required when a lesion is suspected in these areas to afford better definition of soft tissue extension. Radionuclide bone scans are generally more sensitive than standard radiographic examination for detecting osseous metastases and should be used when the roentgenograms are negative as well as to stage the extent of osseous involvement.

Nuclear magnetic resonance imaging (NMRI) recently has been used to visualize the vertebral bodies, discs, neural structures, and extradural structures in the sagittal, axial, and coronal planes. A mass lesion or extradural block can be localized and its extent defined without further contrast studies. The contrast resolution of NMRI scans is equal to or superior to that of CT scans, and multiplanar views are possible without the need for reformatting. Craniocervical junction anomalies or subluxations in the sagittal plane are more easily appreciated on NMRI scans. However, this technology is expensive and not generally available.

In cancer patients who have an obvious myelopathy or a history of an evolving radicular deficit, myelography should be used to delineate the extent of epidural involvement and to detect multiple lesions, which occur in approximately 10 percent of patients. In patients with back pain alone, the indications for myelography are less well defined. In patients with abnormalities noted on plain x-ray studies or with clear evidence of radiculopathy, evidence of epidural disease may be seen in 60 to 80 percent of cases, whereas in those patients with back pain alone and negative plain x-ray films or normal neurologic examination, the probability of finding epidural disease is between 10 and 20 percent.[29] Once the diagnosis of epidural tumor extension is established, patients are immediately treated with a loading dose of dexamethasone (100 mg intravenously); this is repeated every six hours in daily dosages ranging from 16 to 96 mg every 24 hours. In patients with lymphomas, thymomas, and other small round cell malignancies, this regimen alone generally relieves a myelographic block and allows time for other forms of systemic therapy (i.e., chemotherapy) to be instituted. In the majority of patients with solid tumors there is little consensus on management. In patients with advanced cancer, there is general agreement that radiation therapy to the involved spine be given for palliation. Pain relief of varying degrees is obtained for 50 to 80 percent of patients, although this response rate is often sustained for only a few months.

Four groups of patients with metastatic disease to the spine deserve evaluation for possible surgical intervention: (1) patients with pathologic compression fractures as the initial manifestation of malignancy; (2) patients in whom there is a solitary relapse site with a controlled or absent primary site; (3) patients with spinal cord compression secondary to direct extension of a paraspinal malignancy; and (4) patients with spinal metastases and other sites of involvement but with an estimated life expectancy greater than 6 months. For patients in the first three categories, effective treatment of spinal metastases has a direct bearing on the length and quality of survival. In the last group, the major goal is the relief of pain and preservation of neurologic function. Until recently patients with an evolving neurologic deficit and a high-grade myelographic block were considered to have neurosurgical emergencies requiring decompressive laminectomy, since it was believed that neurologic deficits once established were rarely reversible. In a retrospective review, Gilbert et al.[15] showed that the results of decompressive laminectomy followed by radiation were no better than those obtained by treating most patients nonsurgically with radiation and steroids. The ambulatory rate after therapy was used to assess treatment and this was 50 percent in both groups studied. They therefore recommended that radiation and steroid therapy be used to treat all patients with neoplastic epidural cord compression and that laminectomy be reserved for (1) patients who relapsed after radiation therapy, (2) patients who deteriorated neurologically while receiving radiation therapy, (3) patients who could not receive further radiation therapy because the spinal cord had been irradiated previously, and (4) patients for whom no tissue diagnosis was available. Greenberg et al.[16] presented the results of treating spinal cord compression with a more intensive short course of radiation, which produced results comparable with those published by Gilbert. A major secondary finding of this study was that the response rates for patients with radioresistant tumors and patients with nonradioresistant tumors were comparable. The results of laminectomy are equally dismal and have not improved over the past decade. Pain relief is also comparable among patients treated by radiation or by decompressive laminectomy. In addition, laminectomy in patients with advanced cancer is associated with mortality rates of 5 to 10 percent and morbidity rates of 10 to 30 percent, so that recent studies generally recommend radiation as the initial management modality in all such patients.[6,12,18,24,29,30,32,33]

Among patients with a complete myelographic block from spinal metastases who had received radiation therapy, Tomita et al.[40] noted that those patients with significant structural abnormalities of the spine had higher failure rates compared with patients in whom there was no evidence of bone destruction. As a corollary, we noted that patients who relapsed after radiation therapy were often found to have progressive collapse of a vertebral body. The restoration of spinal stability is a major goal in patients with neoplastic disease involving the spine, and loss of stability is a frequent cause of the failure of conservative treatment (Figure 11-1). In the next few sections, we will identify specific stabilization procedures for patients with malignancies involving the spine at different anatomic sites.

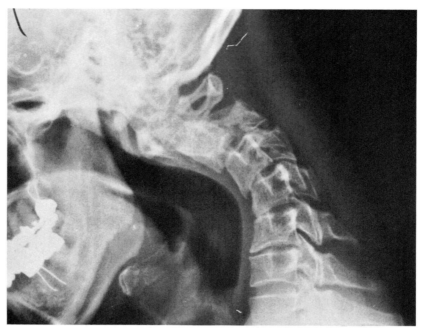

Figure 11-1. "Swan neck" deformity secondary to a cervical laminectomy for metastatic tumor. Treatment options include a posterior facet fusion or an anterior fusion with bone grafting.

POSTERIOR CERVICAL STABILIZATION FOR ODONTOID FRACTURES

In patients with cancer, fractures of the odontoid result from lytic metastases to the axis and represent an important subgroup of vertebral metastases (Figure 11-2). Occasionally a retropharyngeal tumor may involve the spine by direct extension. The resulting instability of the atlantoaxial junction poses the risk of cord transection, and early recognition and treatment is therefore vital. Complicating management is the fact that cancer patients often have involvement of the cervical spine at multiple levels as well as metastases to other organ systems. The presence of associated epidural tumor at the C1-2 level further requires radiation therapy. Although patients with non-neoplastic odontoid fractures may be treated with halo immobilization, our experience suggests that most patients with cancer do not tolerate such prolonged immobilization well. In a previous report of 18 patients with odontoid fractures and atlantoaxial subluxation, we proposed indications for surgery in this population.[36] The majority of the patients in our series complained of severe neck pain and stiffness, signs of spinal cord compression being present in only 4 patients initially. Primary treatment in all patients, except those with myelopathy or gross subluxation, consisted of high-dose steroid therapy and immobilization in a Philadelphia-type collar. Ten patients were successfully treated with radiation therapy, 6 patients underwent surgical stabilization (4 patients before and 2 after radiation therapy), and 2 patients died before completion of treatment. This experience suggests to us that cancer patients with odontoid fractures should be treated initially with radiation and steroids, and the need for

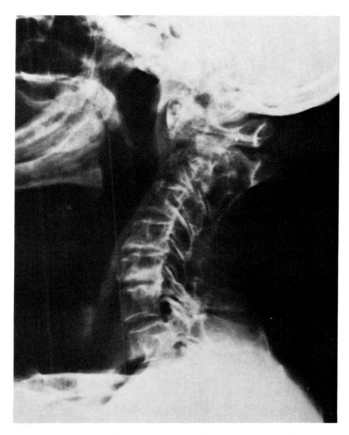

Figure 11-2. Fracture of the odontoid process secondary to metastasis to the axis. For effective palliation, posterior stabilization with methylmethacrylate or bone grafts is indicated after radiation.

surgical stabilization deferred until the end of such treatment. Among these patients, significant pain, gross spinal malalignment, or myelopathy are indications for surgical stabilization if the patient is an otherwise acceptable surgical candidate. The basic surgical technique used in this situation is that originally described by Kelly for acrylic fixation of atlantoaxial dislocations resulting from trauma or rheumatoid arthritis (Figures 11-3, 11-4).[22] This operation is performed with the patient in the prone position. The head is secured with either halo traction or with three-point fixation and the realignment of the spine is checked on intraoperative serial x-ray studies. A series of wires is passed under the lamina of C1 through C3; in the midline, the spinous process of C2 is wired to the arch of the atlas. Methylmethacrylate is then used to reinforce the entire wire matrix. In patients with breast cancer and a longer life expectancy, bone grafts are placed lateral to and in addition to the methylmethacrylate, and the stabilization is designed to include most of the cervical vertebrae, since multifocal involvement in the cervical region is common.

For lesions lower in the cervical spine, Dunn has summarized the various techniques using methylmethacrylate in the stabilization of the cervical spine reported

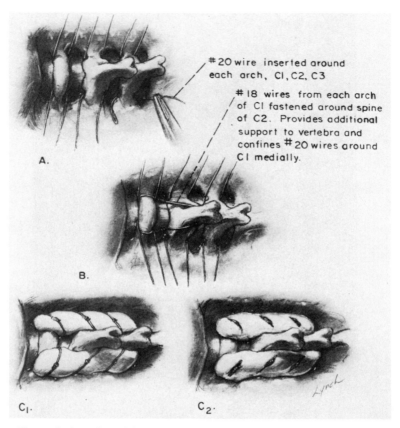

Figure 11-3. The technique for wiring the upper cervical spine as described by Kelly is used for posterior fixation. (Reprinted from J Neurosurgery 36:366, 1972. With permission.)

in the literature.[11] Acrylic may be used alone or in combination with wires, metal plates, or wires placed through holes drilled through the facets. The simplest technique is one in which a laminectomy is performed and then an interwoven mesh of wire and acrylic is used to envelop the lamina and the spinous processes (Figure 11-5). In Figure 11-5B, metal plates are used laterally and wired down and acrylic is used to provide additional reinforcement. As an alternative, acrylic cylinders may be placed laterally after holes have been drilled through the facets. A simple technique in the cervical region is that described by Hoppenstein.[21] After a laminectomy is performed, a stainless steel mesh is molded around the spine above and below, and acrylic is used to reinforce the posterior neural arches after all soft tissue has been removed from the spines included in this matrix.

POSTERIOR STABILIZATION WITH METHYLMETHACRYLATE

In the thoracic and lumbar regions, similar techniques with acrylic supplemented by plates, wire mesh, or heavy gauge twisted wire have also been used.[5,11,17,21] The largest experience with this approach is that of Hansebout, who describes the use of

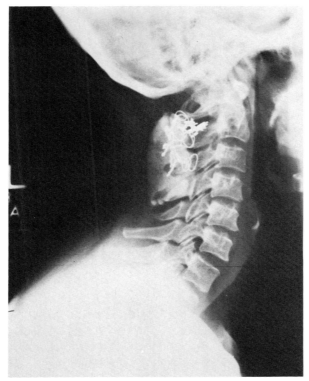

Figure 11-4.   A lateral x-ray film showing normal alignment
of the spine after methylmethacrylate and wire fixation.

acrylic stabilization with a combination of steel plates or wire.[17] A wide laminectomy
is initially performed to decompress the spinal cord or the cauda equina, which allows
resection of epidural tumor. Following neural decompression, vertebrae two levels
above and below the laminectomy site are exposed. A No. 20 wire is then woven back
and forth between the spinous processes of the vertebrae above and below the
laminectomy site (Figures 11-6, 11-8). Two long cylinders of acrylic are then formed
and placed as shown in Figure 11-7. The acrylic is molded to incorporate the wire, with
additional acrylic being added as needed. The spinous processes are exposed to a depth
of at least 1 cm so as not to interfere with closure of the soft tissue. During
polymerization, Gelfoam is placed on the dura and the wound is irrigated with copious
amounts of saline to cool the structures. A drain is then placed in close proximity to the
acrylic and the incision is closed in layers after it is irrigated with antibiotic solution.

In the entire series, a fusion fracture occurred in only one patient in whom the
wires were not crossed and twisted. Hansebout advocated that the wires be carefully
twisted to provide a better matrix for the acrylic. All soft tissue must be removed from
the spinous processes and laminae to allow the acrylic to be molded to the bone over
as large a surface area as possible. The advantages of acrylic stabilization are that pain
relief is immediate and that patients can be ambulated promptly without the prolonged
need for external orthoses. For a grossly subluxated spine, posterior stabilization alone
is unlikely to be effective and the problem may require treatment by a combined

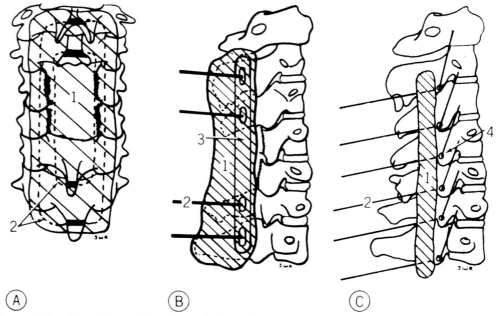

Figure 11-5. Posterior stabilization techniques for the cervical region with (A) methylmethacrylate and wires, (B) metal plates, or (C) facet wiring. (Reprinted from Dunn EJ: The role of methylmethacrylate in stabilization and replacement of the cervical spine. Spine 2:15, 1977. With permission.)

anterior and posterior stabilization procedure. The advantage of posterior stabilization is that bone grafts can be used laterally on the transverse processes or over the facets in the cervical region to provide physiologic fusion as well.[5]

HARRINGTON DISTRACTION INSTRUMENTATION

Acrylic stabilization alone is useful only in the cervical region; in the presence of marked collapse of the vertebral body it cannot be used to restore spinal alignment in the thoracic and lumbar regions. The restoration of vertebral body height and realignment of the spine in such situations is effectively achieved with Harrington rod distraction.[10,27,35] Perrin noted that between 10 and 25 percent of patients who complained of severe vertebral pain have "segmental instability" of the spine and that this pain characteristically was aggravated by movement and improved by skeletal traction. Distraction rod stabilization is effective in treating such patients with intractable pain resulting from osseous involvement of the spine in whom there are minimal signs of spinal cord compression. Three major indications for this procedure are: (1) progressive collapse of a vertebral body as noted on serial plain roentgenograms; (2) after the facets have been removed bilaterally in conjunction with an extensive laminectomy (required for nerve root decompression or access to the anterior aspect of the cord); and (3) pathologic fracture-dislocations with marked displacement in order to reinforce an anterior decompression and fusion. With moderate distraction,

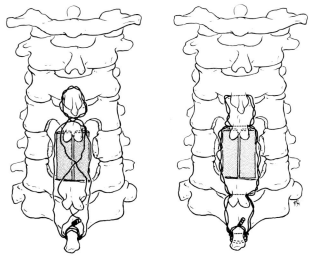

Figure 11-6. Technique for posterior stabilization for the thoracic region. (Left) The wire matrix is passed around the spinous processes of the vertebrae two levels above and two levels below the laminectomy site. (Right) An alternative method of wiring with the wire passed through the base of the spinous processes. Stippled area: Gelfoam protecting the dura. (Reprinted from Hansebout RR, Blomquist GA Jr: Acrylic spinal fusion: A 20-year clinical series and technical note. J Neurosurg 53:60, 1980. With permission.)

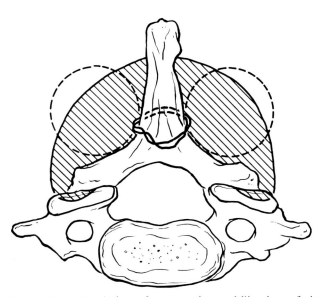

Figure 11-7. Technique for posterior stabilization of the thoracic region. A transverse view showing the original acrylic semihardened cylinders (circles) and the acrylic after being moded to the spine (crosshatched areas). (Reprinted from J Nerosurg 53: 606, 1980.)

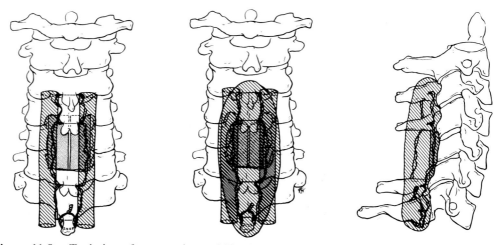

Figure 11-8. Technique for posterior stabilization of the thoracic region. (Left) Placement of semihardened acrylic cylinders over the wire and laminae bilaterally. (Center) Placement of additional acrylic and molding around the spinous processes and wire. (Right) Lateral view of the molded acrylic. Note that the tips of the spinous processes are exposed to facilitate later wound closure. Crosshatched areas: acrylic; stippled areas: Gelfoam. (Reprinted from J Neurosurg 53:606, 1980.)

the Harrington rods themselves exert an anteriorly directed force that is effective in reducing a localized kyphosis. This force is lost if the facets are resected, and progressive tumor growth can then produce late secondary displacement.

After a wide decompressive laminectomy for tumor resection and the removal of all identifiable tumor, the spine above and below the laminectomy sites is exposed. The upper hooks are seated into the facet joints at least two levels above the laminectomy site and the lower hooks are placed underneath the lamina two levels below (Figures 11-9, 11-10). It should be noted that in the lumbar region the lower hook should not be placed on the L5 vertebra; sacral alar hooks may be required in such cases. The distracting rods are then inserted and minimal to moderate distraction is applied in a staggered fashion with the outrigger device. Alignment is assessed on intraoperative x-ray films. The proximal and distal ends of the rods are then wired together with 18-gauge wire; methylmethacrylate may be used to coat the upper and lower ends of the device for more secure fixation. Postoperatively, patients are allowed to ambulate in a molded plastic (Prenyl) jacket.

Although this procedure is effective in the treatment of pain, neurologic deficits were less successfully reversed among our patients who had received prior radiation. Among such patients, a high incidence of wound-related complications (up to 25 percent) were also noted. For these reasons, we believe that the application of the Harrington rod system should be restricted (1) to patients who have not been extensively irradiated, and (2) to selected cases in which more extensive tumor resection has been performed with curative intent to supplement anterior decompression and stabilization (Figure 11-11).

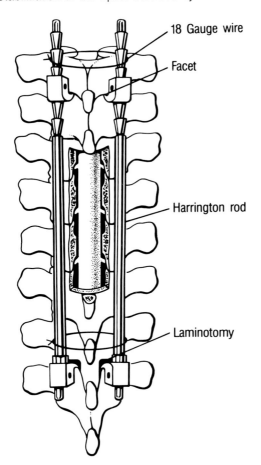

18 Gauge wire

Facet

Harrington rod

Laminotomy

Figure 11-9. Harrington distraction rods. Note the position of the upper hooks on the facets two levels above and under the lamina two levels below the unstable segment.

LUQUE INSTRUMENTATION

The Luque system for spinal stabilization has gained popularity mainly for the treatment of neuromuscular scoliosis and fractures of the thoracolumbar spine, and experience in using the Luque system in the treatment of spinal instability caused by malignant disease is relatively small.[13,23] Flatley has described a series of 7 patients with malignancies involving the spine who underwent Luque instrumentation to reduce pain and to prevent mechanical collapse of the spine or further progression of a neurologic deficit. The 5 patients who had pain noted marked improvement of this symptom after surgery and 3 of the 5 patients with neurologic deficits were improved. In this series, no specific attempt was made to excise the tumor or otherwise provide neural decompression. The heaviest gauge wire (doubled) should be used to fix the Luque rods at each level, and preferentially the fixation should include three levels above and below the level of tumor or of the laminectomized segments. In patients who have undergone wide laminectomies, Flatley suggested wiring not only the laminae above and below the unstable segment but also the transverse processes. Spinal stabilization with Luque

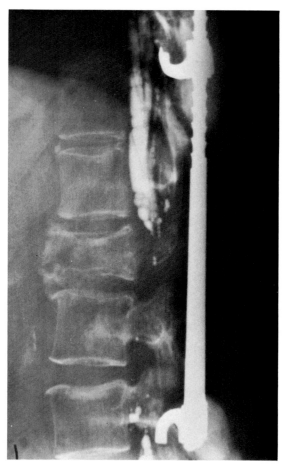

Figure 11-10. A lateral roentgenogram showing realignment of the spine and opening of myelographic block with distraction rods.

instrumentation is a time-consuming procedure; its precise role has not been defined at this time, but the technique of sublaminar wiring is potentially hazardous.

VERTEBRAL BODY RESECTION AND STABILIZATION WITH METHYLMETHACRYLATE

A number of anterior approaches to the spine for benign disc disease, trauma, and tumors are familiar to most surgeons.[4,7,28] In 1965, Hodgson et al.[20] published a report on anterior spinal fusion for the treatment of Pott's disease, and 4 years later followed this with an extensive review of 412 cases. The basic tenents of this approach are full visualization through an extensive exposure, complete excision of all dead bone and diseased tissue, and immediate stabilization of the spine with bone grafts. These basic

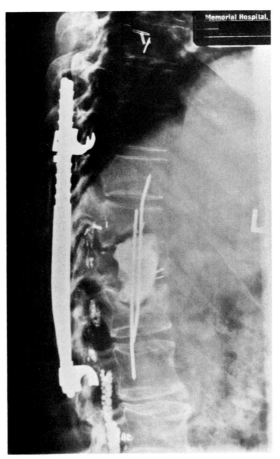

Figure 11-11. Harrington distraction rods to supplement a posterior bone graft and anterior vertebral body resection in the thoracolumbar region.

premises are essentially the same for the treatment of malignancies involving the spine except that in most cases immediate stability is best achieved with the use of methylmethacrylate rather than bone. The original report describing the use of methylmethacrylate for vertebral body replacement in a patient with a lymphoma involving the cervical vertebrae was published by Scoville in 1967.[31] The methylmethacrylate was kept in place with two screws, and a wire mesh was used as a trough over the dura. Since that time, numerous case reports have been published on a variety of techniques for fixing the methylmethacrylate after the resection of tumors involving the cervical spine.[5,9,11,28] Some of these techniques are shown in Figure 11-12A.[12] Harrington recently has advocated the use of methylmethacrylate replacement for pathologically collapsed vertebrae and secondary spinal cord compression in the thoracic and lumbar segments.[19]

The anterior approach is a more effective approach for treating the majority of patients with neoplastic cord compression resulting from an anterolateral soft tissue

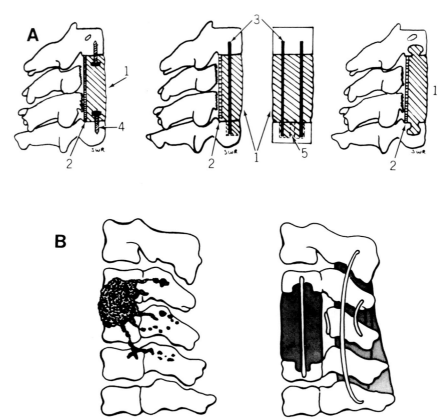

Figure 11-12. (A) Techniques of anterior cervical stabilization according to Dunn. (Left) Screws are used to hold the acrylic in place. (Center) Two Kirschner wires are introduced into the vertebrae above and below. (Right) The endplates above and below are curetted to create an interface between the acrylic cement and cancellous bone. (B) Combined anterior and posterior stabilization is indicated when marked instability exists. (Reprinted from Clark CR, Keggi KJ, Panjabi MM: Methylmethacrylate stabilization of the cervical spine. J Bone Joint Surg 66A:40, 1984. With permission).

tumor mass as demonstrated on CT scans, destruction and collapse of the vertebral body as noted on either plain x-ray films or on CT scans, or an anterior defect secondary to kyphosis (Figure 11-13).[32] Most primary neoplasms of the axial skeleton and the majority of metastatic malignancies fall into this category. Unfortunately, decompressive laminectomy is still being performed on these patients, often with suboptimal results. Approximately 15 percent of patients in our series have undergone such ineffective laminectomies and the loss of posterior stability has aggravated the difficulty of completing anterior decompression and stabilization. Since most patients who have neurologic deficits usually stabilize with high-dose dexamethasone therapy, nonoperative conservative measures are indicated initially while the true extent and the site of compression are being evaluated with radiologic studies. Emergency ill-planned operations have a high rate of failure, as is evident by repeated reports of considerable morbidity in the literature.

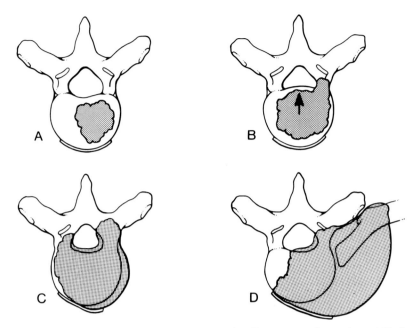

Figure 11-13. Patterns of primary and metastatic disease to the spine. (A) Intraosseous metastasis or primary tumor; (B) with tumor progression; and (C) epidural extension with bilateral involvement of the pedicles; (D) paraspinal tumor with secondary destruction of the spine.

Table 11-1 lists the various anterior approaches for the different segments of the spine. The midcervical region is accessible through a transcervical Cloward or Smith Robinson approach, whereas for lesions involving C1 and C2, an anterior exposure can be performed through a transoral approach.[42] The transoral approach, however, allows only limited exposure for biopsy and decompression. For more extensive tumor resection we prefer a median mandibulotomy, which allows a midline or a paralingual approach to the upper cervical spine. A portion of the soft palate may have to be removed for potentially curable lesions such as chordomas involving the upper cervical spine. At the cervicothoracic junction, the vascular structures of the thoracic inlet and the reversed normal cervicothoracic kyphosis increase the difficulties of adequately exposing the spine. To gain access to the spine we use an operative exposure in which a transverse incision is made 1 cm above the clavicles with a vertical limb in the midline over the body of the sternum. The sternocleidomastoid is detached from the clavicle on one side, along with the medial half of the clavicle and the manubrium. This allows dissection of the subclavian vessels. The prevertebral space can be reached by retracting the trachea and esophagus medially. After the tumor has been resected, fusion is performed using the clavicle as a strut graft. Alternatively, a methylmethac-rylate stabilization procedure as described below can be used. All patients treated in this way eventually require posterior fusion.

Since the majority of the patients with spinal cord compression have involvement of the thoracic or the thoracolumbar region, an extended approach by thoracotomy or a thoracoabdominal incision is required. Access by costotransversectomy allows only

Table 11-1.
Classification of anterior surgical approaches

Cervical and cervicothoracic segments (C1–T2)
Transmandibular median glossotomy
Cloward anterior cervical
Trans sternal
Thoracic Segments (T3–T12)
Posterolateral thoracotomy
Thoracolumbar Segment (T12–L2)
Thoracolumbar with 10–12th rib resection
Lumbar (L2–L5)
Retroperitoneal flank
Transabdominal

limited room for resection of the tumor and rarely allows adequate stabilization to be performed. Resection of the spine for primary and metastatic tumors, especially those from the thyroid and kidney, may be associated with massive blood loss and therefore this operation should be performed under optimal elective conditions. A major clinical consideration is the side of the chest that should be opened for an anterior approach to the spine. Hodgson suggested that the left side be used routinely because he believed the aorta to be more amenable to retraction and dissection than the inferior vena cava. We prefer to open the chest on the right side in the majority of cases or to open the side in which there is a paravertebral tumor mass if one is seen on the CT scans. The incision for the thoracotomy is usually made two levels above the site of spinal compression, since it is easier to work downward in the thoracic cavity because of the slope of the ribs posterior to their angles. Although rib resections have been suggested for additional exposure, it is important to resect only the posterior 4 to 5 cm of the ribs, since this will facilitate closure (Figures 11-14 through 11-23). The resected segment of rib is preserved in one piece if possible for later use as a rib graft. Self-retaining thoracic retractors are placed, and the thoracic cage is opened gradually. A Hurson malleable self-retaining retractor is useful at this stage of the procedure. The visceral pleura is then reflected and the intact discs above and below the site of involvement are palpated. The intercostal vessels are carefully coagulated with bipolar cautery and clipped. The intervertebral discs are removed with curettes and pituitary forceps and the vertebral bodies thus isolated. The vertebral bodies are then removed with a combination of angled curettes and rongeurs. If the patient has not received prior radiotherapy, gross tumor resection is easily accomplished because most solid tumors are soft. In patients with marked sclerosis secondary to radiotherapy, the use of curved osteotomes and a high-speed drill may be necessary. All devitalized bone and tumor is removed to the dura. By extending this approach, it is possible to decompress the dura anteriorly and laterally (by tracing the tumor backward and by removing the lateral masses including the facets and pedicles). Tumor resection should be as radical as possible, especially in those patients who have received prior radiation therapy or those with radioresistant tumors. The anterior longitudinal ligament itself is left in place if possible, but the posterior longitudinal ligament is usually removed to allow the dura to be decompressed. Steinmann pins 1 to 5 mm in diameter are then selected, cut, and bent at either end in the shape of hockey sticks and introduced into the vertebrae above and below

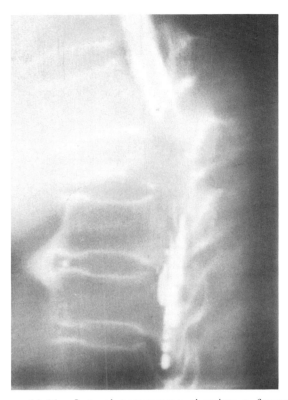

Figure 11-14. Lateral tomograms showing a fracture-dislocation with a pathologic compression fracture and kyphosis. Stabilization is best performed by vertebral body resection and acrylic fusion.

with the aid of two heavy needle holders. This technique allows adequate fixation of the methylmethacrylate and will prevent it from being dislodged in flexion and extension. After the introduction of the Steinmann pins, which usually straddle one vertebra above and one below the resected segment, methylmethacrylate is mixed and injected into the cavity with a 50-mL syringe. The dura is protected with Gelfoam during this procedure. The methylmethacrylate is injected while it is still liquid and it is molded away from the dura with Penfield dissectors. During the polymerization process, the site is irrigated with copious amounts of saline to protect the dura from the heat. Adequate hemostasis is then secured, but no attempt is made to pack the epidural space tightly, which can create a loculated area where blood or fluid could be entrapped. Chest tubes are then inserted and the thoracotomy closed. The postoperative care is similar to that for a standard thoracotomy and the patients are usually allowed to ambulate the next day. A Knight Taylor brace is used for patient comfort and also helps to prevent extreme hyperextension and flexion of the spine.

For the thoracolumbar region, i.e., from T12 to L2, several different approaches may be used. It is possible to approach this segment of the spine either through a thoracotomy with resection of the tenth or eleventh ribs or by an extrapleural,

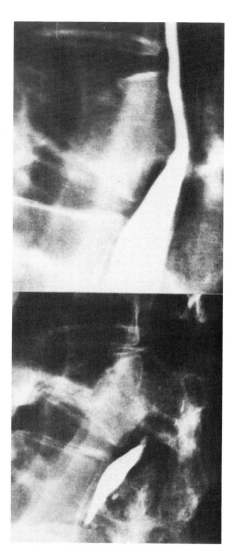

Figure 11-15. Serial lateral views of the lumbar spine showing progressive collapse of the vertebral body secondary to radiation therapy and tumor destruction. This progressive collapse indicates segmental spinal instability.

extraperitoneal approach to minimize morbidity from opening the chest. In the former, the costal origin of the diaphragm is detached posteriorly and the entire thoracolumbar region may thus be visualized. The thoracolumbar junction, especially the T12 and L1 vertebrae, represents a segment of junctional instability and anterior fusion alone may not suffice. Additional stabilization posteriorly either with Harrington instrumentation or bone grafts may be required in potential long-term survivors. The approach to this region is usually made on the left side because the aorta is easier to mobilize at this level than the left lobe of the liver, which is often tethered to the inferior vena cava. Although the artery of Adamkiewicz arises most frequently on the left side. At these levels we have not routinely performed spinal angiography before surgery. Spinal angiography is used to assess tumor vascularity and to perform preoperative embolization in patients

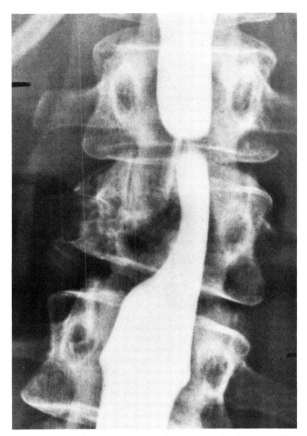

Figure 11-16. A myelogram showing a high-grade block with a pathologic compression fracture in a patient with back pain. Possible primary sites include the lung, kidney, or the thyroid. For symptomatic relief, resection of the vertebral body and stabilization is the best approach.

with extremely vascular lesions. At surgery, intercostal vessels that originate directly from the aorta should be clipped close to their origin rather than at the intervertebral foramina. In the lower lumbar region, a standard retroperitoneal flank approach anterior to the psoas major muscle is used. For the fifth lumbar vertebra, a standard transabdominal approach through a transverse incision in the lower abdomen provides the best access. The fifth lumbar vertebra represents one of the hardest sites to approach anteriorly because it is straddled by both the common iliac artery and veins. In all patients, suction drains are used since postoperative effusions are common. The average operating time for these procedures varies from three to four hours. The postoperative morbidity rate in one series was approximately 10 percent; an additional 6 percent of patients died within a 30-day period secondary to a variety of complications. Permanent neurologic deficits have not been encountered and the ambulatory rate in these patients (80 percent) was superior to that of patients undergoing laminectomy or radiation alone.

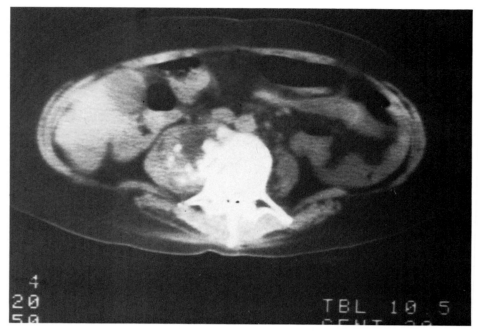

Figure 11-17. A CT scan of the lower lumbar region showing a left paravertebral mass with destruction of the vertebra and pain. Patients with this type of pathologic condition require an anterolateral approach for tumor decompression and stabilization.

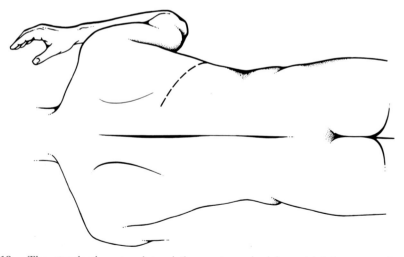

Figure 11-18. The standard posterolateral thoracotomy incision which is centered two spaces above the level of vertebral body compression. (Reprinted from Sundaresan N, Galicich JH, Lane JM, et al: The treatment of neoplastic epidural cord compression by vertebral body resection and stabilization. J Neurosurg 63:676–684, 1985. With permission.)

268

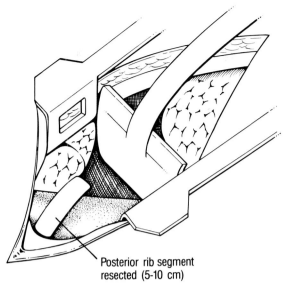

Posterior rib segment
resected (5-10 cm)

Figure 11-19. After thoracotomy, the posterior 5 to 10 cm of rib is resected. This resected rib segment may be used as a graft after surgical resection of the vertebral body. (Reprinted from Sundaresan N, Galicich JH, Lane JM, et al: The treatment of neoplastic epidural cord compression by vertebral body resection and stabilization. J Neurosurg 63:676–684, 1985. With permission.)

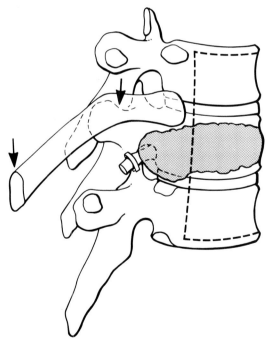

Figure 11-20. The dotted line indicates the amount of pleura that must be reflected to isolate the tumor confined to the vertebral body. The arrows show the extent of rib that must be removed for additional exposure. (Reprinted from Sundaresan N, Galicich JH, Lane JM, et al: The treatment of neoplastic epidural cord compression by vertebral body resection and stabilization. J Neurosurg 63:676–684, 1985. With permission.)

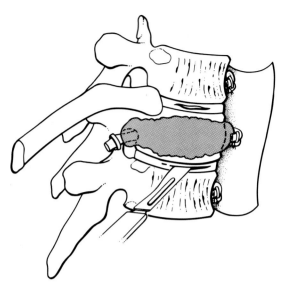

Figure 11-21. After reflection of the pleura and ligation of the intercostal vessels, the intact discs above and below the level of tumor involvement are excised sharply. (Reprinted from Sundaresan N, Galicich JH, Lane JM, et al: The treatment of neoplastic epidural cord compression by vertebral body resection and stabilization. J Neurosurg 63:676–684, 1985. With permission.)

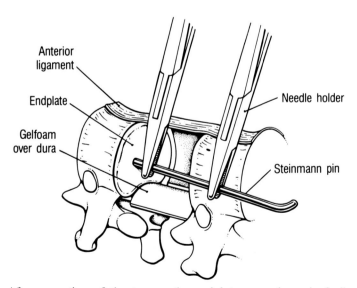

Figure 11-22. After resection of the tumor, the endplates are cleaned of all soft tissue and Steinmann pins are introduced with heavy needle holders. (Reprinted from Sundaresan N, Galicich JH, Lane JM, et al: The treatment of neoplastic epidural cord compression by vertebral body resection and stabilization. J Neurosurg 63:676–684, 1985. With permission.)

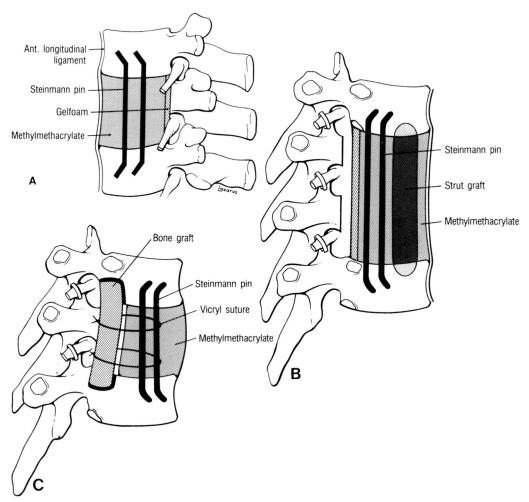

Ant. longitudinal ligament

Steinmann pin

Gelfoam

Methylmethacrylate

A

Steinmann pin

Strut graft

Methylmethacrylate

Bone graft

Steinmann pin

Vicryl suture

Methylmethacrylate

B

C

Figure 11-23. (A) Notice that the space left by the resected vertebra is filled in with methylmethacrylate, which is allowed to polymerize in situ. The anterior longitudinal ligament is left intact and the dura is protected with Gelfoam. (B) In patients with the potential for long-term survival, a rib graft is used laterally to augment the fusion. This rib graft is held in place with Steinmann pins and with heavy Vicryl sutures. (C) An alternative method is to use a strut graft of bone, either from the fibula or the iliac crest. The Steinmann pins are then placed around it and methylmethacrylate is used to surround the entire fusion mass. This provides both immediate stability and long-term fusion. (Reprinted from Sundaresan N, Galicich JH, Lane JM, et al: The treatment of neoplastic epidural cord compression by vertebral body resection and stabilization. J Neurosurg 63:676–684, 1985. With permission.)

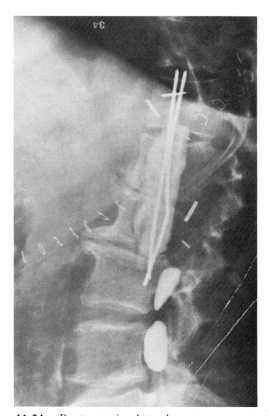

Figure 11-24. Postoperative lateral roentgenograms showing Steinmann pins in place after partial resection of two
adjacent vertebral bodies for tumor involvement. Despite
extensive resection, most patients do not require an external
orthosis. (Reprinted from Sundaresan N, Galicich JH, Lane
JM, et al: The treatment of neoplastic epidural cord compression by vertebral body resection, and stabilization.
Neurosurg 63:676–684, 1985. With permission.)

Timing of surgical intervention in relation to radiation therapy is critical. Patients
who have recently failed to respond to radiation treatment and who are on high doses
of corticosteroids are most likely to develop complications resulting from gastrointes-
tinal hemorrhage or sepsis or both. As a result, we advocate early surgery for patients
who are ambulatory and avoid if possible performing surgery during the critical 6-week
to 8-week period after patients have received radiation or chemotherapy.

There are several modifications of this technique that merit consideration. Harrington advocates the use of anterior Knodt rods to reinforce the methylmethacrylate
(see Figure 11-7), but we have found it difficult to distract the vertebra in cases of
localized kyphosis as he has described. Over an 8-year period, Harrington has used this
technique in 52 patients with spinal instability secondary to pathologic fractures of one
or more vertebrae. There was no late loss of stability over follow-up periods ranging
from 6 to 100 months. Forty patients had major neurologic impairment preoperatively.

Of these, 21 had complete neurologic recovery, 13 others were improved significantly, 5 were unchanged, and 1 patient deteriorated after surgery. Three patients had failure of fixation and 7 others did not benefit from the procedure because of surgical complications or the advanced state of their disease. In our initial 101 cases, improvement in pain was noted after surgery in 85 percent of the patients who had pain preoperatively, and 78 percent of patients maintained their ambulatory status. Of 46 nonambulatory patients, 68 percent improved. Since the majority of patients had undergone prior radiation treatment, up to one half of the patients suffered local recurrence despite initial successful therapy. We believe that this approach should be used in selected patients with neoplastic epidural cord compression before the use of radiation therapy. Local radiation therapy postoperatively is then more effective if used to control microscopic residual disease. In patients with radioresistant tumors, especially those who have a solitary site of relapse, this procedure is indicated even before the onset of spinal cord compression since complete resection can be carried out with minimum morbidity.

ACKNOWLEDGMENT

A portion of this study was funded by a grant from the Greenwall Foundation.

REFERENCES

1. Batson OV: The function of vertebral veins and their role in the spread of metastases. Ann Surg 112:138, 1940
2. Bockman RS: Hypercalcemia in malignancy. Clin Endocrinol Metab 9:317, 1980
3. Boland PJ, Lane JM, Sundaresan N: Metastatic disease of the spine. Clin Orthop 169:95, 1982
4. Clark CR, Keggi KJ, Panjabi MM: Methyl methacrylate stabilization of the cervical spine. J Bone Joint Surg 66A:40, 1984
5. Chadduck WM, Boop WC: Acrylic stabilization of the cervical spine for neoplastic disease: Evolution of a technique for vertebral body replacement. Neurosurgery 13:23, 1983
6. Cobb CA, Leavens ME, Eckles N: Indications for nonoperative treatment of spinal cord compression due to breast cancer. J Neurosurg 47:653, 1977
7. Conley FR, Britt RH, Hanbery JW, Silverberg GD: Anterior fibular strut graft in neoplastic disease of the cervical spine. J Neurosurg 51:677, 1979
8. Constans JP, de Divitiis E, Donzelli R, Spaziante R, Meder JF, Haye C: Spinal metastases with neurologic manifestations. Review of 600 cases. J Neurosurg 59:111, 1968
9. Cross GO, White HL, White LP: Acrylic prosthesis of the fifth vertebra in myeloma. Technical note. J Neurosurg 35:112, 1971
10. Cusick JF, Larson SJ, Walsh PR, Steiner RE: Distraction stabilization in the treatment of metastatic carcinoma. J Neurosurg 59:861, 1983
11. Dunn EJ: The role of methylmethacrylate in stabilization and replacement of the cervical spine. Spine 2:15, 1977
12. Dunn RC, Kelly WA, Wohns RNW, Howe JF: Spinal epidural neoplasia. A 15-year review of the results of surgical therapy. J Neurosurg 52:47, 1980
13. Flatley TJ, Anderson MH, Anost GT: Spinal instability due to malignant disease. J Bone Joint Surg 66A:47, 1984
14. Freeman MAR, Bradley GW, Revell PA: Observations upon the interface between bone and polymethylmethacrylate cement. J Bone Joint Surg 46B:489, 1982
15. Gilbert RW, Kim JH, Posner JB: Epidural spinal cord compression from metastatic tumor. Diagnosis and treatment. Ann Neurol 3:40, 1978
16. Greenberg HS, Kim JH, Posner JB: Epidural spinal cord compression from metastatic tumor: Results with a new treatment protocol. Ann Neurol 8:361, 1980
17. Hansebout RR, Blomquist GA Jr: Acrylic spinal fusion: A 20-year clinical series and technical note. J Neurosurg 53:606, 1980

18. Harper GR, Rodichok LD, Prevosti L, Lininger L, Ruckdeschel JC: Early diagnosis of spinal metastases leads to improved treatment outcome. Proc Am Soc Clin Oncol 6: 1982 (abstr)

19. Harrington KD: The use of methylmethacrylate for vertebral body replacement and anterior stabilization of pathologic fracture-dislocations of the spine due to metastatic malignant disease. J Bone Joint Surg 63A:36, 1981

20. Hodgson AR, Stock FE, Fang HSY, Ong GB: Anterior spinal fusion. Br J Surg 48:172, 1960

21. Hoppenstein R: Immediate spinal stabilization using an acrylic prosthesis (preliminary report). Bull Hosp Joint Dis 33:66, 1972

22. Kelly DL Jr, Alexander E Jr, Smith JM: Acrylic fixation of alanto-axial dislocations. Technical note. J Neurosurg 36:366, 1972

23. Luque ER: The anatomic basis and devlopment of segmental spinal instrumentation. Spine 7:256, 1981

24. Marshall LF, Langfitt TW: Combined therapy for metastatic extradural tumors of the spine. Cancer 40:2067, 1977

25. Mundy GR, Ibbotson KJ, S'Souza SM, Simpson EL, Jacobs JW, Martin TJ: The hypercalcemia of cancer. Clinical implications and pathogenic mechanisms. N Engl J Med 310:1718, 1984

26. Panjabi MM, Hopper W, White AA, Keggi KJ: Posterior spine stabilization with methylmethacrylate: Biomechanical testing of a surgical specimen. Spine 2:241, 1977

27. Perrin RG, Livingston KE: Neurosurgical treatment of pathologic fracture-dislocation of the spine. J Neurosurg 52:330, 1980

28. Raycroft JF, Hockman RP, Southwick WD: Metastatic tumors involving the cervical vertebrae: Surgical palliation. J Bone Joint Surg 60A:763, 1978

29. Rodichok LD, Harper GR, Ruckdeschel JC, Price A, Robinson G, Barron KD, Horton J: Early diagnosis of spinal epidural metastases. Am J Med 70:1181, 1981

30. Rodriguez M, Dinapoli RP: Spinal cord compression with special reference to metastatic epidural tumors. Mayo Clin Proc 55:442, 1980

31. Scoville WB, Palmer AH, Samra K, Chong G: The use of acrylic plastic for vertebral replacement and fixation in metastatic disease of the spine. A technical note. J Neurosurg 27:274, 1967

32. Siegal T, Siegal T, Robin G: Anterior decompression of spine for metastatic epidural cord compression: Is it a promising avenue of therapy? Ann Neurol 11:28, 1982

33. Slatkin NE, Posner JB: Management of spinal epidural metastases. Clin Neurosurg 30:698, 1983

34. Stark RJ, Henson RA, Evans SJW: Spinal metastases. A retrospective survey from a general hospital. Brain 105:189, 1982

35. Sundaresan N, Galicich JH, Bains MJ, Martini N, Beattie EJ: Vertebral body resection in the treatment of cancer involving the spine. Cancer 53:1393, 1984

36. Sundaresan N, Galicich JH, Lane JM, Greenberg HS: Treatment of odontoid fractures in cancer patients. J Neurosurg 52:187, 1981

37. Sundaresan N, Galicich JH, Lane JM: Harrington rod stabilization for pathologic fractures of the spine. J Neurosurg 60:282, 1984

38. Sundaresan N, Shah J, Foley KM, Rosen G: An anterior surgical approach to the upper thoracic vertebrae. J Neurosurg 61:686, 1984

39. Tang SG, Byfield JE, Sharp TR, Utley JF, Quino LL, Seagren SL: Prognostic factors in the management of metastatic epidural spinal cord compression. J Neurooncol 1:21, 1981

40. Tomita T, Galicich JH, Sundaresan N: Radiation therapy for spinal epidural metastases with complete block. Acta Radiol Oncol 22:135, 1983

Index